HEALTH LIBRARY

WOMEN'S HEALTH

HEALTH LIBRARY

WOMEN'S HEALTH

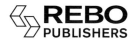
REBO
PUBLISHERS

© 2006 Ars Medica, Grupo Ars XXII, Barcelona, Spain
© 2006 Rebo Publishers

Book conception and management: Jordi Vigué
Editors of original version: Myriam Cañas, Gustavo Villalobos, Jordi Vigué
Correction: Ramon Aymerich
Medical adviser: Dr Gonçal Folch
Photographs: Gorg Blanc Photographic Archive, Capsa Mágica Studio
Illustrators: Ana Journade, Roger Tallada, David Navarrot, Daniel Martínez
Image processor: Rosa Rigau
Special collaborators: Canica Estudio, Laumar Estética
Graphic designer: Celia Valero
Dummy production: Gloria Badia, Manuel Guirado, Marta Ribón, Martín Riveiro
Editorial coordinator: Miquel Ridola

Layout: AdAm Studio, Prague, The Czech Republic
Typesetting and pre-press services: A. R. Garamond, Prague, The Czech Republic
Translation: Jennifer Forbes for First Edition Translations Ltd, Cambridge, UK
Editing: Lin Thomas for First Edition Translations Ltd, Cambridge, UK
Proofreading: Sarah Dunham

ISBN 13: 978-90-366-1906-6
ISBN 10: 90-366-1906-8

C O N T E N T S

WOMEN'S TROUBLES AND ILLNESSES

Infancy

Infancy is the period between birth and puberty, a time when an important development process takes place both physically, with growth and organic maturation, and psychologically.

Infancy

Infancy is defined as the series of periods or phases through which a human being passes until the end of adolescence.

The development of the human being from birth until adulthood is a slow, continuous, and

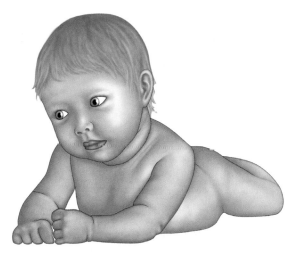

complex process that begins at the moment of conception and is determined and influenced by many biological and psychosocial factors. When the little girl is born she has an organism that already possesses all the structures of a human being and is capable of some deliberate movement, but acts basically through automatic reflexes. In the following few months, her body will undergo a series of changes:

- **Physical changes.** Her organism will grow, change, and acquire the physiological characteristics of an adult.

- **Psychomotor changes.** These include the maturation of her psychic functions, the acquisition of voluntary control, and the coordination of her movements.

Some achievements

- She reacts to the voice between the 2nd and 3rd month.

The phases of infancy

- *Intrauterine period:* Fetal growth and development begins. Early fetal period: the first 28 weeks of pregnancy. Late fetal period: from 28 weeks until birth.

- *Neonatal period:* From birth until the first month of life. Early neonatal period: the 1st week of life (first 7 days). Late neonatal period: from the end of the 1st week until the end of the first month.

- *Lactating period:* From the end of the first month until the end of the first year.

- *Infant school / nursery school / pres-chool period:* From the first year until the age of 5–6 years.

- *Primary school period:* From the ages of 6 to 12 years.

- *Adolescence:* From 12 or 14 years until 18 years. It begins at puberty.

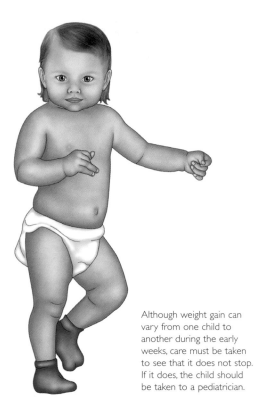

Although weight gain can vary from one child to another during the early weeks, care must be taken to see that it does not stop. If it does, the child should be taken to a pediatrician.

- She smiles from the 2nd month.
- She is capable of upward ocular perception as from the 3rd month.
- From the age of 3 months, a little girl can lie on her front supporting herself on her forearms and raising her head.

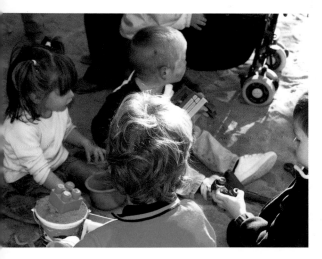

■ Female genitals

In a newborn girl, the labia majora almost completely cover the labia minora and the clitoris, although individuals differ. During the first days of life, a whitish, mucous, and milky vaginal secretion can be observed which can, in some cases, contain blood. This is called pseudomenstruation. It results from the rush of hormones caused by the effect of her mother's hormones during birth. It is a normal and passing phenomenon.

- 180° horizontal optical perception by the 4th month.
- She bursts out laughing from the 4th month.
- She can sit up with support from the 5th month.
- By the age of 5 or 6 months, a little girl discovers her feet.
- She can sit up unaided between the 6th and 8th month.
- She can turn herself round as from the 7th month.
- Her first teeth appear between the 6th and 8th month.
- She babbles from the 8th month.
- She recognizes her name between the 10th and 11th month.
- She manages to stand upright from the 11th month.
- She can walk with help, holding on to furniture and so on for support at 12 months.
- She uses her index finger to point from the 12th month.

Growth and weight gain in the infant

Immediately after birth, a baby normally loses 5 to 10 percent of its weight. However, at the age of 2 weeks it should begin to grow and gain weight rapidly. The perimeter of the skull increases in size as the brain develops. Thus, during the first six months, the perimeter grows 0.3937 inch (1 cm) a month and, as from the 7th month, about 0.1968 inch (0.5 cm) a month until the first year of life.

From the age of 4 to 6 months, a baby doubles its birth weight.

During the second 6 months of life, growth begins to slow down. Little girls will usually start

VACCINATIONS RECOMMENDED BEFORE THE AGE OF 2 YEARS			
Name of vaccine	**Illness prevented**	Number of doses	Vaccination guide
Hepatitis B	Hepatitis B	3	0 m, 1–2 m and 6 m or 2 m, 4 m and 6 m
DTP	Diphtheria	4	2 m, 4 m, 6 m and 15-18 m
	Tetanus		
	Pertussis (whooping cough)		
Hepatits A	Hepatits A	2	12 m, 18 m
Hemophilus	Meningitis by H. influenzae type b	4	2 m, 4 m, 6 m and 15-18 m
Inactivated polio	Poliomyelitis	4	2 m, 4 m, 6 m and 15-18 m
Triple virus MMR	Measles	1	12-15 m
	Rubella (German measles) Mumps		

Physical development

The preschool girl becomes more slender, her arms, legs, and trunk lengthen and her head is more in proportion to her body. Her muscles and bones develop. During this period, she gains weight more regularly at between about 4½–5½ lb (2–2.5 kg) a year. Up to the age of 3 years, the little girl's height continues to increase very fast. By the age of 2 years she may have grown by about 4½ inches (12 cm) and at 3 by some 3¼–3½ inches (8–9 cm) more.

Sexual development

At the age of about 2 years, little girls demonstrate curiosity about their own bodies. At the age of 3 their interest in the differences between the sexes awakens and the process of sexual identification and modesty begins. Little girls generally imitate the sexual stereotypes of their own sex: they usually play at dressing up like Mom and looking after their dolls.

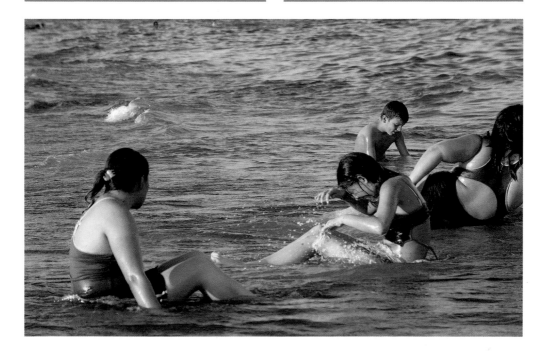

VACCINATIONS RECOMMENDED BETWEEN THE AGES OF 3 AND 6 YEARS			
Triple virus	Measles	1	3–6 years
	German measles (rubella)		
	Mumps		
DTP	Diphtheria	1	4–6 years
	Tetanus		
	Whooping cough		

walking between the first 12 to 24 months and their weight will increase by about 4¾lb (2.2 kg).

The preschool period covers the ages of 2 to 6 years and is characterized by the need for individual and social physical activity. Autonomy is consolidated and the child's initiative develops as she carries out a multitude of actions. The passage from total egocentricity to socialization is important and is accompanied by a little girl's desire to describe, invent, and investigate things. There is a marked development of her personality that lets her express her opinion to adults, interact, and learn to separate from her parents. All these changes will prepare her to start school.

Some achievements

• She learns to walk from the age of one.
• She walks more than 5 steps from 13 months.
• She becomes better at using her index finger to point.
• She can jump clumsily.
• She says "dada" and "mama" meaningfully from the 14th month.
• She can use a few words.
• She can run, spin round, and walk backward.
• She can eat unaided and use a spoon and fork.
• She can turn the pages of a book between the ages of 16 and 18 months.
• She can say the names of commonplace objects and indicate parts of the body.
• She walks faster.
• She imitates others, repeating their words.
• She obeys orders and says "no" by the 20th month.

• At about the age of 15 or 16 months, a little girl can move about completely independently and can even climb the stairs on all fours.
• She starts to pedal.
• She recognizes and classifies colors.
• She can distinguish men from women.
• From the age of 2 she starts to draw lines.
• She starts to dress herself unaided.
• She learns to share toys.
• She starts to throw, kick, and play with a ball.
• She can stand briefly on one foot.
• She can climb on recreation ground installations.
• She can operate door handles and turn on faucets.
• By the age of 3 she has developed a preference for one hand over the other—demonstrating right or left-handedness.
• She has good thumb and finger control.
• She starts to achieve bladder and bowel control.

The preschool phase

This is the phase when physical and psychosocial skills are consolidated and expanded, and play is one of the main ways of learning them.
• She is capable of drawing a circle and other geometric shapes.
• She speaks her mother tongue perfectly.
• She can learn other languages.
• She can draw linear figures with two or three personal features.
• She can balance while standing on one leg with more stability.
• She can catch a bounced ball.

- She understands concepts of size.
- She can jump.
- She likes acting independently and managing without help.
- Her balance improves and she can start to ride a bike.
- She understands the concept of time.
- She learns to read and write.
- She starts to recognize written words and becomes good at reading.
- She starts school.

Physical development

Between the third and fifth year of life, weight and height increase is fairly constant. Every year, the little girl will gain some 4½–6½ lb (2–3 kg) and grow some 2¾–3¼inches (7–8 cm).

Throughout this period, her face will grow more than her cranium and her jaw will broaden. The cephalic perimeter grows only 1¼ inches (3 cm) in total and reaches 19½–21½ inches (50–55 cm) by the age of 5 years.

Primary school age, which extends from 6 to 11 or 12 years of age, is a phase when the little girl learns about the outside world and becomes increasingly independent of her parents. She developlops a conscience or sense of responsibility and begins to take an interest in subjects that seem important to her. This is a period when she comes into contact with the culture of her society, especially through her school.

The Electra complex

It is common in infancy for little girls to express their first feelings of love for their mother, but when they grow older they transfer them to their father, a person of the opposite sex. Their increasing dealings with other people—for example in the infants' school—makes them feel like a separate being from their mother: a little woman in love, who does everything possible to attract the attention of the person she loves.

All fathers like seeing their little girl behaving in a feminine and flirtatious way. And mothers usually seem pleased too, thinking that the little girl is trying to behave like them. As a rule, neither parent realizes that in fact she is trying to show her father that she, the daughter, would be a much better wife than her mother. This kind of innocence on the part of parents is explicable, as the little girl's romance with her father is usually less visible than that of a little boy with his mother, primarily

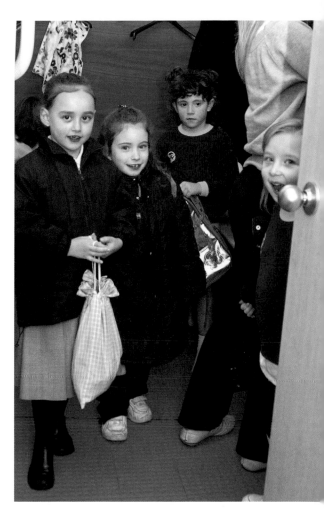

Sexuality

As a rule, girls of 7 are already aware of the fundamental anatomical differences between the sexes and to begin to demonstrate remarkable reserve and shyness about showing their bodies. It is natural for the little girl's curiosity to appear in games that allow sexual exploration. Gradually, the most usual sexual actions will be genital self-stimulation and showing or looking at her sexual organs and those of others. Like heterosexual approaches, homosexual games between little girls form part of the child's normal development.

because the object of the little male's love is much more accessible to him than is the object of the little female's love.

In modern society, mothers tend to spend more time at home than fathers do, so the little girl has to experience her romantic feelings toward her father more in fantasy than in reality. This rivalry with her mother makes the little girl feel bad. In a normal family, she learns in time that her daddy belongs to her mummy and that she cannot have him. Gradually, she gives up her romantic feelings for her father and directs them toward another male figure. At the same time, she begins to identify with her mother who sets her the example of the woman she will be when she grows up.

Some achievements

- From 6 to 7 years of age:
- She enjoys many activities and keeps herself busy.
- Her vision is as sharp as an adult's.
- She practices her skills to perfect them.
- She jumps rope.
- She rides a bike.

- From 8 to 9 years of age:
- Her movements and skills become more elegant.
- She dresses and washes herself completely independently.
- She can use tools (a hammer, for example).

- From 10 to 12 years of age:
- Her adult dentition is complete.
- She likes manual activities, sewing, and painting.

The schoolgirl's increasing weight and height

Although every little girl grows at a different rate, the average per year from the age of 6 to 12 years is usually a weight increase of approximately 4½ lb to 6½ lb (2 to 3 kg) and a height increase of some 2½ inches (6 cm). During later childhood between the ages of 10 and 11, the physical changes in girls are more noticeable than in boys. The secretion of female hormones—estrogen and progesterone—occurs, preparing the organism for the changes of puberty. As a consequence of this, the breasts can begin to appear, sometimes as early as the age of 8, and menarche can occur from the age of 10 years.

Up to the age of 10 years, growth will be constant, and with the arrival of puberty a sudden spurt of growth will occur.

AGE	Weight (lb / kg)	Height (inches/cm)
1st month	9 lb / 4.25 kg	55 cm / 21½"
2nd month	11 lb / 5 kg	57 cm / 22½"
3nd month	12 lb /5.75 kg	61 cm / 24"
4th month	14 lb / 6.35 kg	62 cm / 24½"
5th month	15 lb / 6.95 kg	63 cm / 24¾"
6th month	16¾ lb / 7.55 kg	64 cm / 25½"
7th month	17¾ lb / 8 kg	66 cm / 25¾"
8th month	18¾ lb / 8.45 kg	68 cm / 26¾"
9th month	19¾ lb / 8.9 kg	69 cm / 27"
10th month	20½ lb / 9.35 kg	71 cm / 27¾"
11th month	21 lb / 9.65 kg	73 cm / 28¾"
12th month	21¼ lb / 9.8 kg	75 cm / 29½"
18th month	24 lb / 10.97 kg	80.66 cm / 31¾"
2 years	26 lb / 11.92 kg	85.14 cm / 33½"
3 years	30¼ lb / 11.92 kg	93.58 cm / 36¾"
4 years	35 lb / 16.07 kg	100.13 cm / 39½"
5 years	39¼ lb / 18.03 kg	106.40 cm / 41¾"
6 years	43¼ lb/ 19.91 kg	112.77 cm / 44¼ "
7 years	48½lb/ 22.00 kg	118.50 cm / 46½"
8 years	52 lb/ 23.56 kg	122.86 cm / 48¼"
9 years	58 lb / 26.40 kg	128.50 cm / 50½"
10 years	63 lb / 28.73 kg	132.94 cm / 52¼"

Puberty

Puberty is distinguished by the growth of the genital organs and the development of the secondary sexual characteristics. The more general word "adolescence" refers to the period of life from the end of infancy until the beginning of adulthood, with all the physical, psychic, and psychosocial aspects that implies.

Puberty

The period of adolescence, also called the *juvenile state*, is considered a period of transition between two phases: childhood and adulthood. The age limits vary for the start and completion of puberty. From the biological, psychological, and social point of view, it is divided into three stages: early adolescence (10–12 years), mid-adolescence (12–14 years) and late adolescence (15–19 years). Others refer to prepuberty (10–12 years), puberty (12–16 years), and adolescence (16–24 years). During puberty, biological changes take place in the physical and endocrinal spheres, implying a series of insecurities and self-esteem problems that can extend into adulthood. Social changes also occur which bring with them a greater need for independence: a critical phase occurs regarding relations with parents and a transition from attachment focused on the family to one focused on a member of the opposite sex.

What is puberty?

It is the phase of development of the human body when the maturation of the sexual organs begins and the secondary sexual characteristics start to appear.

The average age at which these changes occur is between 10 and 14 years.
- Height increases by 2 to 10 inches (5–25 cm).
- Weight increases by 15½ to 19¾ lb (7–9 kg).
- The body grows, lengthens and widens, particularly the hips.
- Growth of the nose, ears and jaw, growth of hands, feet, arms, and legs.
- Hormonal changes occur.
- Fat is redistributed.
- The breasts start to grow and the mammary areola develops.
- Hair appears in the armpits and on the pubis.
- Perspiration increases all the time and body odor appears.
- The hair and skin can become more oily and acne may appear.
- The menarche occurs, that is to say the first menstruation, also called "period," usually between the ages of 10 and 16 years.
- A rebellious reaction to parental authority occurs, as a way of opposing the process of growing up.

When an adolescent girl ovulates, a mature egg, that is to say one capable of being fertilized, is released by one of the ovaries. If an egg passing through the fallopian

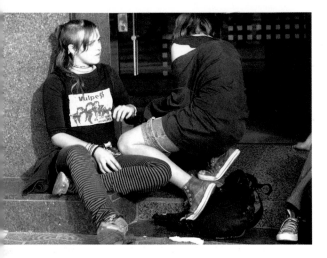

There is great variation in the speed of the changes that occur in puberty. Some adolescent girls can experience these signs of maturity earlier or later than others. It must be remembered that these variations occur at different times for each person.
A phase of ingenuousness and innocence is being left behind and the bodily changes induce new feelings.

tubes is fertilized, pregnancy occurs and it adheres to the lining of the uterus (womb) until the placenta develops. If, however, the egg is not fertilized, the endometrium (the uterine lining) is eliminated through the vagina, a process called *menstruation*.

An average menstrual cycle lasts 28 days. It starts on the first day of a menstrual period (which lasts about 6 days and involves only a very small loss of blood in some women and a more profuse loss in others) and ends on the first day of the following menstrual period. However, the duration of menstrual cycles varies, especially in the first two years following the menarche (the first menstrual period). Women can have cycles as short as

21 days or as long as 35, but anything outside those limits could be considered abnormal and requires medical attention.

As from the first menstrual period, every month one of the two ovaries will release an egg, in turn. In a normal cycle of 28 or 29 days, ovulation occurs on about the 14th day. In the first two years, menstrual cycles are irregular— longer or shorter—and later become more regular. This cycle will be repeated throughout the woman's fertile life, that is to say while the woman's body remains capable of ovulating, except during pregnancy. The fertile phase ends with menopause, which occurs at about the age of 50, when the

When does puberty begin in young girls?

Puberty usually begins in girls a year earlier than in boys, that is to say at around 10 to 11 years of age. Some girls can show the first signs at 8 to 9 years (precocious puberty) and in other cases these signs do not appear until the age of 17 (late puberty). Whether it starts early or late, this phase of growth usually lasts 4 to 6 years. A varied diet rich in vitamins influences the fact that young people today reach sexual maturity earlier than in generations past.

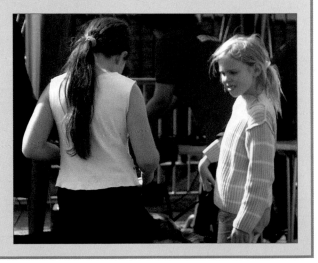

Although the physiological changes of puberty are the same in all young girls, they do not all occur at the same time for each girl. What is clear is that, by the age of 17, a girl should have experienced all the changes in her body.

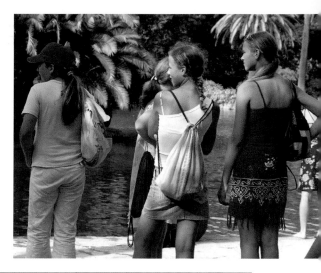

ovaries cease to be capable of producing estrogen and progesterone. With menopause, the menstrual cycle first becomes irregular again and then ceases altogether. This is often accompanied by other symptoms and disturbances, such as breathlessness, depression, and vaginal atrophy.

Where are the hormones that cause all these transformations located?

The hormonal changes that induce puberty begin in girls aged about 8. The hypothalamus, the

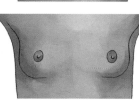

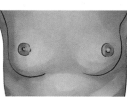

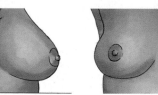

TUNNER PHASES. MAMMARY DEVELOPMENT

Phase 1. The breasts still have a prepubescent appearance. There is no mammary tissue. The areola is not developed and a slight rise in the nipple can be observed.

Phase 2. An increase in the diameter of the areola can be observed and a degree of prominence caused by the initial development of the mammary tissue below it. The areola and nipple both project. This is the mammary bud phase.

Phase 3. Following the appearance of the mammary bud, the whole breast grows in size and, at the same time, the nipple becomes more prominent. Pigmentation of the areola begins.

Phase 4. The breast size increases, the areola becoming more pigmented and prominent and projecting from the surrounding breast, three areas becoming distinguished: the nipple, the areola, and the breast.

Phase 5. The breasts acquire the appearance of those of an adult woman and only the nipple protrudes from the surrounding breast.

TUNNER PHASES. THE DEVELOPMENT OF PUBIC HAIR

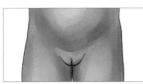 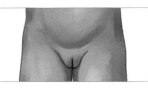 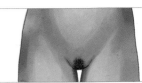

Phase 1.
Corresponds to the prepubertal phase when there is no pubic hair.

Phase 2.
A fine, soft, and pale colored down appears, covering the edges of the labia majora.

Phase 3.
The hair becomes darker, coarser, and curlier and stars to extend over the pubic area.

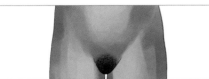

Phase 4.
The hair acquires adult characteristics, but the area it covers is still small and it does not reach the thighs.

Phase 5.
The hair covers the mound of Venus. Its shape is triangular and it extends to the inner side of the thighs.

The action of hormones, which are especially active during puberty, as well as the physical changes the body undergoes, lead to psychological changes ranging from emotional instability and odd behavior to feeling lonely and inclined to depression.

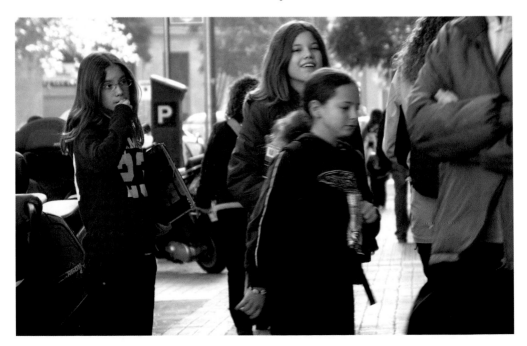

Menarche

When a girl reaches puberty she begins to ovulate. On average, the first menstrual period, or menarche, occurs between the ages of 12 and 14 years, usually two years after the breasts start developing and in most cases shortly after the appearance of the pubic and underarm hair.

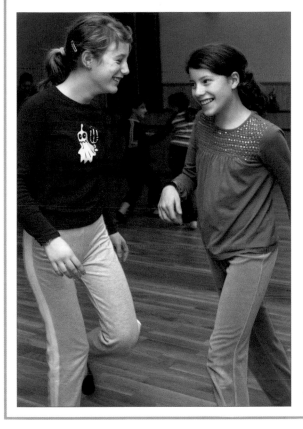

Several factors influence the early or late occurrence of sexual maturity:

- *The climate. The menarche occurs earlier in warmer climates. In hotter geographical zones and in the tropics it can occur as early as 10 to 11 years of age. Conversely, in arctic zones it can be delayed until the age of 17 or 18 years.*

- *Inheritance and the environment. There is a correlation between the age at which the menarche occurred in the mother and the age at which it occurs in the daughter. An urban environment makes the menarche occur earlier.*

- *Stress, various kinds of exhausting exercise and even diet can affect the start of menstruation and the regularity of the menstrual cycle.*

It is recommended that a girl who has not started to menstruate by the age of 16 should consult a doctor or if she has not yet shown any signs of breast, pubic or underarm hair development by the time she reaches the age of 13–14 years.

organism's control center, starts to secrete the substance that releases gonadotropine, which acts on the hypophysis [pituitary gland] to make it secrete various hormones. The first is the follicle stimulant (HFS) which acts on the female gonads, the ovaries, causing the follicles containing the eggs to start growing and produce estrogen. This hormone stimulates the growth of the breasts, the widening of the pelvis, and the development of the vulva.

The increasing level of estrogen in the bloodstream makes the hypothalamus order the pituitary gland to reduce its secretion of luteinizing hormone (HL). This makes one of the follicles burst open and release an egg (ovulation) for possible fertilization.

The remains of the follicle, now called the *corpus luteum*, stay in the ovaries secreting estrogen and a second hormone, progesterone, which prepares the lining of the uterus, the endometrium, to receive and nourish a possible zygote, or fertilized egg. If fertilization does not occur, the levels of estrogen and progesterone decrease. The lining of the womb comes away and, together with the mucous matter and the unfertilized egg, is expelled via the vagina. This involves bleeding which lasts three to seven days, a hemorrhage that constitutes the menarche or first menstruation.

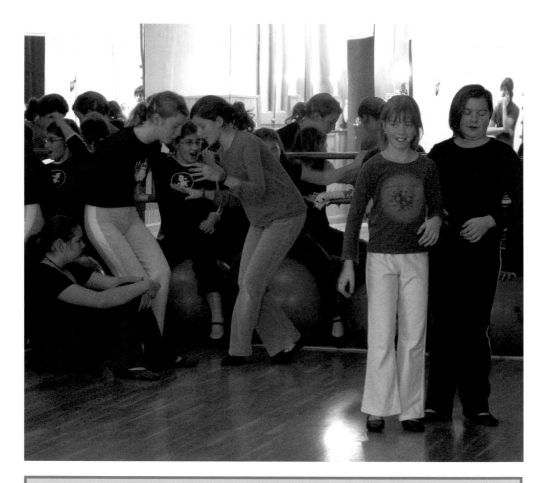

Premenstrual syndrome

Premenstrual syndrome is a series of physical and psychological symptoms that appear regularly 7 to 14 days before a menstrual period. They are not caused by any demonstrable physical or mental illness, but are intense enough to change the woman's habitual behavior. They usually disappear during the rest of the cycle. They are mainly observed in women aged between 20 and 35 years. As a rule, it can be affirmed that the more children a woman has had, the less likely she will be to suffer pre menstrual syndrome.

Symptoms
- Headaches, abdominal and muscular pain, painful breasts.
- Hot flushes, sweating, nausea, vomiting.
- Swelling of the abdomen, breasts, hands and ankles.
- Skin problems: acne, brown marks, pimples.
- Tension, irritability, aggressiveness.
- Tendency to be emotional, mood changes, apathy.
- Depression, tiredness, weakness, torpor.
- Difficulty in concentrating, social withdrawal.
- Increased appetite and/or eating candy, etc.

Adolescence

Adolescence is the phase that marks the transformation of the little girl into the adult woman, a period of transition with its own particular characteristics. It is called adolescence because those it concerns are young people with a clear identity and definition who are no longer entirely little girls but are not adult either. They are a kind of hybrid with foretastes of adulthood and remnants of childhood. The development adolescents experience during this phase causes them to experience a crisis, as they find themselves seeking their own identity in the process of configuring their personality.

The characteristics of adolescence

During adolescence, girls grow and mature rapidly. These changes usually start at the age of 11 years. The hormonal changes responsible for them really begin years earlier and can cause periods of anxiety and bad temper. Girls experience these changes earlier than boys and therefore seem to mature much more quickly. Young girls can already be as physically mature as their parents, and capable of having their own children. It is not surprising that, due to the speed of these changes, some adolescent girls become so preoccupied by their appearance that they have to be subdued, particularly if they do not grow or mature as fast as their female friends.

Adolescent girls start to think and feel differently. This is the time when they begin to form close relationships outside the family circle with friends of their own age. Relations with the family change too. Parents become less indispensable when adolescents develop their own lives outside the family.

The first disagreements usually arise when adolescents start to develop their own points of view, which are frequently not those of their parents. As a way of achieving a sense of identity different from that of their relatives, adolescents usually spend a lot of time with people outside the family or talking to friends on the telephone. This is another aspect that can annoy parents, but it is an important way for them to achieve a sense of own identity, independent of their family. These friendships form part of the girl's apprenticeship in how to get on with others.

During this phase, clothes, fashion, and physical appearance become very important, either as a way of expressing their unity with friends or as a way of declaring their growing independence from the family.

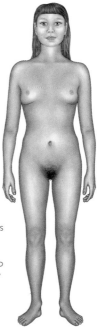

Adolescence is a process, without temporal limits, in the cycle of human life. The World Health Organization defines adolescence as the phase that occurs between the ages of 10 and 19 years, establishing two stages, early adolescence (10–14 years) and late adolescence (15–19 years). Adolescence begins with puberty, that is to say, a series of fairly rapid physical and physiological changes that end with the full maturity of the sexual organs and the capacity to reproduce and have sexual relationships. However, adolescence is not confined solely to those changes, but is typified also by important psychological and social transformations.

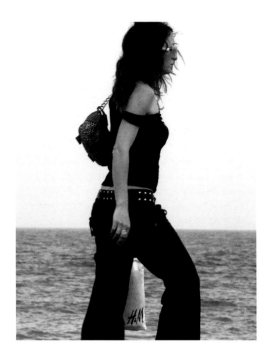

Parents often feel rejected, and to some extent they are. But this apparent rejection is necessary for the young girl to become an adult with her own identity. Although confrontations and quarrels may be frequent, adolescents usually have a high opinion of their parents. The rejections and disputes do not usually have anything to do with the personality of the parents, but rather concern the fact that it is precisely from their parents that they must become independent if they want to have their own life.

While they are striving to be more independent, adolescents also want to achieve new objectives but, when they find themselves in difficulty, they may admit that they have little past experience to rely on. This can lead to rapid switches in their self-confidence and behavior, so they may appear very mature one moment and very childish the next. The feeling of being overwhelmed or losing self-confidence can make them feel childish, and this is often expressed in moods and grumpiness rather than disagreement.

Parents have to be flexible about this behavior, although they may well find it quite stressful.

Sexual development

Falling passionately in love is a phenomenon that acquires some especially strange characteristics in adolescence and is intensely, but delicately, linked to interpersonal relations at this age.

In early adolescence, what is called love at first sight can occur, and not only may such love not be reciprocated but the beloved person may also be totally unaware of it. The loved one then becomes an idealized figure incarnated in the form of a movie star, famous sportsperson, etc. who may also have the characteristic of being, in some way, a substitute parent figure.

In adolescence, sexual relations with people of the opposite sex are more frequent than is generally believed, although as a rule they are only exploratory learning exercises. During this phase, we clearly see sexual development, which customarily begins with autoeroticism. This is the phase of discovering the opposite sex through dances, sport, games, and petting, and also of sexual curiosity expressed as the interest in pornographic magazines that is frequent in many adolescent boys.

Certain aspects characteristic of masculine behavior are sometimes seen in girls and feminine behavior in boys, although as a rule these are only normal expressions of an as yet incompletely resolved sexuality.

During this phase, idealizations of the mother appear. The mother acquires positive and powerful characteristics and the teenage girl accepts her feminine physical attributes and identifies herself with the positive aspects of her progenitor. The same occurs between teenage boys and their fathers.

By adequately combining the acceptance of their physical characteristics and their identification

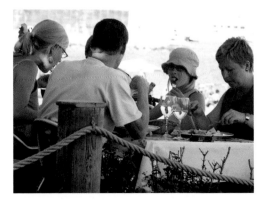

with the corresponding feminine and masculine figures, adolescents form a sexuality that will enable them to assume their responsibilities.

Changes in adolescence
• Emotional instability and fluctuation in self-image. Variations occur in the adolescent's state of

Advice for parents

• Adolescents must be guided so that they learn and know how to profit from their mistakes. Instead of subjecting them to interrogations that will only exasperate them, the best way is to ask: "Why do you think you made a mistake?" "What do you think you should have done?"

• Instead of giving them instructions, let them assume responsibilities and ask them "What do you think you'll do now to sort the situation?"

• Avoid forcing them to do things the way their parents do. Instead of trying to convince them, give them a chance to judge and experiment—for example, in the case of their clothes.

• Help them to discover what is admirable in their person. Make them aware that they are valued for what they are, not for what they wear or what they own.

• Give them the opportunity to live their own experiences in situations that do not imply any great risk. For example, in the case of money, they can be allowed a certain sum to manage as they like.

• Make sure that at home there are clear rules and that they know what they are and the reason for them, to help and train them. There must be clear but reasonable limits set down for their security.

• Be watchful about what your children see and read, as a basis for reflection rather than repression. You could make or take the opportunity of going to a movie or watching a television program with them and then discuss and assess it, to help them form standards.

Emotions

There is a strong tendency to melancholy. Adolescents are inclined to extend the consequences of a failure to all their plans, tending toward fatalism and obsession when faced by small and passing physical problems, such as acne, obesity, growth anomalies, etc.

In many cases they keep an intimate diary, which is nothing more than a conversation with themselves, as they feel they cannot converse with another person they trust.

The movement toward others and the creation of cliques or gangs is an expression of the desire to make themselves known or to be recognized, the desire for approval and understanding, which are essential during this phase.

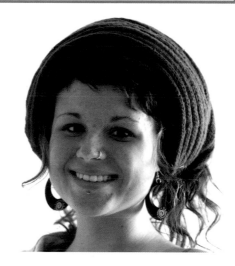

mind without apparent reason. Sometimes they are full of energy and at others they fall into lethargy.

• Insecurity. The adolescent girl finds herself in a no man's land, as she has ceased to be a child but does not yet feel like an adult. The disproportion between the goals she is pursuing at this age and the means and experience necessary to attain them makes her feel discouraged and even like a failure on occasions.

A time of personal insecurity. The changes the adolescent girl undergoes during this time, her aspirations, which sometimes become a veritable obsession, through constructing her own world, make her feel great insecurity and uncertainty about the future, but she wants to emerge by her own efforts. Nevertheless, this is the time when adolescent girls most need affection.

Reactions can be contradictory, but they are always objectively exaggerated. The immature personality of an adolescent girl can make her react disproportionately to difficulties and even lead her to take a self-affirming attitude, systematically opposing her parents, as well as adopting forms of rebellion that in reality are defense mechanisms.

• Lack of determination. The adolescent girl finds it difficult to do things and can feel a degree of dejection when faced with the problems of ordinary life. She devotes herself enthusiastically to the things that interest her personally and makes huge efforts in that respect, but not to daily obligations or family requirements. Adolescents usually want to achieve things right here and right now. They tend to want immediate and easy satisfaction, and lack the perseverance to finish what they have begun.

Adolescent situations

- *The desire to make herself independent from her parents.*
- *Ascertaining her own personality.*
- *Sexual behavior with the development of her sexual identity.*
- *Group tendency.*
- *Importance of the influence of her female friends and their acceptance.*
- *Relations with companions become more accentuated.*
- *Possibility of falling in love.*
- *Possibility of forming a committed long-term relationship.*

• Sexuality. More than half of adolescent girls will have their first complete sexual experience before the age of 16. Those who start sexual relations as early as this are at greater risk of unwanted pregnancies and health problems such as sexually transmitted diseases. Moreover, the adolescent girl may not be certain of her sexual orientation and have doubts about whether or not she is attracted to her own sex.

• Tendency to gregariousness. Distinctive signs, group standards, and a particular jargon are adopted, giving the adolescent girl the feeling of belonging to a group and of unity with friends. She is no longer so dependent on the family and, conversely, becomes more dependent on the group. Moreover, having this group of friends also allows the integration of the sexes and greater familiarity with the opposite sex. The adolescent girl seeks friends to whom she can express everything she feels and wants. Very few people will be considered worthy of this.

• A time of change. During this time, the young girl starts to notice changes in her body, her state of mind and sensitivity, and doesn't know how to deal with them. She feels new instinctive tendencies and does not yet have the capacity to rationalize them or the temperamental balance to confront them.

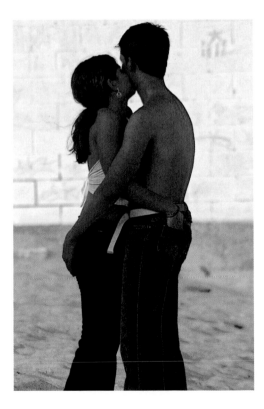

The principal risk factors

- Family problems.
- Poor performance at school and even abandoning school altogether.
- Eating disorders.
- Drinking alcohol and taking drugs.
- Sexually transmitted diseases associated with risky behavior.
- Unwanted pregnancies.

Genital anatomy

- Vulva or external genitals. Situated in the bottom of the pelvic cavity. Two pairs of lips start below the mound of Venus—which is the area where the pubic hair appears at puberty—and end at the anus.
- Labia majora These lips surround and protect the external orifices of the reproductive and urinary systems, the clitoris and the labia minora, which are inside them and smaller.
- Clitoris. This is the most sensitive part of the female sex organs. It is like a little button that varies in length from ¼ to 1 inch (0.5–2.5 cm). It is formed of two hollow pieces of spongy tissue, which grow harder and increase in size during sexual arousal.
- Urethra. The outlet orifice of the urethra, by means of which urine is evacuated from the urinary bladder, is located between the clitoris and the entrance to the vagina.
- Vagina. A highly elastic muscular tube, 4 to 6 inches (10–15 cm) long. It is partially blocked by a membrane called the hymen, which is usually broken when a woman begins her sexual life. It accommodates the penis during coitus and is the

channel through which the baby emerges in natural childbirth.

- Uterus. Also called the womb, the uterus is situated behind the bladder and in front of the rectum. It is a hollow, muscular pear-shaped organ with a thick and elastic wall 2¾–3¼ inches (7–8 cm) long. Its function is to nourish the developing embryo until birth. It reaches adult size at the age of 15 years and shrinks after the menopause.
- Uterine or fallopian tubes. These tubes emerge from the top of the uterus, one on each side. Their lower part, known as the neck or cervix, is attached to the vagina. The tubes are two channels some 4 inches (10 cm) long which extend from the ovaries to the uterus. Their task is to receive the eggs released from the ovaries and conduct them to the uterus. Inside, each tube contains microscopic hairs which, when they vibrate, help

Sexually transmitted diseases (STDs)

Also known as venereal diseases, these illnesses are spread by promiscuous sexual contact, which is very frequent in adolescence. The sexual partner may seem healthy but may have the infection asymptomatically and pass it on. The risk of most of the common and treatable infections is progression to inflammatory pelvic disease with its fearful consequence: infertility. These are the infections caused by gonococcus, chlamydia, papilloma virus and trichomonas. Others, such as syphilis (treatable), hepatitis B and the human immune deficiency virus [HIV], cause disease in different parts of the body and to the baby in pregnant women. Although it is not the most frequent, HIV infection may be the most dreaded at present because it is incurable and frequently fatal.

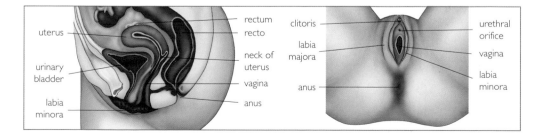

■ Sexuality in adolescence. Adolescent pregnancy

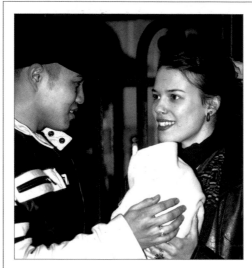

Sexuality in adolescence is typified by curiosity and anxiety about one's own body, which is developing and changing abruptly, and about the sudden increase in sexual hormones, sexual feelings, and the sexual instinct. As a result of this revolution that is being unleashed in the adolescent, masturbation occurs, the causes of which are biological.

It should be pointed out that masturbation is just another sign of the adolescent's sexual development and is completely natural. Adolescents are very curious. This quite natural adolescent curiosity in many cases leads them to start sexual relations early, but it is not simply an indication of freedom and can often lead them to lose the capacity to be free.

Unwanted pregnancy is one of the principal risks associated with sexual relations in adolescence. The factors that increase the risk are:

- *Lack of accurate information. More than 70% of young people think they are well informed about sexuality. However, certain myths are still widespread among young people today. This is not surprising, considering that almost half of all young people obtain their information either from friends or from magazines and movies. On the other hand, many young people who decide to inform themselves do not know where to go, or feel embarrassed about doing so.*

- *Another factor is lack of social skills or self-control or the failure to require their partner to exercise self-control. The idea that it is normal for young people to have sexual relationships is very widespread. Adolescents feel themselves pressurized by their friends, or by television programs showing young actors who are sexually active. This is known as group pressure and may trigger them to do something even though they are not fully convinced it is right, simply by believing that the rest of the group is doing it. And again, they feel they are ready to maintain this type of relationship although they are not so from the social point of view.*

- *In some cases, another factor is ambivalence about a pregnancy as the fruit of an idyllic and marvelous adolescent love affair. Added to this is the eagerness for risk and the low self-esteem that are characteristic of adolescence, which helps us understand the situation of many girls who end up with an unwanted pregnancy.*

to move the egg on its way to the uterine cavity. It is on this journey that the egg is fertilized.

• Ovaries. These are the sex glands that contain the eggs and produce the sexual hormones. They are oval in shape, measuring about 1 ½ inches (4 cm), and are situated at the ends of the fallopian tubes. The woman does not manufacture her sexual cells—when she is born she already has about 400,000 oocytes, that is to say, immature eggs, which are stored in bag-like follicles. Some

400 of them will mature during the woman's fertile life, which begins at puberty and ends with menopause.

Maturity

At the end of adolescence, about the age of 18, a woman completes her physical development and embarks on the period of life called maturity or *adulthood*. During this time, therefore, a series of anatomical and physiological changes occur in the organism which constitute the culmination of the complex process of growth and development that has been going on during childhood and puberty. During this period, which lasts from about the ages of 20 to 40, the woman makes many decisions which will affect the rest of her life: she becomes more emotionally stable, more autonomous and independent of her parents, starts work, finds a partner, has children and brings them up. The achievement of all her plans will determine the rest of her life.

The mature woman

The young woman finds herself in a period of apprenticeship, adjustment and decision-making that will lead her to commit herself and define her lifestyle. Biologically, she is an adult, but that does not mean that she has made career, family, and work commitments. Psychologically, she is waiting until she has overcome the changes of adolescence and achieved emancipation, emotional and sexual stability, her complete identity, and the capacity to make commitments.

As far as social development is concerned, it is possible that most of the differences between early maturity and middle-maturity are due not so much to physical or cognitive changes as to the course of life itself: working, forming a couple, having children, establishing new relationships, etc. It could be said that there are two basic facts that distinguish maturity: the need to establish emotional relationships and productivity. For most adults, emotional links are focused on family commitments with one's partner, parents, and children. Work is the person's other productive activity, including

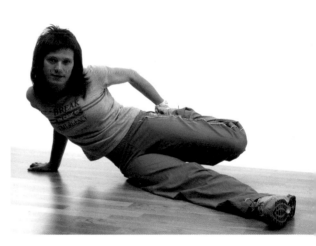

From the point of view of physical development, a woman's capacities reach their highest point at the beginning of adulthood. Her capacity to react, the acuteness of her senses and her cardiac efficiency, for example, reach their peak at about the age of 25.

the professional career. Many women start their adult lives through work rather than marriage these days.

The family has changed a great deal recently. Nowadays, there are very diverse family units, but in spite of everything, most young adults marry or find partners. The beginning of life as a couple means facing responsibilities and a form of apprenticeship involving a sharing of roles or tasks, something which is not always easy.

Characteristics of the adult woman

- The typical adult woman is characterized by her strength, energy and stamina.

- From the age of 20, when most of the body is fully developed, until the age of 50, the decline in physical capacities is usually so gradual as to be unnoticeable.

- She is usually taller than her mother because of progressively improving diet and health care. Between the ages of 30 and 45, her height remains stable, but later begins to decrease.

- Her muscular strength reaches its peak at between the ages of 25 and 30, following which 10% of it is gradually lost between the ages of 30 and 60. Most of the weakening occurs in the back and leg muscles. The decline is less marked in the arm muscles.

- Manual dexterity is most efficient in the young woman. Finger agility and hand movements begin to decline from the age of 35.

- The capacity to react and the acuteness of the senses reach their peak at the age of about 25.

- There is a gradual loss of hearing which typically starts before the age of 30. Once past that age, hearing loss becomes progressively more marked.

- The senses of taste, smell, and sensitivity to pain and temperature do not usually show signs of decline until about the age of 45 to 50.

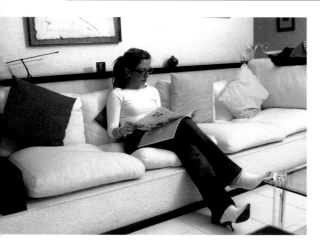

complain or feel anxious about their lack of time to devote to motherhood, because of other responsibilities. Few women today operate only as wife-mother-housewife—the great majority of

At present, women play an active role in the family, and the division of duties between the couple is usually more adapted to the work requirements of each of its members. The role of the mother is usually one of the most important for an adult woman and a great satisfaction to the couple. However, many mothers nowadays

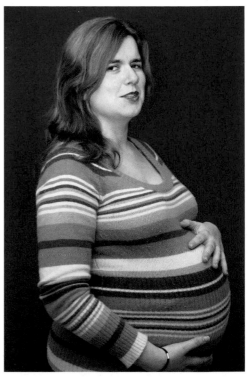

As regards motherhood, the birth of a child is usually a happy event and, generally, this experience makes a woman mature. Pregnancy, birth, and bringing up the baby are indisputably feminine functions.

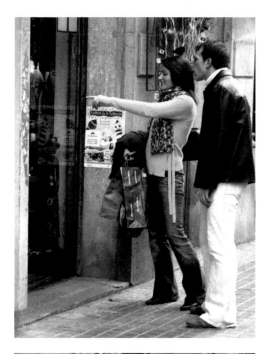

As regards cognitive development, early maturity represents the years of greatest interest in certain kinds of learning and memory. It is not known whether problem-solving and creativity suffer a decline in middle-maturity. Other factors have to be borne in mind when assessing these functions: the teaching imparted, personal circumstances, and the state of mind.

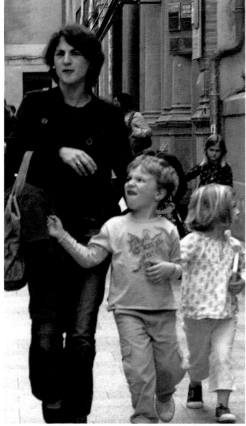

them work, study, or carry out other activities, so they have less energy to dedicate to the family.

Gradually, women have fallen into what could be called the *superwoman syndrome* in an accelerated and competitive society. Women spend their lives trying to be good wives, good mothers and good professionals, not to mention, in many cases, the commitment also to be good daughters caring for elderly parents. It is not surprising that women frequently suffer from stress.

Sexuality and the couple relationship

The capacity to feel erotic pleasure starts at birth and is maintained throughout life. However, age models the biological dimension of sexuality, and the intensity and quantity of response vary considerably from one phase of life to another.

Age influences the sexual cycle of men differently from that of women. Men achieve the maximum level of sexual response at about the age of 18 and show a slow and progressive decline from then on. Conversely, women experience the maximum capacity for sexual response at around the age of 30 to 40, after which the sexual impulse declines, but more slowly than in men.

These days, women see the sexual relationship as an act of gratification and not merely an act of procreation, which has caused eroticism to be accepted in everyday life. For women, their sexuality has become a form of play. It is not possible to

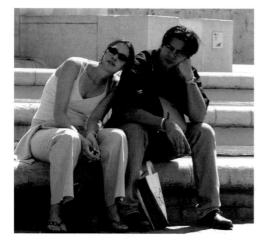

Almost all couples experience problems about the frequency of their sexual relations. This is inevitable, but these difficulties need not necessarily threaten their life together. Each partner must be reasonable and surrender a little of their terrain to the benefit of their partner.

Upbringing considerably affects a person's sexual instinct. Severity, the repression of instincts and their assimilation with sin can produce a conscious or unconscious reaction in the adult, reducing his or her sexual appetite or, on the contrary, increasing it considerably.

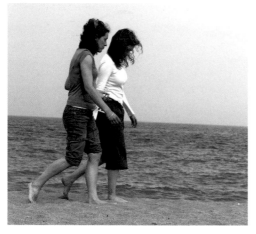

generalize and say that all women find their sexuality gratifying, but nevertheless more than 60 percent of women today admit that they masturbate, which would have been unthinkable only a few decades ago.

The personality of a woman, her intellectual motivations, sensitivity, and previous education are very important factors in the enjoyment of full sexuality. Women are becoming increasingly active and less conformist, which has changed the stereotypical roles played by the man and by the woman herself in their sexual relations. Moreover, women are becoming ever better informed and have more reliable methods of birth control, which has given them greater freedom and security to enjoy sex.

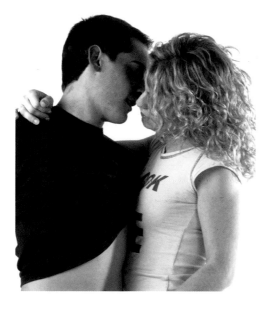

A woman's sexual instinct oscillates enormously because of conditioning factors in her environment, such as children, the family, financial problems, the amorous indifference of the man or differences in understanding between the couple.

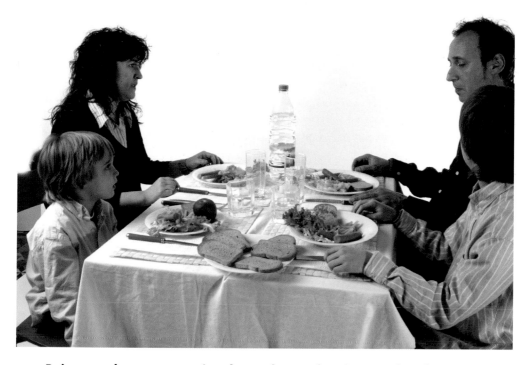

Being good parents requires large doses of patience, a lot of serenity and a well-ordered list of priorities. Children need great dedication.

Relations between parents and children

Relations with children must not be rigid or cold. Common sense should guide parents about how to react at the right moment and with the right degree of intensity. Cheerfulness, calm, patience, firmness, attentiveness, acknowledging limitations and highlighting virtues are important in winning the trust of children. The authority of the mother and father must be imposed with the aim of each helping the other with respect to the child. A parent must be firm, but moderately so. Children were not born knowing everything and everything in life requires a period of apprentices-

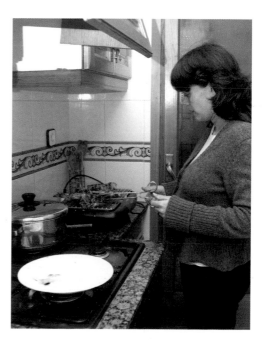

Modern society, the pace of life and today's demands oblige women to play a difficult role with many facets and various responsibilities, both in the family and at work.

▟ The patience of parents

All parents lose patience now and then, although the most likely to do so are those who are experiencing work or domestic problems.

Several types of impatience can be distinguished, such as giving a smack in a certain situation, not listening to the child when she wants to talk, never playing with her or not showing the least interest in her school or out-of-school activities, and always justifying it with not having time. These attitudes are negative for both the child and the parents, who will later feel a sense of guilt.

Probably the worst attitude is that of parents who continually shout at their children, belittling or ridiculing them, behavior that will lead to reducing their self-esteem.

There are also some parents who are over-demanding and harsh with their children when they do not attain the standards required of them.

hip. Sometimes, only the negative is stressed, but the positive should also be pointed out, and children must be allowed peace and tranquility within parental requirements.

Always, in any situation, it is best to act serenely and calmly. Life is usually very hurried and so it is easy to be unhinged, but, for the good of the children, it is best not to lose one's balance, to talk with them, make them think, and de-dramatize the situation as much as possible. If two people try to be serene parents, it will be easier for children to grow up mature and happy, because, irremediably,

for children their parents are and will continue to be the model to follow, for good or ill.

Whatever may be the model of a parent that appeals to you, if you really want to be a patient parent, you will have to make an effort to put your priorities in order. It is important to spend some of your spare time with your children, and it must be remembered that children should be treated with respect, just as you expect respect from them. Good manners are necessary for everyone, be they young or old.

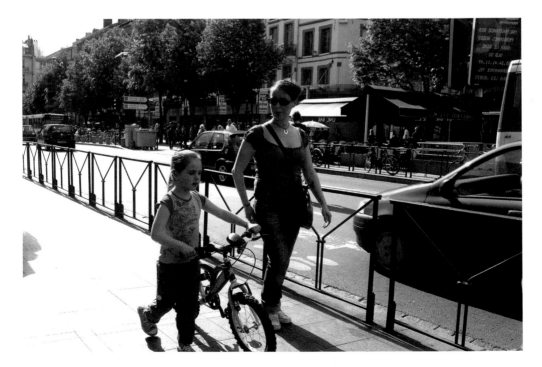

Old age

Aging is a process inherent in all living things. It is just one more biological process that forms part of life. It begins at the moment of birth, as it is nothing more than an accumulation of years. Aging is not pathological in itself, so it should be viewed positively and the negative aspects usually attributed to it should be rejected.

Important changes in the various systems that should be borne in mind

Changes in appearance

• With age, height declines at just under a ½ inch (1 cm) a decade from the age of 40 to 50, owing to the wear of the vertebral column. The trunk becomes stouter and the extremities thinner. There is increased curvature of the vertical column, cyphosis, which produces a bent look typical of old age.

• The stride changes, arm movements growing smaller, and the support base increasing.

• The skin loses flexibility and elasticity and lines appear. The woman's sweat glands grow smaller and she perspires less, predisposing her to erratic temperature changes.

• The hair can lose the cells that produce the pigment called melanin and white hairs appear.

As her life proceeds, the woman approaches maturity and achieves it fully when her physical faculties (agility, stamina) and intellectual capacities (analysis, skill, memory, knowledge, etc.) are in perfect balance. The moment when one of these faculties starts to decline initiates the aging process. This change occurs very slowly. We do not at present know exactly what causes aging in living things. It is known that the life of each species is directly linked to the length of time that particular species take to reach reproductive maturity.

THE PRINCIPAL COMPLAINTS OF OLD AGE IN WOMEN

Vision
• Reduction in capacity to focus.
• Loss of visual acuteness.
• Loss of capacity to adapt to darkness.

Hearing
• Overall loss of hearing.
• Loss of discrimination.

Heart and arteries
• Fibrosis of the blood vessels: hardening of the arteries, high blood pressure, reduction in circulation.
• Cardiac fibrosis: calcification of the heart valves, loss of myocardial elasticity, diastolic diminution.

Respiratory system
• Reduction in pulmonary elasticity.
• Reduction in ciliary activity.
• Deterioration of the pulmonary vessels.
• Reduction in respiratory movements.

Digestive system
• General reduction in motility.
• Loss of teeth. Poor mastication.
• Reduction in gastrointestinal secretions.

Kidney function
• Sclerosis of the renal vessels.
• Reduction in intrarenal circulation.
• Reduction in overall functioning.

31

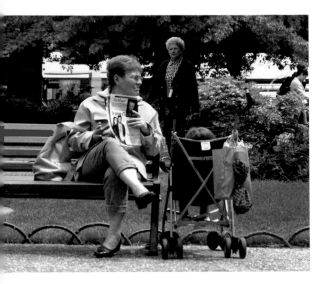

The fact that the arrival of menopause coincides with a series of changes in the woman's body in no way means that she cannot lead an absolutely normal life, both physically and socially.

Changes in the composition of the body

• With aging, muscular mass is lost and thus the strength and capacity to exert maximum physical effort.

• Bodily water in the organism lessens. In a young person, water accounts for about 60 percent of body weight, but declines to 50 percent of body weight in old people. This loss occurs mainly through loss of water in the cells. This means a greater tendency to dehydration in the old.

• The muscle mass reduces and bodily fat increases, redistributing itself mainly on the trunk.

• Bone mass is lost, favoring the appearance of osteoporosis and fractures.

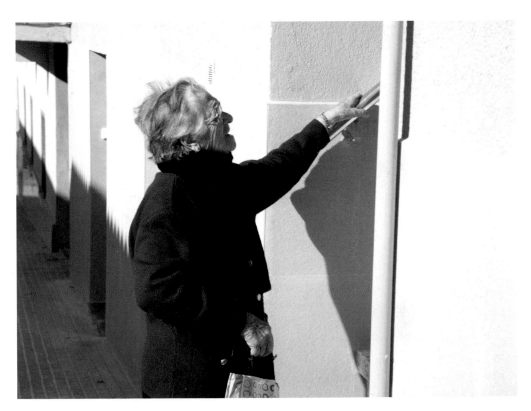

In recent years life expectancy has increased and will go on increasing thanks to improved medicines, better laboratory tests, and technology for making earlier diagnoses of many of the ailments that used to be incapacitating and/or fatal. It is thought that in the near future the old-age threshold of 60 years will be modified.

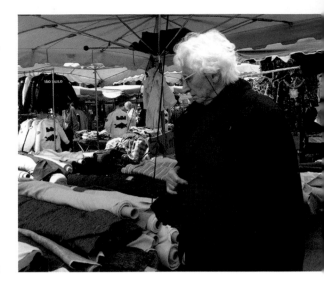

Changes in the sense organs

• With age, taste buds are lost, especially those that perceive sweet tastes.

• There is a reduction in the *capacity* to hear high frequency sounds because of the degeneration of the inner ear in a phenomenon called *presbycusis* or *deafness*, due to aging. This makes it difficult to hear high notes or consonants and can make them unintelligible.

• The crystalline lens of the eye becomes denser, thicker, and less elastic, losing the capacity to focus on close objects, in a process called presbyopia or *long-sightedness*. Those suffering from it start to have difficulty reading the small print in a newspaper held at a normal distance and can only

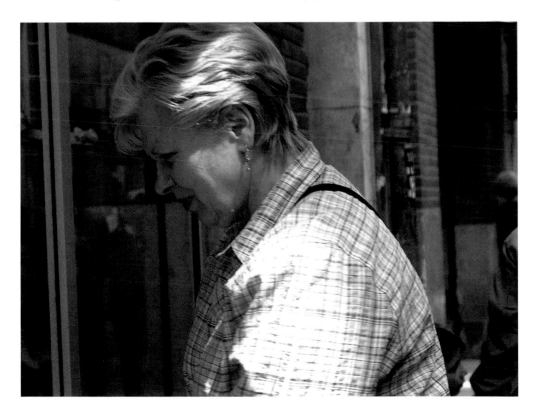

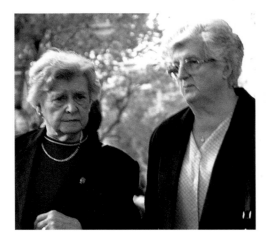

focus on it by holding the paper farther away. Sharpness of vision also declines with age and the deterioration of the receptive cells of the retina may contribute to this.

Changes in the circulatory system

• The arteries become more rigid due to the increased thickness of their internal or intimate layer. This occurs independently of any arteriosclerotic disease, which is generally universal in developed societies and is favored by these changes.

• The heart suffers a loss of internal or intimate lining that controls the increase in the heart rate in response to exercise. The functioning of the heart does not change when at rest but does change as regards the mechanisms that adapt to effort.

Changes in the respiratory system

• A stiffer and less mobile thorax and a lessening of pulmonary elasticity causes the respiratory system to lose vital capacity, producing a reduction in the volume of respiratory reserve and an increase in the residual volume which does not move within the lungs.

Changes in the digestive tract

• In addition to tooth loss and less efficient mastication, the most important changes in this system have two aspects:
- Reduced motor function, making the stomach slow to empty and causing a tendency to strain in the bowel.
- A reduction in the secretion of gastric juices which makes some things difficult to absorb. The

secretion of certain gastrointestinal hormones is also reduced.

Changes in the kidneys

Renal function is generally reduced because of a reduction in the size of the kidneys, a reduction in the flow of blood to them, and a reduction in the functioning glomerular cells which filter the blood. A reduction in the clearance of substances occurs and a loss of capacity to dilute and concentrate the urine.

Nevertheless, this renal aging still allows adequate maintenance of the internal environment, although it makes this purifying system more vulnerable to any kind of attack.

Changes in the endocrine system

As a general rule, some hormones behave very differently from others. There is a marked reduction in glucose tolerance with lower sensitivity to normal insulin secretion. This phenomenon is attributable to greater peripheral resistance to its action in the tissues, contributing to sugar intolerance and the fact that diabetes is more frequent among older people.

Changes in the immune system

The immune system undergoes changes that tend to reduce its defensive capability against infections and tumors. With age, the thymus involucrates and changes occur in the number of lymphocytes and the response to antibodies.

As well as these changes in its defensive role, the immune system's capacity to recognize foreign material deteriorates, leading it to react against what is wanted and to favor the development of autoimmune illnesses.

Changes in the nervous system

As regards the aging of the nervous system, and specifically of the brain, it is very difficult to separate what is normal from what is pathological. Many of the changes that are observed under the microscope in ailments such as Alzheimer's disease or Parkinson's disease are also observed in the normal brain. In many cases, the difference is only a question of quantity. The brain atrophies with age. There is a reduction in its weight and an increase in the furrows between the cerebral convolutions and in the internal cavities. From infancy onward, there is a loss of neurons that is offset by an increase in the connections between them.

THE PARTS AND ORGANS AFFECTED BY MENOPAUSE

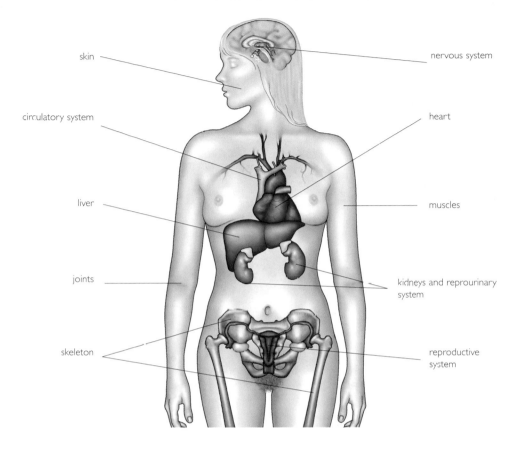

skin

circulatory system

liver

joints

skeleton

nervous system

heart

muscles

kidneys and reprourinary system

reproductive system

Changes also occur in the neurotransmitters produced in the central nervous system. All these changes to the aging nervous system mean that the old person becomes less sensitive to touch and vibrations. As regards movement, the capacity for muscular coordination and control declines leading to a slowing of psychomotor function. The speed at which the peripheral nerves operate decreases, leading to slower reflexes.

Menopause

Menopause is a medical term meaning the last menstruation in a woman's life. The word comes from the Greek word *mens*, meaning monthly, and *pausis*, meaning cessation. Menopause is a natural phase in the aging process, due to a decreased production of the estrogen and progesterone hor-

mones, accompanied by the loss of the capacity to reproduce.

Unlike the menarche, the start of menstruation in youth, the changes that lead to the cessation of the menstrual function and to a metabolic adjustment last for several years, corresponding to the period called the climacteric. It varies from woman to woman, but usually occurs between the ages of 42 and 56. A woman is considered to be menopausal when she has not menstruated for a year without being pregnant and is not suffering from an illness causing an absence of menstruation.

Menopause is a normal process. In no case is it an illness or a pathological process. However, some women go through difficult years because of hormonal changes.

The symptoms of menopause are many and each woman experiences or suffers them differently. Many women have few or no symptoms,

Symptoms that can appear during menopause

- Weight gain.
- Breathlessness or sudden hot flushes.
- Insomnia.
- Night sweating.
- Vaginal dryness.
- Joint pain.
- Fatigue.
- Small memory losses.

- Intestinal troubles.
- Dryness of the eyes.
- Itchy skin.
- Mood changes.
- Greater proneness to urinary infections.

while for others they are very intense and troublesome.

The most obvious symptoms of the start of menopause, in reality the perimenopause, are changes in the rhythm of the menstrual cycle (monthly periods very close together or very far apart) or changes in the quantity of blood loss (excessive or slight).

It has been suggested that 30% of women have ceased menstruating before the age of 45 and about 2% are still menstruating after the age of 55. Among the factors that affect the arrival of menopause are heredity, socioeconomic level, race (Mediterranean and Nordic women experience it earlier), and smoking. These advance the age at which it occurs. There are changes in the amount and distribution of body fat, wrinkles increase, the skin becomes flabby, and osteoporosis occurs.

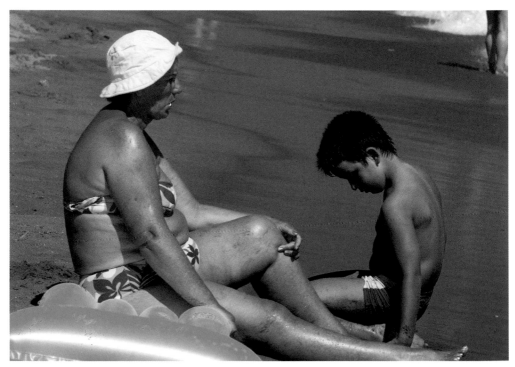

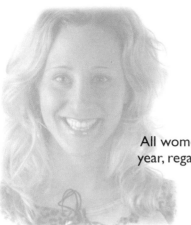

Medical checkups

All women need to undergo medical checkups at least once a year, regardless of their age or state of health, to eliminate the possibility of an illness or prevent it in good time.

General checkup

There are various reasons for routine medical checkups: to check the woman's present general state of health, to ensure that she has not caught any transmissible disease, or in the case of a hereditary condition. Whatever the reason, a series of different analyses are made in order to establish a complete diagnosis. These checks are also advisable to discover various serious ailments in their initial stages, facilitating their treatment.

TEST	FREQUENCY	WHY?	MORE FREQUENTLY
Weight	At any medical examination	Weight variations are related to many illnesses.	When there are sudden weight changes and they are not deliberate.
Blood pressure	Annually, for an adult woman	To check the state of health of the heart and blood vessels.	At least once a year, or more often if contraceptive pills are being taken, if there are problems, or if the doctor so prescribes.
Urine	With any other medical examination	To reveal the state of health of the kidneys, whether there is an infection of any kind or if the patient is diabetic.	In the case of suspicious symptoms.
Blood sugar	In any blood analysis	A high level of sugar in the blood can be a symptom of diabetes.	If the patient is diabetic.
Cholesterol	Once every five years	Indicates the probability of heart problems and/or heart attack.	If the patient's clinical history includes high cholesterol levels, or depending on the medication being taken.
Cervical smear test, also called Papanicolau test	Annually. For every woman between the ages of 18 and 64 who has had sexual relations.	Reveals the existence of abnormal cells that could indicate cancer of the cervix.	If there are gynecological problems or if the doctor requests it.
Mammogram	Once a year as from the age of 40–50.	Early detection of breast cancer	If there is a family history of breast cancer.

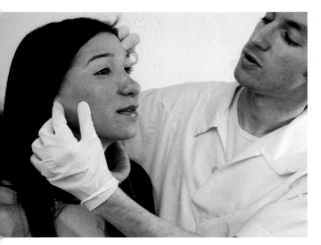

If you think you can't hear properly, consult your doctor. Above all, don't put off visiting a specialist: there is an easy solution to many hearing problems.

The World Health Organization (WHO) defines health as *"the complete state of physical, psychic, and social well-being, and not only the absence of infections and illnesses."* This means that, to achieve optimum health, each person must play an active and responsible role regarding his or her beha-

What is glaucoma?

Glaucoma is a disease of the eyes which is usually hereditary. Abnormally high blood pressure inside the eye can lead to blindness. Therefore if there has been any case of glaucoma in the family, the eyes should be examined regularly. Early and correct treatment and, in more severe cases, surgery, can prevent or delay the more serious problems caused by glaucoma.

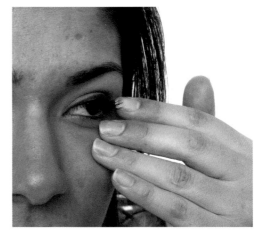

vior and habits, which are what mainly determine their total level of well-being.

What is included in a medical examination

Before any physical medical examination, the woman is asked a series of questions about her medical antecedents, whether there is any illness in the family, and about her general way of life, for example whether she smokes or suffers from insomnia.

Sight tests, dental care, and hearing
The eyes

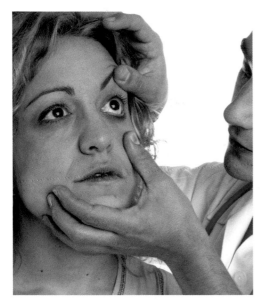

• The eye examination is very important, especially in infancy, as it is at that stage that defects can still be corrected, before they become irremediable problems. In adulthood, especially in people

THE NORMAL VALUES OF BIOCHEMICAL PARAMETERS MOST FREQUENT IN WOMEN	
BIOCHEMICAL PARAMETERS	NORMAL VALUES
Glucose in blood	70 and 105 mg per deciliter; in children, 40 to 100 mg/dl
Uric acid	Adult women: 2.5 to 7.5 mg/dl Little girls: 2.5 to 5 mg/dl
Urea	7 and 20 mg per deciliter Little girls: 5 to 18 mg/dl
Creatinine	Adult women: 0.5 and 1.2 mg/dl Little girls: 0.2 and 1 mg/dl
Direct bilirrubine	0.1 to 0.2 md/100 ml
Total bilirrubine	0.3 to 1.0 mg / 100 ml
Indirect bilirrubine	less than 1.0 mg/ml
Alkaline phosphatase	30 to 120 U/L
Gamma GT	Women: 5 to 120 U/L
GOTS	5 to 32 mU/ml
GPT [glutamic pyruvic transaminase]	7 to 33 mU/ml
HDL [high-density lipoprotein level]	Women: more than 55 mg/100 ml
Total proteins	6.4 to 8.3 gr/dl
Albumen	3.5 to 5 gr/dl
Calcium	8.5 to 10.5 mg / 100 ml
Potassium	3.5 to 5 mmol/L
Sodium	135 to 145 mEQ/L
Phosphorus	2.9 to 5.0 mg / 100 ml

aged over 40, the eyes should be examined once or twice a year to try to detect sight deterioration due to age and to give adequate treatment so as to retain the maximum possible visual capacity. If the patient is suffering from an illness, such as diabetes or abnormally high blood pressure, she should visit the ophthalmologist once a year, as those conditions also affect the sight.

• If a patient is suffering any problem, stinging, double or blurred vision, or black spots and colored circles around lights, she should immediately consult an ophthalmologist.

Teeth and gums

• Daily cleaning using a toothbrush and dental floss is essential to keep the teeth and gums healthy and strong.

• To maintain a healthy mouth, the dentist should be visited at least once a year. Early treatment of cavities and unhealthy gums avoids greater damage. The wisdom teeth must be extracted if the jaws are too small.

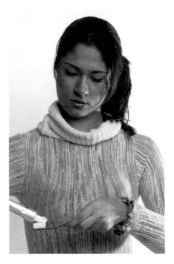

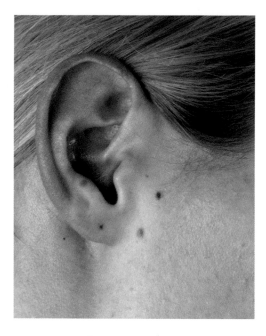

Even if your health is good and you feel well, you should never neglect visits to the doctor.

Normal values in a urine analysis

- The color of the urine should range from transparent to dark yellow.
- The pH balance of the urine must be between 4.6 and 8.0.
- No glucose, ketones or proteins should be present.
- No red corpuscles should be present.
- No hemoglobin should be present.
- No bilirrubine should be present.
- There may be traces of urobillinogen in normal urine.
- No nitrates should be present.
- No leucocytes should be present.

Hearing

Hearing loss is one of the commonest health problems. The risk of hearing loss increases after the age of 50.

Blood analysis

Blood analysis is a very important factor in the diagnosis of many illnesses, because the blood is

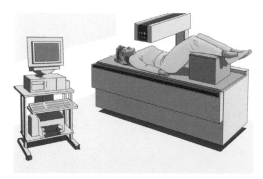

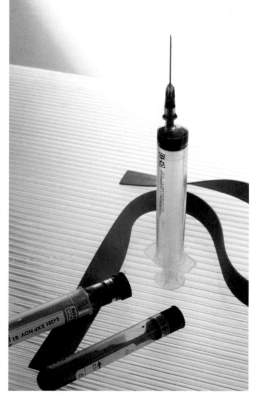

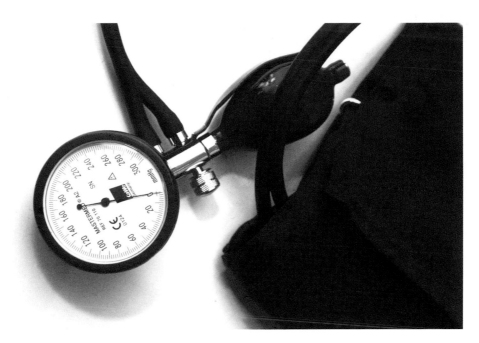

composed of hundreds of different particles whose concentration or appearance is modified during an illness. This indicates that something may be wrong with an organ of the human body, or there may be a hormonal imbalance, infectious disease, or defect in the immune system.

Urine analysis

Urine analysis helps to confirm the existence of an infection, a kidney disease, or pregnancy, and can check the presence of diabetes.

Blood-pressure check

Approximately one in every four people in the Western world suffers from abnormally high blood pressure, even when at rest. If the right medicines are not taken, there is a risk of suffering a heart attack, stroke, or other circulatory disease. As these conditions do not produce any symptoms, it is advisable to check the blood pressure regularly.

Bone density check

Osteoporosis reduces the density of the bones, making them more fragile and susceptible to fractures. Women are especially vulnerable after menopause when the ovaries stop producing the female hormone, estrogen, which affects bone conservation.

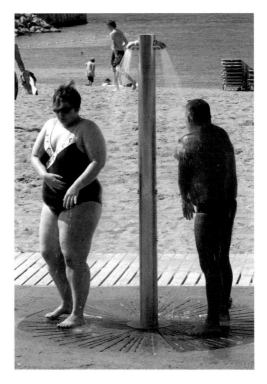

The gynecological checkup

Every woman should undergo a gynecological checkup when she starts to have sexual relations and, of course, when any problem of gynecological origin arises.

Gynecological checkup

First of all, a woman should choose a doctor to whom she can talk with absolute confidence, as she will have to discuss certain subjects, such as sexuality, birth control, and pregnancy. The woman should not be shy or embarrassed, as the gynecologist is an experienced professional who is duly prepared to deal with family problems and with physical and emotional abuse and drug-taking. All the information he or she receives will be confidential.

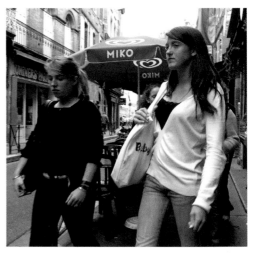

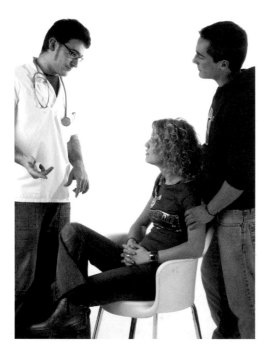

Based on a review of the history of gynecological diseases, a complete medical and surgical history can be compiled which will include health problems that are not strictly gynecological. The doctor needs to know all the pharmaceuticals the woman is taking, including prescribed or over-the-counter medicines, as well as drugs, tobacco, and alcohol, because many of them affect gynecological function and general health. Questions about mental, physical, or sexual abuse now or in the past are extremely important.

Gynecological examination

Some women may feel uncomfortable about a gynecological examination. The doctor should be told about this beforehand so that she can take more time and make sure that she reassures the patient about any doubts she may have and makes

Questions about the woman's gynecological clinical history

- A complete gynecological clinical history includes questions about the age when menstruation started, its frequency, regularity, duration, and flow, as well as the dates of the last two menstrual periods.

- Questions are also usually asked about any abnormal, excessive or sparse blood loss, or episodes of abnormal menstruation.

- The doctor may also ask about the woman's sexual activity in order to determine the presence of gynecological infections, injuries and the possibility of pregnancy.

- The patient is asked if she uses birth control methods, or wants to use them, and if she is interested in receiving advice or other information.

- A record is made of the number of pregnancies, the dates when they occurred, the result and any possible complications that may have arisen.

- The doctor asks the woman if she feels pain during menstruation, coitus or in other circumstances, how intense such pain is and how she controls it.

- Questions are also asked about any breast problems or pain in the breasts and whether the patient has noticed any changes or detected any lumps or anomalies.

- Lastly, she is asked whether and how often she examines her breasts herself and whether she needs instructions in how to do so.

her feel calm. As a rule, the woman is asked to urinate before the physical examination and bring a sample with her for laboratory testing. The breasts may be examined before or after the pelvic examination. With the woman seated, the doctor examines her breasts to discover any irregularities, skin retractions, lumps, or secretions of any kind. Then, with the woman still sitting up or lying down, with

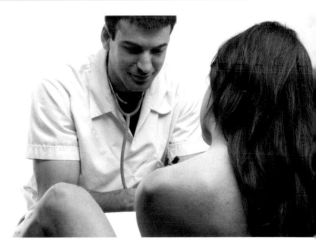

Cervical smear test or Papanicolau test

This is a simple and painless test facilitating the immediate detection of any anomaly in the cells of the surface of the cervix. These changes in the cervical cells, known as *displasia*, are easy to detect and treat, thus preventing cancer from developing. An abnormal smear does not necessarily mean cancer is present. The most frequent anomaly is a small *displasia* in which the anomalous cells disappear after a few months. If this happens, no treatment is needed but if the condition persists most doctors insist on the application of adequate treatment.

her hands on her hips or her head, the doctor feels each breast and examines each armpit to check for any enlarged lymph glands. The doctor also examines the neck and the thyroid gland, looking for lumps and anomalies.

During the pelvic examination, the woman lies face up with the hips and knees bent and the buttocks on the edge of the couch. Most examination couches are fitted with stirrups to hold the heels or knees, helping her to maintain this position. Then, the genital area is visually inspected and attention is paid to the distribution of the pubic hair and any other anomaly, alterations in color,

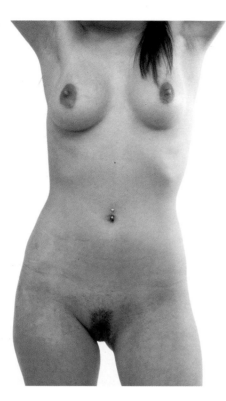

Wearing gloves, the doctor opens the lips to examine the opening of the vagina. Using a speculum (a metal or plastic instrument which separates the walls of the vagina), which is at a suitable temperature and lubricated, she examines the deepest parts of the vagina and the neck of the uterus (womb). This is explored carefully to detect signs of irritation or cancer.

To conduct a cervical smear test, cells are scraped from the surface of the neck of the uterus using a small wooden applicator similar to a spatula, so as to obtain some cells. Then, a small brush can be used to obtain a sample of cells from the neck of the uterus. The patient can feel something, but these procedures are not painful.

After removing the speculum, the doctor makes a two-handed examination, that is to say she inserts her index fingers and half a hand into the vagina and places the fingers of her other hand on the lower part of the abdomen above the pubic bone. In this position, the uterus is felt as a smooth and consistent pear-shaped structure and it is also possible to determine its position and whether feeling it causes pain.

Then, she tries to feel the ovaries, moving her hand over the abdomen from the middle to the sides and pressing a little more. As the ovaries are small and much harder to perceive than the uterus more pressure is needed, and the woman may feel a somewhat unpleasant sensation. The doctor determines the size of the ovaries and whether

flow or inflammation. This examination can confirm that everything is as it should be or, conversely, can indicate hormonal disturbances, cancer, infections, injuries, or physical abuse.

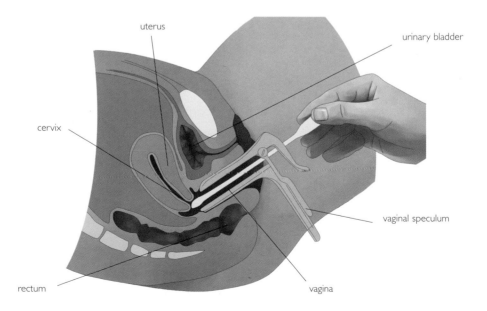

▪ Tests to detect vaginal infections or other sexually transmitted diseases

- A simple vaginal exudate, or culture, is taken if vaginal secretions are present and the patient is sexually active.

- If these symptoms are not present, the patient should speak to the gynecologist to determine whether she should take this test.

- The gynecologist should also tell the patient whether she needs to undergo other tests to detect sexually transmitted diseases.

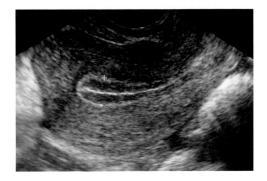

It is sometimes necessary to conduct certain complex tests so as to examine the internal genital organs. Several methods are used, including instruments that apply fiberoptic technology: thin and flexible glass or plastic strips that transmit light. With a fiberoptic cable connected to a visualization tube, or laparoscope, it is possible to examine the uterus, fallopian tubes, and ovaries, without the need to make a large incision. The laparoscope also enables surgical procedures to be carried out on the genital organs.

the area is painful. She also looks for irregularities or painful areas in the vagina.

Lastly, the doctor puts her index finger into the vagina and her middle finger into the rectum to make a rectovaginal examination. Thus, she examines the rear wall of the vagina to detect lumps or swellings. She also examines the rectum, looking for hemorrhoids, injuries, polyps and lumps, and the feces are examined to ascertain the presence of blood that is not perceptible from a simple visual examination. The woman may also be given an appliance to enable her to check at home that no blood is detectable in her feces.

Colposcopy

A colposcope is a kind of microscope or magnifying lens that enables the tissues to be seen enlarged and is used to detect both benign and malign lesions in the cervix, vagina, vulva, etc.

Colposcopy is a medical procedure consisting of the microscopic observation of the epithelium of the cervix and vaginal walls, as well as the entrance to the vagina, enabling precancerous lesions to be identified very precisely. This procedure enables the cervical smear test to be carried out more precisely and safely, or biopsies if suspicious lesions are revealed in the cervix.

Colposcopy is not painful and does not cause bleeding. It takes only a few minutes, is safe, it does not require hospitalization and, once the test is over, the patient can return home.

The breast examination

A lump in the breast, whether benign or cancerous, feels the same, even to an experienced doctor, so other tests are recommended, such as an ultrasound test, X-rays, and a biopsy. If the tests reveal a benign tumor, no subsequent treatment is needed, but if it is malign or if doubt persists, the lump is surgically removed and radiotherapy, chemotherapy, and occasionally other hormonal therapies are applied.

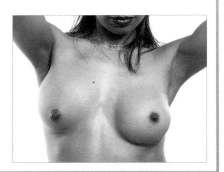

It is conducted with the patient lying on her back with her feet in the stirrups of the gynecological examination table. A speculum (an instrument used to keep the vagina open and to visualize and examine the cervix) is inserted. A chemical solution (acetic acid) is applied to the cervix to take a sample of the mucus that covers its surface and help highlight any abnormal areas. The colposcope is placed into the opening of the vagina and the area is extensively examined. Photographs can be taken. If the doctor considers it necessary, she can use this appliance to take a sample of tissue for a biopsy.

When should this examination must be carried out?

• In any woman who has started sexual relations.

• In patients with an abnormal cervical smear result (presence of displasia or cervical intraepithelial neoplasia (CIN).

• To monitor patients with a human papilloma virus infection or cancer.

• In patients with abnormal vaginal bleeding.

• In patients with a vaginal flow that does not clear up with the usual treatments.

• In the presence of external lesions (warts, condyloma, ulcers, skin lesions).

• As an examination preceding uterine surgery.

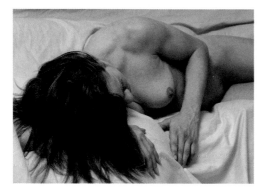

Many adolescent girls feel a mixture of anxiety, embarrassment, and fear when confronting their first gynecological examination. It is very important to play down this event and explain that it is in no way traumatic. On the contrary, they must attend the examination calmly, with a positive attitude, and ask for all the information and explanations they need to clarify any doubts they may have about it.

■ Recommended gynecological checkups

• On starting to have sexual relations. One of the principal reasons for these checkups is the early diagnosis of sexually transmitted diseases and gynecological cancer. The young woman will also be guided about contraceptive methods and the principal points regarding unwanted pregnancies and sexually transmitted diseases, as well as the risk factors: not using a condom, having numerous sexual partners, sexual relations which present a high risk of sexually transmitted diseases (a partner who is a drug addict, anal penetration) and starting sexual relations very early in life.

• Changes in vaginal flow (itching of the vulva or vagina, excessive increase in genital discharge).

• Menstrual upsets (severe pain during menstruation, very irregular periods, very heavy periods, late menstruation).

• Changes in the breasts (appearance of mammary nodules, mammary secretions, painful breasts).

• Suspected pregnancy (absence of menstruation).

• Abdominal pain (when nongynecological causes have been ruled out).

• Appearance of vulvar or abdominal lumps.

• Disturbances in pubertal development; Mammary or genital injuries.

• Excessive pubic hair.

• Sexual attack or rape.

Food and nutrition

Unlike men, whose nutritional requirements do not vary, female nutrition must be matched to the special times when her organism is undergoing considerable hormonal, metabolic, and physiological changes: adolescence, periods, pregnancy, lactation, the practice of sport, and menopause. To maintain vitality, control weight, prevent disease and disorders, and avoid nutritional deficiencies, the woman's diet must be balanced, varied, and complete. It must contain the right proportions of all the necessary vitamins, minerals, and nutrients and regularly include different types of foods, as is recommended generally to everyone.

What is a diet?

The diet is formed of the food, the organism's fuel, which provide the energy necessary to be able to carry out all the daily functions.

The nutritional pyramid

The nutritional pyramid is the method generally used to suggest the variety of foods that should be consumed in the diet every day. The pyramid proposes eating the products that compose it in proportions similar to those of its steps.

• The lower steps propose mainly complex carbohydrates.

• The central steps suggest foods that contain fewer carbohydrates, more proteins and fats, and a high vitamin content.

• The upper steps, from bottom to top, contain proteins and fats.

• The top step contains mostly fats and simple carbohydrates, all foods that supply mainly calories.

• We should not forget to drink plenty of water.

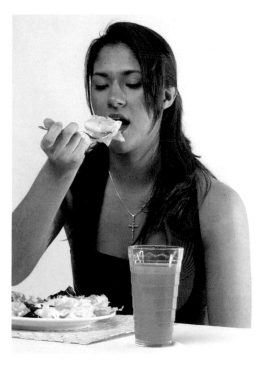

Every day you want and need to eat, but the important thing is to know how to vary your food so that what you eat is nutritious, balanced, does not become boring or cause secondary problems if you have any health problems.

NUTRITIONAL PYRAMID

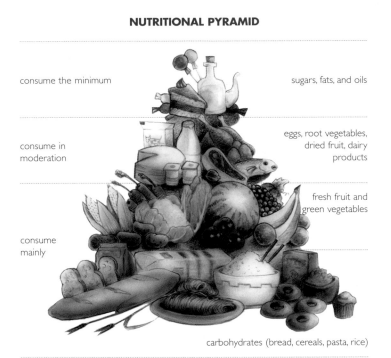

consume the minimum — sugars, fats, and oils

consume in moderation — eggs, root vegetables, dried fruit, dairy products

— fresh fruit and green vegetables

consume mainly

carbohydrates (bread, cereals, pasta, rice)

drink plenty of water

According to the nutrition experts, a woman's diet needs to be more specific and controlled than a man's, as it must suit the various stages a woman goes through throughout her life, which significantly change her nutritional requirements.

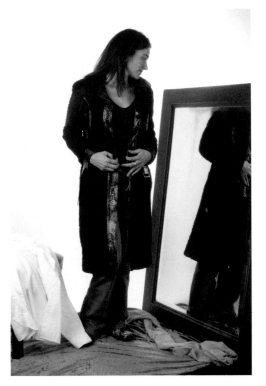

Food and nutrition

Food is what provides the energy necessary for the body to work properly and that energy can be expressed in different units.

For all the organism's biochemical processes to be carried out, an exchange of energy is necessary. This energy is derived from the carbohydrates, fats, and proteins in the food ingested. A woman's energy requirement is the quantity of energy she must ingest in order to offset the energetic or calorific she expends.

There are four elements that can supply energy to the organism, but only three of them are nutritious: carbohydrates, proteins, and fats. The fourth element is alcohol, which does not supply any nutrition, except energy in the form of actual calories.

Proteins. These are some of the nutrients contained in food that are formed of long chains of smaller units called *amino acids*, and these in turn are composed of carbon, hydrogen, oxygen, and nitrogen. They are the principal structural components of the cells and, therefore, constitute the basis on which the tissues of the organism are formed. Proteins are essential for growth and deve-

The word kilocalories is used in nutrition. In thermodynamics, from where this unit originates, a calorie is defined as the amount of energy required to raise the temperature of 1 gram of water by 1°C. In the case of the human body, which uses a lot of energy, large figures are used and therefore the kilocalorie is used (often wrongly called calories).

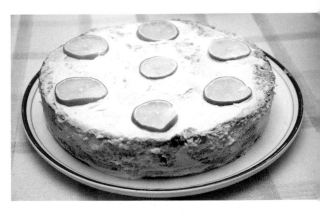

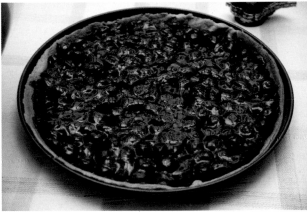

lopment. They maintain and repair the tissues and intervene in the production of enzymes that participate in metabolic and digestive processes. They are the essential constituents of certain hormones and participate in the defense mechanisms, as they are a structural part of the antibodies of the immune system and also intervene in the processes of coagulation. Proteins are contained in meat, eggs, fish, and some root vegetables.

Carbohydrates. Classified as carbohydrates are sugars and starches, as they are organic substances composed of carbon, hydrogen, and oxygen, in combination with molecules of water.

When ingested, most starches, which are considered to be complex carbohydrates, and most sugars, called simple carbohydrates, are converted into glucose, an element that is incorporated into the bloodstream and provides the organism with the energy it needs.

A second group of complex carbohydrates is composed of cellulose, which, although it is not absorbed by the human organism, has beneficial properties for health.

Carbohydrates, hydrates of carbon or sugars are very important in the diet because of their energy-giving properties, their sweetening capacity, and their high fiber content. The most important source of carbohydrates is food of vegetable origin. Thus, glucose is found in fruit and green vegetables; fructose in fruit and honey; sucrose in sugar beet, cane sugar, or fruit and green vegetables; starch in cereals, tubers, root vegetables, fruit and green vegetables.

Fats. Fundamentally, fats or lipids provide the organism with energy and are essential for its proper functioning: they form part of the structure of the cellular membrane, transport liposoluble vitamins (A, D, E, and K) to the cells and

Energy contributed by each of these dietary components is as follows:

- Proteins: 4 kilocalories / gram.
- Carbohydrates: 4 kilocalories / gram.
- Fats: 9 kilocalories / gram.
- Alcohol: 7 kilocalories / gram.

It should be pointed out that the grams of these chemical components must be considered as dry, and not directly related to the weight of a food. All foods contain water and therefore their content of the three nutritive elements is mixed, and not in proportion to the weight of those components.

Unsaturated fatty acids help reduce LDL cholesterol levels (known as *bad cholesterol*) and increase HDL levels (*good cholesterol*). This type of fat is linked to the prevention and cure of diseases such as cancer, inflammatory illnesses, and skin problems. Unsaturated fatty acids are recommended and are very important in pregnant women, small children, and old people.

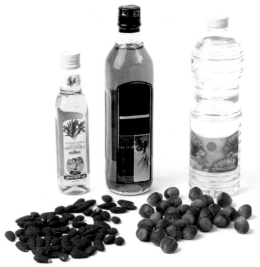

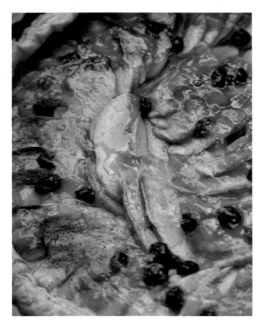

diet. They are found mainly in oily fish, some green vegetables, and enriched foods.

Vitamins and minerals. These are essential for the organism, but necessary in small quantities. A shortage of them causes illnesses and, conversely, they help prevent many problems such as cardiovascular diseases, cancer or

aging. A healthy diet must contain all the food groups and sufficient quantities of nutrients for the body to be able to carry out all its functions. Excessive amounts of food should not be consumed, as this causes imbalances, such as an increase in cholesterol or a drop in blood pressure.

store energy. However, depending on the type and amount of fat ingested, lipids can be friends or enemies for health.

• Saturated fatty acids. These are derived mainly from animal fats, such as butter, cheese, fatty meat and some vegetable oils. Excessive consumption of this type of fat raises the cholesterol level and the triglycerides and is a cardiovascular risk.

• Unsaturated fatty acids. These are in turn divided into:

- Monounsaturated fats. These are found mainly in olive oil, dried fruit, and seeds.

- Polyunsaturated fats. These are essential fatty acids because the organism cannot synthesize them, so they must be obtained through the

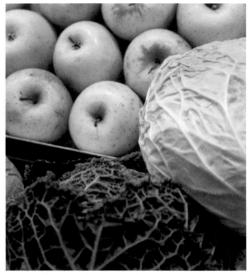

Interesting information about fats

- Cholesterol is a fatty substance found in animal products (meat, chicken, egg yolks, full-fat milk, ice cream, butter). Check your cholesterol level and ascertain what it should be from your doctor.

- High-density lipoprotein (HDL) is a kind of cholesterol whose real role is to protect the body against heart diseases (it is also known as *good cholesterol*).

- Low-density lipoprotein (LDL) is cholesterol that is deposited on the walls of the arteries and thus increases the risk of heart diseases (*bad cholesterol*).

- Monounsaturated fats are a type of unsaturated fat that reduces blood cholesterol. They are found in olive oil and peanut oil.

- Polyunsaturated fats are vegetable fats that reduce blood cholesterol. They are found in cottonseed, soya beans, and sunflower oil.

- Saturated fats are fats of animal origin that raise the blood cholesterol. They are found in hydrogenated vegetable fats, coconut oil, cocoa butter, the fat of meat, full-fat milk, cream, and full-fat cheeses.

- Triglycerides are blood fats that can increase the risk of heart diseases.

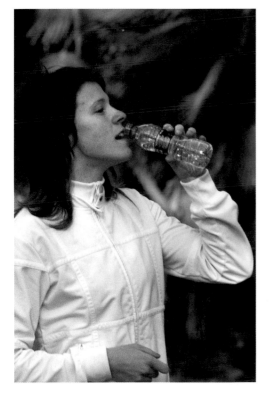

Avoid eating too many fats of animal origin. Eat more fruit, green vegetables and foods rich in fiber. People of any age and both sexes are also recommended to reduce the amount of sugar they eat and moderate the amount of alcohol they drink.

◾ The World Health Organization (WHO) establishes the following proportions:

- Carbohydrates should constitute at least 55–60% of the total calorie contribution.

- Fats should not exceed 30% of the total calories ingested.

- Proteins should supply the remaining 15% of the diet.

It is vital to drink and drinking should be an important component of the daily diet. Sixty percent of the human body is composed of water and it is indispensable for a multitude of organic processes. The body loses water constantly, through urine, sweat, the humidity of the air we breathe and, to a lesser extent, through the feces. The water we lose is made up for by the water we drink and ingest with our food. Many foods, such as fruit and green vegetables, contain water. However, the body is also capable of producing water by metabolizing carbohydrates, fats and proteins.

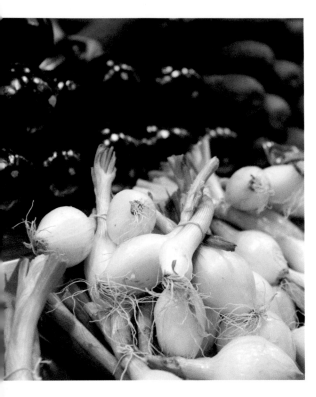

Types of diet

Food influences health and also helps prevent heart disease and some types of cancer; it is therefore advisable to check that foods are low in fat and sugar and high in fiber.

Healthy eating is the basis of good health and a key element in reducing the risk of suffering any ailment related to nutritional deficiencies. Food, that is to say the diet followed, must include all the natural products that provide the necessary carbohydrates, fats, proteins, fiber, vitamins, and minerals.

The risks of poorly planned vegetarian diets

• If it is not well planned, the ovo-lacto-vegetarian diet can be deficient in some of the nutrients contributed to the traditional diet by meat and fish. These nutrients include easily absorbed iron, zinc, and vitamin B12, which are especially necessary during pregnancy (anemia) and during growth and development (to prevent infantile rickets), periods when greater quantities of those nutrients

▪ The Mediterranean diet

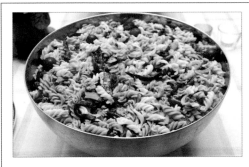

• Specialists in nutrition recommend following the diet of Mediterranean villages, as its typical dishes are perfectly balanced as regards their content of proteins, fats and carbohydrates, as well as fiber, vitamins, and minerals.

• Foods rich in protein, such as fish and shellfish, lean meat, chicken, and lamb, have a low level of saturated fats.

• They are usually cooked in vegetable oil, and olive oil is used in mayonnaise and salad dressings, so most of the fats are unsaturated and do not raise cholesterol levels.

• Fish is eaten as often as meat, thus increasing the consumption of polyunsaturated fats over saturated fats.

• Very few carbohydrates in the form of processed sugars are eaten. Most of them come from unrefined starches such as rice, pasta, dried beans, potatoes, and lentils, all of them products rich in fiber and essential nutrients.

• The Mediterranean diet also involves eating a large amount of fresh fruit and green vegetables, supplying a lot of vitamins, minerals, and fiber.

• Moreover, Mediterranean dishes include spices that assist digestion.

are needed. The intake of calcium and vitamin D can also be threatened if the diet does not include milk or milk derivatives.

• The cereal diet is very unbalanced. The quality of the protein this diet provides to the organism is insufficient, as cereals are deficient in essential amino acids.

• There is also the risk that vitamin deficiencies may occur: vitamin A (skin and eye lesions), vitamin D (rickets), vitamin B12 (anemia), and vitamin C (scurvy). The reduced absorption of calcium and iron of vegetable origin is worsened by the presence of phytic acid or phytates in the husks of cereals, which increases the risk of rickets and anemia. Moreover, by limiting the intake of liquids, the normal functioning of the kidneys is compromised.

• Another deficiency of a strict vegetarian diet is the difficulty the person has in acquiring iron of the quality found in meat or eggs. It should be remembered that vegetable iron is not absorbed as efficiently.

Eating away from home

Modern working hours oblige many women to eat outside the home, but eating out does not have to be synonymous with growing fat or not following a balanced diet. Firstly, there is the alternative of bringing food from home, which is usually complete and appetizing. But this is not always

▪ The vegetarian diet

• There are several vegetarian tendencies with well defined principles, as well as the ovo-lacto-vegetarian diet (the most complete of all the alternatives from the nutritional point of view), which includes milk and eggs, or its nearest derivatives, the ovo-vegetarian or lacto-vegetarian diets.

• Another group of vegetarian diets are those of people who eat green vegetables only, and consider that honey is an animal by-product so do not eat it, or root vegetables either (except for soya).

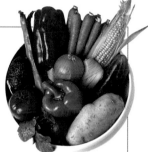

• The vegan variant of vegetarianism allows leguminous plants to be eaten.

• Other trends are fruitarians who eat only fresh and dried fruit, crudivores who eat only fruit and raw green vegetables and cerealists (macrobiotic diet) who eat only cereals and restrict their intake of liquids.

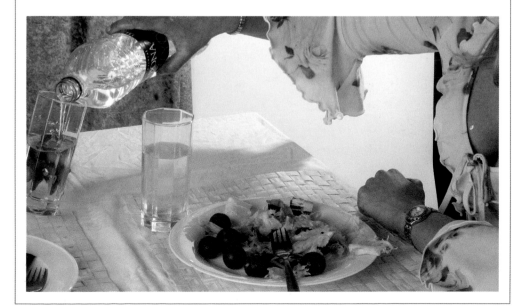

possible and, if you have to eat out, it is wise to follow the advice of nutrition experts, which can be summarized in the following points:

• Variety. Choose a different menu every day, and even a different establishment, if possible.

• Quantity. Eat the calories you need—neither more nor less.

• Balance. Proteins, fats, carbohydrates, and fiber must be included in adequate proportions, as already indicated several times.

• Time. Always try to eat at the same time of day and devote at least 40 minutes to your meal. You should eat slowly and masticate thoroughly. Otherwise, the food will not be correctly chewed and salivated and digestion will be less efficient. Moreover, psychologically you will not fully ingest what you have eaten and, on reaching home, you will tend to eat more because your midday meal "was only a snack."

• Alcohol. Drink it only in moderation, if at all.

• Proteins. Experts recommend eating the same amount of fish as meat, so it is wise to alternate them. For preference, choose meat with less fat: chicken or steak is better than lamb or hamburgers. Don't eat too many eggs.

• Cooking methods. Choose few fats. Eat grilled food rather than a stew.

• Side dishes. Substitute the most filling (fried potatoes, various fritters, pancakes and so on) with other lighter foods such as rice.

• Desserts. Although you can allow yourself a treat now and then, it is healthier to eat fruit than a pastry.

Food in relation to the time of life

• For a new-born baby, mother's milk is the best food;

• Milk and its derivatives (yogurt, custard, cheese) are basic foods for children.

• They should drink whole-fat milk. Only give them skim milk on the recommendation of a doctor.

• Growth requires a lot of proteins. Meat, liver, fish, eggs, and cereals are important, as well as green vegetables and fruit.

• They should eat few fats and few sweetened foods. These cause dental cavities and spoil the appetite.

• It is better not to put too much salt in their food.

• Children should be given healthy snacks instead of candies.

• Avoid stimulating drinks (coffee, tea) and fizzy drinks (colas).

• They should have a good breakfast before

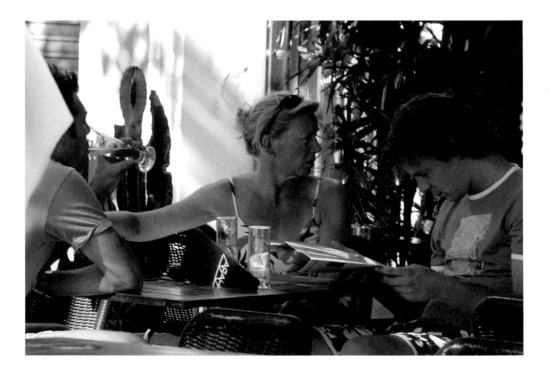

Recommended daily quantities

- Two or three glasses of milk and milk derivatives.
- Three eggs a week, a portion of meat and another of fish.
- Between one and three portions of bread a day.
- One or two portions of rice or pasta a day.
- Two to four pieces of fruit a day,
- Three to five portions of green vegetables.

going to school.

• Avoid high-calorie diets and don't let them overeat. Fat little girls are more prone to certain illnesses and are likely to be obese all their lives.

• During the early years of life, the growth rate is very fast and nutritional requirements are similarly high. Any deficiency can cause illnesses.

• Schoolchildren are recommended to eat foods from each group of nutrients and control the intake of fats caused by eating too much deep-fried food that raises their cholesterol level.

Adolescents

A series of changes occur in adolescence (very rapid growth, distribution of the fat and muscular tissue and sexual maturity), so they must be sure of a healthy, complete, and balanced diet.

• During growth, little girls gain more in fat tissue, but their bone growth is less—compared with little boys—and takes less time. Nutrition is very important during this time and is therefore different for each sex. More proteins should be eaten, as tissue growth is also greater. Between 12 percent and 14 percent of a person's energy must be provided by proteins. This contribution must be gradually reduced in girls, as in them tissue development is faster between the ages of 11 and 14, and slower between the ages of 19 and 24.

• The proportions of fats and carbohydrates they need are the same as for adults.

• Special attention should be paid to minerals during this phase of life, especially calcium, iron, and zinc. The World Health Organization recommends some 0.21–0.245 oz (600–700 mg) per day for adolescents between the ages of 11 and 15 and some 0.017–0.21 oz (500–600 mg) per day for

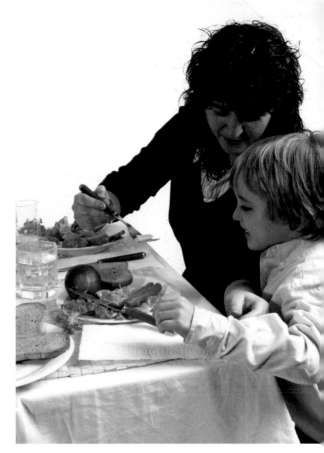

those between the ages of 16 and 18 years.

• To calculate these amounts, it is assessed that a glass of milk measuring 0.42 US pint (200 ml) provides some 0.008 oz (250 mg) of calcium, and that cheese and yogurt supply the same amount. It must be remembered that substances such as sugar, caffeine, and fiber hinder calcium absorption, whereas vitamin D, magnesium, lactose, and proteins facilitate it.

• Iron is necessary for forming the blood and muscular tissue. The recommended intake of iron is 0.0005 oz (15 mg) per day for young girls, remembering that menstruation involves iron loss and a risk of anemia. The body absorbs 20 percent of the iron originating from meat and 5 percent of the iron originating from fruit and green vegetables. Some foods rich in iron are animal organ meats, sesame seeds, egg yolk, lentils, chickpeas, almonds.

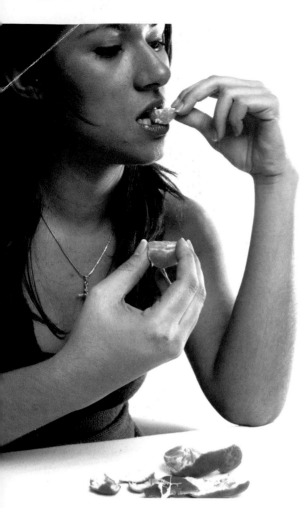

Adults

- Adults must monitor their weight and avoid getting fat. Less energy is consumed with age and, therefore, the amount of food eaten at each meal must be monitored.
- Avoid animal fats and high-cholesterol foods such as butter, fat cheese, sausages, eggs, etc.
- Drink more milk (preferably skim) and milk derivatives: calcium reduces osteoporosis.
- Eat little salt to avoid high blood pressure.
- Eat fruit, green vegetables, and cereals.
- Fish is preferable to meat. It provides the same proteins and is more digestible.
- Avoid bowel straining caused by physical inactivity, taking whole cereals and fiber-rich foods (chickpeas, spinach, cherries).
- If there are problems with chewing, eat soft meals: purées, croquettes, and meatballs.

The pregnant woman

- Eating the right food while pregnant is perhaps the best gift a woman can give her baby. A good diet for pregnancy should be varied and well balanced. It should include enough fresh fruit and green vegetables, whole grains, dairy products, proteins, some fats, and eight cups of liquid a day.
- Eating large amounts and foods rich in calories is harmful to the health of both mother and baby. Overeating only leads to excessive weight gain, resulting in complications at the end of pregnancy and during birth.
- During gestation, a woman should eat:
- Proteins: meat, fish, eggs, poultry, green beans, nuts, cheese, milk, lentils.

- Zinc is very necessary for tissue development and a shortage of it causes skin lesions, falling hair, slow healing of wounds, etc. The daily zinc intake should be 0.0042 oz (12 mg) for young girls. Some foods rich in zinc are: oysters, veal, shellfish, dried fruit, carrots, corn, tomatoes, bananas.
- Vitamins are also recommended as at other stages of life. The most important are those related to protein-synthesis and cellular development, such as vitamin A (involved in the growth, differentiation, proliferation, and reproduction of cells), vitamin D (related to calcium and phosphorous metabolism) and the vitamin B complex (involved in energy metabolism).

> The adolescent girl's rapid growth demands an adequate diet. She must have basic knowledge of nutrition and take responsibility for what she eats.
>
> As far as possible, avoid them eating too many hamburgers, pizzas and fast food. If what they eat away from home cannot be controlled, healthy and appetizing dishes should be prepared so they can eat them when they come home. Pay special attention to the drastic diets some young girls adopt who want to be slim above all else.

- Vitamins, minerals, and fiber: fresh fruit and green vegetables, whole-grain cereals, and bread. A moderate salt intake is necessary for both mother and baby. Only in very special cases should it be restricted. Iron, folic acid, and calcium must be taken as prescribed by the gynecologist.
- Calcium: dairy products.
- Iron: green vegetables, dried fruit, green beans, and almonds.
- Liquids. It is important to drink plenty of water, fruit juice, and other liquids to provide the necessary amount of fluid.
  - Foods to avoid:
- Fats: butter, margarine, fried foods, oils.
- Sweetened foods: sugar, syrups, desserts, sandwiches and snacks, cakes, cookies.
- Caffeine: coffee, tea, cocoa, cola drinks, chocolate.
- Alcohol and Tobacco: The enormous harm caused to adults by tobacco has been amply demonstrated and even more so for the developing fetus: miscarriage and low birth weight. Cot death is three times more frequent in the children of mothers who smoke, as are premature birth, premature detachment of the placenta, premature rupture of the membranes, hare-lip, microcephaly, increased irritation of the nervous system, lower intellectual coefficient, attention

- The pregnant woman should increase her daily diet by some 300 kcal, and when she is breastfeeding, by some 500 kcal.
- It is a myth that she should eat for two. Her weight should increase by only about 22 lb (10 kg).
- She should follow a healthy, nutritious, and varied diet. When a pregnant woman is not properly nourished she runs a greater risk of having a weak or sickly child.
- She should not smoke or drink alcohol.
- She should consult a doctor before taking any kind of medicine. He will probably recommend her to take iron and other minerals.

deficiency, antisocial behavior, allergies, bronchitis, asthma, etc. It is hardly necessary to say that it should be avoided.

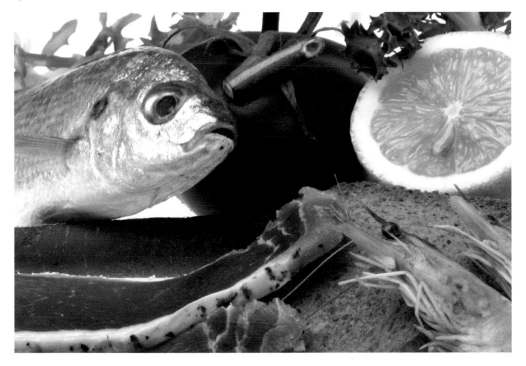

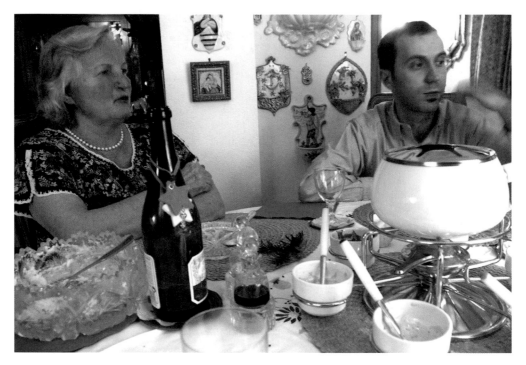

The elderly

• The need to follow a balanced diet is the same for an old woman as for a mature one, although some aspects change.

• She should eat three to five portions of green vegetables a day with an average weight of between 5½ and 7 oz each (150 and 200 grams), raw weight.

• The number of calories needed declines, so she should avoid foods with high fat or sugar content to prevent obesity.

• It is wise to moderate the intake of vegetable fats instead of animal fats to maintain adequate cholesterol levels.

• Quite the reverse occurs with proteins, more of which are needed. Dairy products, fish, and eggs should be eaten frequently.

• Above all, the diet must be personalized and adjusted to suit each individual. In those who are overweight or have high cholesterol levels, skim or semiskim milk should be taken.

• Many women have high blood pressure. In those cases, less salt should be eaten and less alcohol, black coffee, and tea drunk.

• At least 2 quarts (2 liters) should be drunk, and its ingestion monitored, as the risk of dehydration is greater in old people.

• If a special diet is being followed because of diabetes or some other condition, that diet should be balanced to make sure it includes all the required nutrients.

Food-related problems and diseases

People do not eat only in order to satisfy hunger or stay alive. They should do so also with a view to maintaining good health and preventing disease. Eating a varied and balanced diet (with the right amount of individual necessities) is, among other factors, one of the principal ways of promoting health and the quality of life. On the one hand it covers the basic biological necessities so that the body will function completely normally every day and, on the other, it is a way of preventing and treating certain diseases and/or organic irregularities.

Food-related problems and diseases

Gaining or losing weight

Women follow diets, perhaps because of the importance to a woman of her physical appearance and her greater preoccupation with health and its preservation. However, it should be remembered that diets can be difficult to follow. It is important for her to set a target, know why she wants to lose or gain weight and how far she should go.

If you want to go on a diet, the first thing you should do is consult a medical specialist to determine whether there is any reason why you have gained or lost weight and whether there are any contraindications or pathologies. If there are none, you simply need to be disciplined, change your habits and eat what will nourish you while enabling you to achieve your ideal weight.

Some specialists define the ideal weight as "the weight at which an individual feels at ease, allowing all the biological functions to develop normally." It

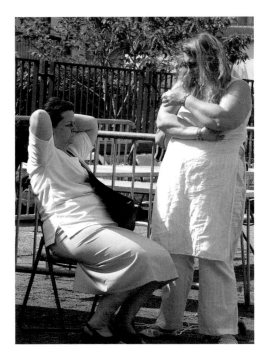

There are two determining factors that have important consequences for health: choosing the wrong foods and the resulting nutritional imbalance. Illness is certain to result when the food ingested does not satisfy the body's requirements, inducing imbalance.

should be pointed out that, with the same height and weight, one person may feel well and another overweight. This fact has certain physiological foundations: all individuals are different; there are differences in the relationship between lean mass and fat mass, hormonal secretions, muscular innervation, etc.

The body-mass index (BMI) is an index of the weight of a person compared with their height. Although this index makes no distinction between the fat and nonfat components of the total body mass, it is the most practical way of assessing the degree of risk associated with obesity.

The body-mass index is a reasonably reliable way of estimating the body weight. The formula is: BMI = weight in pounds, divided by height in inches squared, multiplied by 703. (Weight in kg, divided by height in meters squared.) [A search for BMI on the Internet will do your calculation for you.]

Figures of under 18.5 indicate excessive thinness, between 18.5 and 24.9 indicate a healthy weight, between 25 and 29.9 indicate that the person is overweight and above 30 mean obesity.

When starting a diet, it is very important not to be over-strict, because the diet needs to be maintained for quite a long time and, if it is impossible to follow, it will be practiced only intermittently, making it increasingly difficult to achieve the desired weight loss or gain.

Controlling obesity

Here is some advice to follow for a balanced diet that will enable you to lose several pounds or kilos, make a vigorous start and regain your figure.
• Eat better

The key to a good diet is to eat better, which does not mean eating less or following a strict or restrictive diet. There are no good or bad foods, only healthier foods and foods containing fewer calories, and those are the ones that should predominate in your daily diet. Treats must be admitted too, but only occasionally. It is preferable to allow yourself to make the odd exception than to prohibit those small, irresistible mouthfuls. It won't do any harm just for one day.

A varied diet is a healthy diet and taste lies in variety. That is why it is recommended to include foods from all groups in it, choosing seasonal food because it is fresher, tastier, and reasonably priced. Seasonal green vegetables and fruit, oily fish (fresh sardines, fresh anchovies, tuna, etc.), shellfish and mollusks, poultry, are all very healthy foods that can be prepared in a wide variety of ways.
• Healthier cooking

Certain cooking methods can convert a light and balanced food into a heavy, hypercalorific dish that is hard to digest. The most recommended cooking methods are those that add the least fat to the food and maintain its nutritional and organoleptic value. These include: broiling, oven baking, steaming, wok cookery, cooking en *papillotte*, etc.

It is important to choose the right seasonings too: avoid sauces based on oil, cream, butter, and meat concentrates, and go with virgin olive oil, lemon juice, and balsamic vinegar. Vary the flavor of your dishes, seasoning them with aromatic herbs (parsley, dill, oregano, basil, etc.) and spices (cumin, pepper, chilli, curry, etc.).

Is it best to eat "light" or precooked food?

Some studies have shown that a third of "light" foods cannot be considered as such, because the reduction in calories compared with their approved component of reference is less than 30 percent. Also, others described as "low fat," "integral," "less fat," "sugar-free," "6.5% fat," "0% fat," "diet," "light," "fat-reduced," or "low in calories" do not usually reduce your calorie intake. Some examples are: breakfast cereals, chocolates, light fried potatoes, cookies, etc.

The most important thing in this respect is to be clear that, even if a food is described as light, this does not mean that it does not contain plenty of calories and, therefore, you should not increase the amount of it you habitually eat. The recommended light foods are dairy products that reduce your caloric intake, e.g. made with skim milk.

And what about precooked foods? Are there healthier options?

You should try to avoid foods that are prefried, battered, covered in sauce, have added fat, etc. However, supermarkets are now offering a range of precooked products that fulfill balanced diet parameters. These include sautéed green vegetables and rice, fish dishes, poultry dishes, preserved root vegetables, etc.

Slimming is not always a matter of willpower. Excess pounds, your medical history, your objectives, the pace of your life and even your lifestyle affect the way you will lose weight.

Some causes of obesity
- Weight problems in the family.
- Eating when you feel lonely, sad, or stressed.
- Feeling pressurized to eat by friends or family members.
- Taking medicines that make you feel hungry.
- Having a slow metabolism (that is to say the speed at which you burn calories).
- Having hormonal problems

How to follow a healthy but effective slimming diet:

- Eat three meals and two snacks a day instead of spending hours without eating, which makes you feel hungry and gobble your food.
- Eat a varied but balanced diet: cereals, meat, fish, fruit, green vegetables, dairy products, and fats.
- Eat fruits and vegetables of various colors. Dark green vegetables are rich in calcium and folic acid, orange ones contain carotene.
- Choose whole wheat and whole-grain rice products, as they contain more fiber and minerals.
- Drink at least 2 quarts (2 liters) of water a day. It improves your appearance, makes you feel better and gives a feeling of fullness.

▪ Every woman is a world

- There are many criteria for choosing a diet.
- Each woman is a world in herself, and a method that works perfectly for one woman may be hopeless for another, because she doesn't have the time to cook, leads a very sedentary life or is hyperactive.
- If you have a serious obesity or medical problem, it is advisable to consult your family doctor.
- If you have gained only the few pounds that prevent you doing up a pair of pants or if your eating habits are not the best, a multitude of diets are available to you.
- Although the Mediterranean diet is the healthiest and most recommendable, you may find it easier to maintain your weight by following a vegetarian diet.
- It is very important to find out all about each diet before following it, or to visit a specialist.

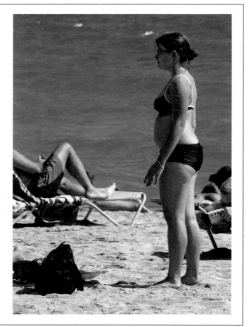

Eating disorders

Eating disorders are extreme manifestations of a variety of worries about weight and eating experienced by many women, and by many men too. These disorders include anorexia nervosa, bulimia nervosa, and obesity. All these are serious emotional problems which can have lethal consequences.

Anorexia nervosa

This is a mental illness that consists of a loss of weight derived from an intense fear of obesity and a distorted body image. The inadequate consump-

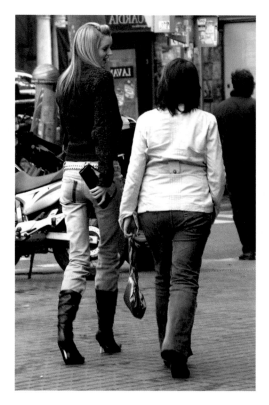

tion of calories or the excessive expenditure of energy causes a severe loss of weight achieved by the person on her own initiative and making her ill as a result of a series of behaviors.

It most often affects adolescent women.

The most frequent symptoms are:

• Intense fear of gaining weight, keeping it below the minimum normal figure.

• Eating very little food or following severe diets.

• A distorted body image.

• Feeling fat when they are in fact thin.

• Feeling of guilt or self-disgust when they have eaten.

• Hyperactivity and excessive physical exercise.

• Loss of menstruation.

• Character changes (irritability, sadness, sensitivity to cold).

Obviously, the treatment of these problems is not easy and requires psychological and dietary help for prompt recovery.

Bulimia

This is a mental problem characterized by repeated episodes of excessive eating in a short space of

Anorexia is most common among girls between the ages of 14 and 18. This group accounts for 90% of cases. The remaining 10% of anorexics are adolescent girls, little boys, little girls and mature women.

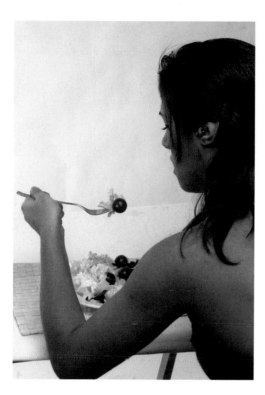

Bulimics cannot control the impulses that lead them to eat, but the feeling of guilt and shame after eating a lot of food makes them fast, take purgatives and make themselves vomit to prevent weight gain. Bulimics have about 15 episodes of gorging and vomiting per week and, as a rule, their weight is normal, so the condition is difficult to detect.

• Inappropriate behavior to make up for the excessive intake of food so as not to gain weight: excessive use of pharmaceuticals, laxatives, diuretics, and self-induced vomiting.
• High level of tooth enamel erosion, which can lead to losing teeth due to repeated vomiting.
• Character changes, including: depression, sadness, feelings of self-blame and self-hatred.

Obesity

This is a chronic treatable illness. It occurs when there is an excess of adipose tissue (fat) in the body. As well as the problem it represents in itself, experts warn that its most negative effects occur because it acts as an agent that soon and evidently exaggerates and aggravates serious complaints such as diabetes, high blood pressure, cardiovascular complications (especially ischemic cardiopathy), and even some types of cancer including gastrointestinal cancer.

time, as a form of gorging, and an exaggerated preoccupation with weight control which leads the affected person to adopt inappropriate behavior and endanger her health.

It also mainly affects young women, usually a little older than with anorexia. It is more difficult to detect. Nutritional problems are not as serious as with anorexia. In addition to vomiting, dysfunctions arise in the distribution of liquids that can lead to a heart attack. Its treatment is psychological, as the bulimic person suffers from depression and anxiety.

The most frequent symptoms are:
• Compulsive eating in the form of gorging when alone.
• Constant preoccupation about eating and weight.

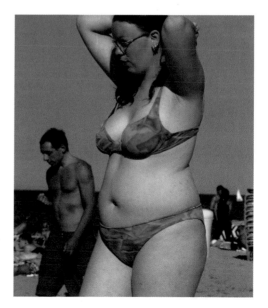

Obesity has become a public health problem in all developed countries. As well as being a cardiovascular risk, obesity in women is associated with an increased risk of breast and endometrial cancer, ovarian polycystosis, and infertility. Women are strongly motivated to control their weight for esthetic reasons and diet is a highly emotive matter to them.

Morbid obesity

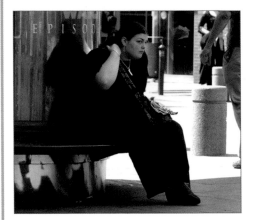

• Morbid obesity is one of the most serious diseases of our time, especially because of the number of complications that accompany it. It has to be treated with surgery, as diets are ineffective. Two methods are used: surgical removal, designed to induce poor absorption, or restriction. The second method is less drastic, as nothing has to be removed. It suffices to reduce the size of the stomach so that the patient cannot eat.

• A surgical procedure is the only way of getting the patient to lose weight in many cases of morbid obesity. Reducing techniques produce fewer side effects, but weight is not lost so easily. There are three surgical techniques for morbid obesity: vertical gastroplasty, gastroplasty with an adjustable gastric band, or the gastric bypass.

Obesity is classified into two types:

• **Central or android obesity and peripheral or gynoid obesity.** The first is more serious and can involve severe pathological complications. Central obesity localizes the fat on the trunk and predisposes the sufferer to metabolic complications (especially type 2 diabetes and dislipemias).

• **Peripheral or gynoid obesity.** This accumulates the fat deposits from the waist downward and causes problems by overloading the joints.

• Many causes are implicated in the appearance of the problem. As well as a bad lifestyle (eating disorders and lack of exercise), genetic and organic factors can play a part in its appearance.

• The best way of treating the problem is preventive, identifying it early in patients who start to gain weight from the age of 20 to 25.

Doctors consider that obese people should be seen as chronically ill and in need of long-term treatment, with eating rules, behavior modification, physical exercise, and pharmacological therapy.

Modern therapeutic attitudes are based on promoting weight loss with programs to control these illnesses and their associated problems, because they give rise to vascular, cardiac, and metabolic problems

The expression "ideal weight" is being replaced by "recommended weight." The obese person does not need to lose pounds or kilograms, but fat, with small and progressive losses over time, implying metabolic improvement.

On the subject of losing weight, the patient's loss needs to be consolidated in the long term and the risk of premature death, heart disease, and metabolic and vascular problems needs to be reduced.

In certain cases, doctors may decide to prescribe pharmaceutical treatment as well as physical exercise and a change of diet. The pharmaceutical prescribed will be Orlistat (Xenical), an intestinal lipase blocker that inhibits the absorption of fats and has to be combined with a moderately hypocaloric and balanced diet.

Food-related diseases and pathologies

A correct, varied, and complete diet on the one hand enables the organism to work properly and, on the other, reduces the risk of suffering certain conditions or diseases in the short or long term. Abnormally high blood pressure, obesity, diabetes, heart diseases, and even certain types of cancer are linked to an unbalanced diet. There is not usually a direct cause–effect connection, but eating the wrong foods can be one of the factors that help increase the risk of the appearance and development of such diseases.

Orthorexia: addiction to eating healthy food

• Orthorexia is an obsession or extreme preoccupation with health, focused on eating as healthily as possible. It can become a serious problem. People suffering from orthorexia end by focusing almost exclusively on what they eat. Meals are the center of their thoughts and their life.

• As a rule, they reject meat, fats, foods grown using pesticides or herbicides, and those containing artificial substances, but their obsession with healthy eating goes far beyond that and they even worry about the way their food is prepared and the containers in which they cook it.

• They devote much time to planning menus and preparing food. Each small eating transgression is accompanied by ever-increasing feelings of guilt and frustration. Everything that is not "natural," healthy or controlled is rejected, which has a very negative effect on the person's social life. Eating out in a bar or restaurant becomes unthinkable to them.

• As a rule, orthorexia sufferers are very strict, controlled, and demanding of themselves and others. Women, adolescents, and people dedicated to sport are the most vulnerable groups, as they are usually highly sensitive to the nutritional value of food and its effects on their figure or body image. Their personality is usually extremist—it's all or nothing, either obese or thin.

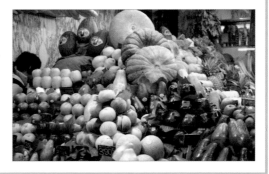

Diabetes

Diabetes is a chronic disease in which sugar is poorly absorbed due to a partial or total absence of the hormone insulin, or because that hormone is not performing as it should. Insulin enables sugars to enter the cells so they can be used as a source of energy. If it is in short supply, or if it is not working properly, sugars accumulate in the blood, producing what is called *hyperglycemia* (excessive levels of sugar in the blood).

There are two main types of diabetes:
• Type I, dependent on insulin, sometimes called juvenile diabetes, because it usually begins in infancy (although it can also occur in adults). As their bodies are not producing insulin, people with type I diabetes have to inject themselves with insulin in order to live. Less than 10 percent of diabetics suffer from type I diabetes.

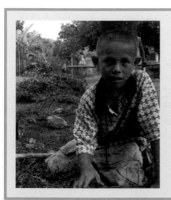

Malnutrition

This is the condition that occurs when a person's body is not receiving sufficient nutrients. It can result from eating an inadequate or unbalanced diet, digestive or absorption problems, or other medical conditions. Depending on which food is deficient, a woman will be more or less affected to a greater or lesser degree.

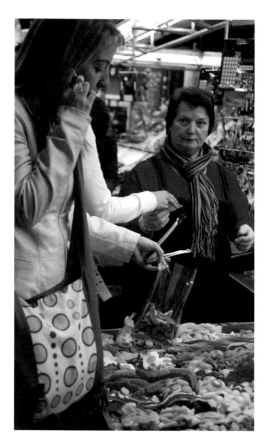

Many people with this type of diabetes do not even know they have it, although it is a serious problem. This type of diabetes is becoming increasingly common, due to an increase in old the number of people, increasing obesity and lack of exercise.

• In Type II, which occurs in adults, the body does produce insulin but either does not produce enough of it or cannot use what it produces. The insulin cannot accompany the glucose into the cells. This type usually occurs mainly in people over the age of 40.

Hyperlipemias: cholesterol and triglycerides

Hyperlipemias are a group of fat metabolism problems that cause an increase in one or more lipidic fractions in the blood. The two most important types are triglycerides and cholesterol. They originate from the diet and synthesis by the liver. Both types fulfill different physiological missions in the organism, especially as regards structure and energy but, when their production is excessive or their metabolism deficient, the resulting accumulation can become a factor in the risk of developing hardening of the arteries.

The fats in the blood circulate in combination with protein particles forming lipoproteins. There are different types of lipoprotein. The most important are kilomicrons, VLDL, LDL, and HDL particles. The LDL particles are the ones that carry cholesterol to the tissues and, when the cholesterol level is high, it is known as *bad cholesterol*, in contrast to the HDL particles that carry cholesterol to the liver and are known as *good cholesterol*.

Although there are various classifications of hyperlipemias, to simplify the matter, we can refer to hypertriglicerydemias, or the increase in the concentration of triglycerides, hypercholesterolemias and mixed hyperlipemias in which both the cholesterol and the triglycerides increase.

Primary hyperlipemias are transmitted by heredity with greater or lesser penetration, meaning that this possibility should be assessed when there is a family history of hyperlipemia. This type includes family-linked hypercholesterolemia, family-linked hypertriglyceridemia and combined family-linked hyperlipemia. Many diseases are conveyed with hyperlipemia, such as discompensated diabetes mellitus, hypothyroidism, nephrotic syndrome, obstructive ictericia, anorexia nervosa, lupus erythematosus, alcoholism, and treatment with gestagens, beta blockers, etc.

In most cases, the high level of fats in the blood does not produce acute symptoms, so it is necessary to carry out a blood analysis for diagnosis. When, exceptionally, the triglyceride figures are very high, they can cause episodes of abdominal pain due to pancreatitis, an enlarged liver and spleen, and the

Hyperlipemia

There are two types of hyperlipemia, primary hyperlipemia which is due to a problem with the metabolism of fats itself, and secondary hyperlipemia which occurs as a consequence of another disease or of taking certain medicines.

Recommended foods

- Milk and dairy products. Skim or semiskim milk, according to individual needs, but it is particularly recommended to eat yogurt and other low-fat dairy products more often, unsweetened, of course. Some are flavored with saccharine, etc., and can be eaten without causing problems (always read the label).
- Meat, fish, eggs and their derivatives, all as often as recommended in a balanced diet.
- Cereals and potatoes (starch). Combine them with green vegetables, rice, pastas and, as regards other cereals, prefer whole grain (bread, cereals and whole-grain cookies without sugar) to refined products.
- Legumes. Lentils, chickpeas, beans, broad beans, peas. It is advisable to combine them only with potatoes or rice and green vegetables.
- Leaf vegetables and greens. All of them, preferably one portion of them per day raw (salad).
- Fruit. Fresh, if possible unpeeled, and well washed, in a smoothie, or baked in the oven without sugar, except those indicated under "restricted foods."
- Drinks. Water, soups, infusions, natural unsweetened fruit juices.
- Fats. Olive and other seed oils (sunflower, corn, soya), butter, vegetable margarines.

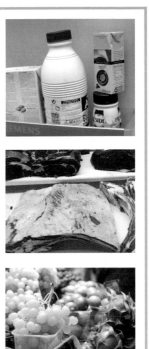

appearance of fatty skin eruptions called *xantomatosis eruptiva*.

If the increase in cholesterol and/or triglycerides is chronic, there is a risk of developing hardening of the arteries. Therefore, especially in the case of hypercholesterolemias, it may give rise to coronary insufficiency (angina pectoris, myocardial infarction), strokes, and circulation problems in the legs. The damage to the large blood vessels happens as a consequence of the accumulation of cholesterol in what are called the *spongy* cells, constituting the basis for the development of the ateroma plate, the basic element in hardening of the arteries. The ateroma plate progressively obstructs the passage of blood, resulting in a poor supply of oxygen to the tissues, or ischemia, which can cause irreversible lesions.

Hypercholesterolemias cause deposits of cholesterol, called *xantomas*, on the skin and in the tendons. When they occur on the eyelids they are called xantelasmas. In some patients, hypertriglyceridemia is associated with a reduction in HDL, cholesterol, and other complications such as high blood pressure, diabetes mellitus, obesity and hyperuricaemia, producing what is called *metabolic syndrome* and causing a high risk of heart disease.

People suffering from hyperlipemia should take proper dietetic treatment based on the restriction of saturated fats or fats of animal origin. They should also maintain as normal a weight as possible, avoiding both being overweight or obese and excessively underweight. Regular physical exercise is highly recommended as it helps improve lipidic metabolism. If, after these measures have been applied for at least three months, the hyperlipemia persists, pharmacological treatment will be necessary.

Primary hyperlipemias require regular treatment throughout life. Secondary hyperlipemias can disappear once their cause has been eliminated. However, the pharmacological treatment of hyperlipemias often has to be given permanently. The treatment of hyperlipemias has been shown to be effective as regards the development of ateroma plates.

Anemia

Ferropenic anemia is characterized by a reduction in deposits of organic iron, at the same time causing a reduction in the number of red corpuscles. The organism contains some 4 grams of iron, most of which (2.5 grams) are combined with a

Restricted foods

A person suffering from hyperlipemia should consume the following only occasionally or in small quantities:

- Whole and condensed milk, dairy products enriched with cream, custard, baked custard, full-fat and blended cheeses (slice or portion) and cheese spreads, cream.
- Fatty pork, veal and beef, duck, smoked or cured meats, organ meats, delicatessen meats (sausages, liver and other pâtés), pickled, salted and smoked fish, fish marinades.
- Sugar and chocolate-coated cereals, potato chips and similar snacks. Beans and peas cooked with fatty ingredients (chorizo sausage, etc.).
- Greens prepared with butter, cream, cheese and other excessively fatty sauces.
- Dried fruit (figs, dates, plums, etc.), in syrup, candied and preserved.
- All alcoholic drinks.
- Butter, mixed margarine, lard, bacon and suet, coconut and palm oil, cocoa butter and products containing it. Dried fruit, olives, avocado pears and coconuts.
- Sweet foods: sugar, fructose, glucose syrup, jelly, honey, chocolate and its derivatives, deep-fried products, confectionery and pastries, sugary drinks. Products containing egg yolk (mayonnaise, croquettes, fritters, battered food).

LDL is the type of cholesterol of which there is the greatest proportion in the blood. If too much of it is circulating in the bloodstream, it is dangerous because it is deposited on the walls of the arteries and, together with other substances, can start to form ateroma plates. This is known as aterosclerosis.

protein, transferian, forming hemoglobin. This is the molecule that transports oxygen from the lungs to all the cells. Therefore, iron is essential for the formation of hemoglobin.

- In the liver, spleen and bone marrow, it is stored in the form of ferritine, constituting the body's iron reserve.
- Every day, an adult loses about 1 milligram of iron through the skin, mucous membranes, feces and urine.
- A fertile woman loses more through menstruation.
- During pregnancy, there is a degree of anemia caused by an increased demand for iron by the fetus accompanied by an increase in the volume of blood in the circulatory system.
- In adults, the most frequent cause of anemia is the reduction in the absorption of iron due to diseases that affect the duodenum—the part of the intestine close to the stomach where iron absorption takes place (ulcers, hemorrhoids, intestinal inflammatory disease, etc.)
- Children often suffer from this type of anemia during periods of rapid growth and development because of their increased need for iron.

Ferropenic anemia

- This is caused by an inadequate intake of iron, called a nutritional deficiency, the most frequent in our environment and one that is likely to increase.
- Inadequate or monotonous food can mean customarily consuming insufficient iron.
- The symptoms are similar to those of other forms of anemia: tiredness, pallor, and weakness.
- It usually starts insidiously.
- The skin, mucous membranes, and nails are pale because they are short of hemoglobin.
- If this form of anemia has been developing for some time, it can cause the taste buds of the tongue to atrophy.

Constipation

Constipation is characterized by a reduction in the number and normal weight of the feces and often by feces of harder consistency. It is difficult to diagnose because of the subjective nature of the problem and the difficulty of establishing what the patient's normal bowel habits are, clearly influenced as they are by sociocultural and dietary differences. In a healthy general population, the normal frequency of defecation varies between three times a week and three times a day, and feces are elimina-

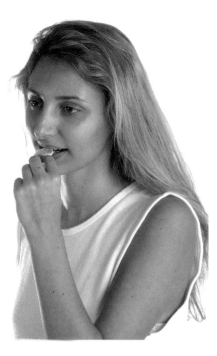

Anemia causes a series of general complaints that are not actually a specific disease and can be summed up as:

- Tiredness.
- Reduced sexual desire.
- Heart disease symptoms.
- Palpitations.
- Fatigue following effort.
- Low blood pressure.
- Swollen ankles.
- Headaches.
- Nausea, giddiness.
- Sleepiness, confusion, irritability.
- Noises in the ears.
- Menstrual upsets.
  - Pallor.
- Fragile nails.
- Hair loss.

In severe and/or acute cases:
- Cold, damp skin.
- Reduction in volume of urine.
- Chest pain.

ted without difficulty in 75 percent of cases. According to this criterion, constipation can be defined as difficulty in defecating on more than 25 percent of occasions and/or a frequency of less than three times a week, sometimes associated with abdominal cramps and flatulence after defecating, a hard fecal consistency, or feces in the form of little pellets which can be well below the normal weight.

Other symptoms can also occur, such as headaches, irritability, and lack of appetite. A person suffering from constipation can present all or only some of these symptoms.

ANEMIA	
According to the World Health Organization, anemia is present when the concentration of hemoglobin in the blood is below the following figures	
Girls aged between 6 months and 6 years	11 g/dl
Girls aged between 6 and 14 years	12 g/dl
Adult women, not pregnant	12 g/dl
Adult women, pregnant	11 g/dl

The most common causes of this acute or chronic complaint include:

• A shortage of foods rich in fiber (green vegetables and pulses, fresh and dried fruit, and wholegrain cereals) in the daily diet, combined with a low intake of liquids, making the feces small in size and very hard.

• The weakness of the muscles of the abdominal wall and pelvic floor that are involved in defecation.

• The effect of certain medicines (codeine taken for colds, analgesics, sedatives, oral iron, and antidepressants, among others), which cause a reduction in intestinal peristalsis. This also occurs in conditions such as diabetes, hyperthyroidism, Parkinson's disease, and natural processes such as pregnancy.

• Some people's genetic predisposition to constipation.

• Age. Constipation is very common in people aged over 65, because of changes in the intestinal tract, sometimes aggravated by immobility, taking many types of medication, and mental deterioration.

• Anal and rectal diseases. Fissures or hemorrhoids that make defecation painful, leading the sufferer to avoid all intestinal movements.

• Irritable bowel syndrome, diverticulosis or other causes, including the absence of intestinal training in people with strokes and neurological diseases, mental deficiency, muscular diseases, stress or depression, and people who travel, associated with prolonged storage of the feces in the final part of the colon.

• Stenosis (narrowing of the intestine), polyps, or cancer of the colon, in which the large intestine is obstructed.

Treatment must be etiological, that is to say, it must depend on the cause of the complaint (improved diet, increased physical exercise, retraining bowel habits, health and hygiene recommendations, treatment with laxatives in specific cases, etc.). Diet plays an important part, not only in preventing constipation but also in treating it and resolving its symptoms.

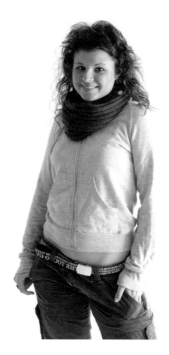

Constipation is three times more frequent in women and can be due to their biological predisposition to the complaint (hormonal factors, pregnancy, and multiple births) and their more sedentary lifestyle (women practice less sport than men), or even generally incorrect dietary habits (not eating enough green vegetables, legumes, and fruit). It is also influenced by psychological factors (women suffer from anxiety and depression more often than men) and psychosocial factors, ranging from suffering ill-treatment to taking on a social and family-oriented role that leaves them little time for themselves and may lead them to resist the urge to defecate and postpone going to the toilet when they feel the need.

Emotional health

These days, everyone knows the part emotions play in overall health and, hence, in the development of disease. The World Health Organization (WHO) affirms that a high percentage of diseases have a psychosomatic origin. In fact, each person's character and self-control and the way they manage emotions and combat stress, conflicts, failures, and frustrations can empower or aggravate various illnesses.

Anxiety and depression

Anxiety

Anxiety is a normal reaction to a tense and stressful situation and only becomes a pathology if the sufferer loses control of it.

Anxiety problems affect a significant number of the population. Young adults suffer them more frequently. Anxiety becomes an illness when worry, fear, or the sense of imminent threat appears without any obvious reason, if such reactions are out of all proportion to their cause, or when psychological and physical symptoms start to influence or affect daily life.

Four clinical forms of anxiety are described:

• Generalized anxiety disorder. Generalized anxiety is associated with a constant and somewhat unreasonable preoccupation with many areas of a person's own life. Preoccupation over things such as physical safety or the financial stability of the family can persist in spite of efforts to convince the sufferer that everything is as it should be. People with generalized anxiety feel worried, have difficulty sleeping, are irritable and physically tense to an extent that interferes with their daily lives.

• Panic attacks. Clinical panic involves sudden and unexpected attacks of intense terror. Its symptoms include agitated breathing, heart palpitations, chest pain, breathlessness, trembling and feeling nauseous. Panic attacks can occur at any time, which distinguishes them from natural reactions to real danger.

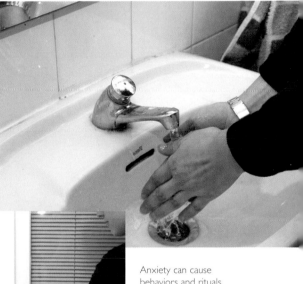

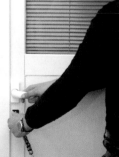

Anxiety can cause behaviors and rituals such as repeatedly washing the hands or checking over and over again that doors and windows are closed. This type of repetitive action is usually done to lessen anxiety.

• Phobias. Many people suffer from minor phobias such as fear of heights, snakes or spiders. These phobias can cause temporary upsets but do not affect the possibility of leading a totally normal life. However, some types of phobia are so incapa-

Most patients respond well to treatment and the success indices of those treated are usually very high, enabling them to live full and productive lives again.

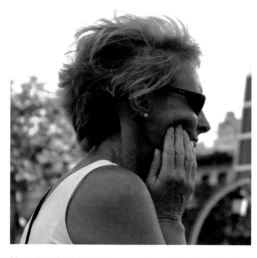

Nowadays there is a wide range of medicines to relieve the extensive symptoms that accompany anxiety.

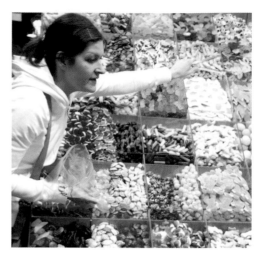

It appears that women are more inclined than men to suffer depression.
One woman in every seven consults a doctor, compared with one man in every nine. It has not been determined whether there are differences between the sexes in this respect. Possibly, women are more inclined to express their hopes and fears to a doctor, while men resort to other ways of expressing their feelings, such as violence or alcohol.

citating that the patient feels he or she cannot possibly leave the house.

• Obsessive compulsive behavior. Many people show a degree of obsessive and compulsive behavior, such as, for example, checking again and again that a window is closed or repeatedly washing their hands. This is problematical if these behaviors and rituals seriously interfere with daily life.

Depression

Depression is the most frequent mental illness and is characterized by a feeling of uncontrolled despair. At some time in their lives, about 5 percent of the population will suffer a depressive state so severe that it requires professional treatment. Although depression can occur at any age and affects both sexes, it is more frequent in women between the ages of 35 and 55.

The way depression is suffered varies greatly from one person to another. For a state of mind to be considered depressive, the symptoms must be severe enough to interfere with the sufferer's daily life or work. A person suffering four or more of the nine symptoms described below for two weeks or longer requires professional attention:

• A marked change in sleep pattern.
• A marked change in appetite.
• A reduced capacity to feel pleasure, for example, loss of interest and enjoyment in things that previously induced great pleasure.
• Feelings of worthlessness, despair, and helplessness.
• Inappropriate feelings of guilt.
• Problems with thinking, concentration, and attention.
• Recurrent thoughts of death or suicide.
• Crushing sorrow and grief.
• Physical symptoms: fatigue, or loss of libido.

Certain situations predispose people to depression

- Loneliness.
- Pain.
- Marriage problems or divorce.
- Job loss or overwork.
- Retirement.
- Financial difficulties.
- Relocation.
- Having suffered traumas in infancy.

People suffering from depression describe the following symptoms:
- Reduced capacity to make decisions.
- Low spirits.
- Physical pain and suffering.
- Discouragement.
- Lack of motivation.
- Isolation.
- Restlessness and negative thoughts.
- Self-blame.
- Drinking excessive amounts of alcohol.
- Confused thoughts.
- Anxiety.
- Irrational fears and phobias.

■ Treatment of depression

With adequate help, depression can be overcome.

- **Antidepressants.** These are drugs that reestablish energy, sleep patterns, and appetite. The disadvantage is that they can cause giddiness and sleepiness and can take weeks to produce results.

- **Psychotherapy.** This is a very effective treatment for depression caused by traumatic life experiences or personality problems.

- **Cognitive-behavioral therapy.** This therapy helps sufferers to think positively and increase self-esteem.

- **Support.** The best help for people suffering depression is their family's support and understanding.

Addictions

Although drug addiction is a serious and recurrent health problem for men and women of all ages and social conditions, in females drug abuse can present special problems and require different methods of treatment.

There are drugs (medicines, alcoholic drinks, tobacco, marijuana, cocaine, etc.) and activities (gambling, slot machines, the Internet, etc.) that can be harmful to health and lead to addiction. Not all use is addiction. There have to be some distinctions.

Many mothers go through a period of slight depression after giving birth to a child. This type of depression makes them feel unhappy and more emotional than normal, as well as suffering frequent bouts of weeping. The symptoms occur between four and five days after the birth and last about a week. Their origin can be hormonal. However, there are other factors such as fears, small worries that become exaggerated panics, about the baby's health, initial difficulties with feeding the baby, stress, irritability, physical exhaustion.

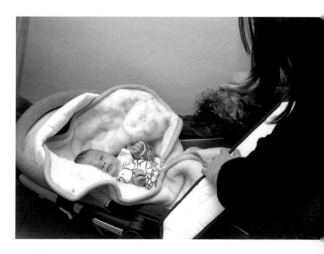

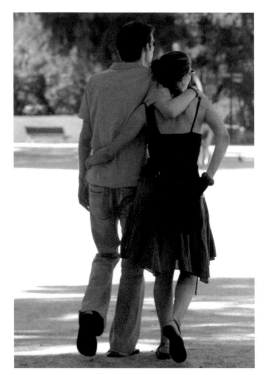

When a close relative is depressed, it alters the whole balance of family life. At first, it is difficult to understand what is happening, and family members become irritated or angry, pay little attention to the depressed person, and reject the way he or she is behaving. It is important to remember that affected people cannot change their behavior and are very disturbed by what is happening to them. It is vital to pay affectionate attention so as to be of help to people suffering depression.

• **Use.** The substance is used or the activity practiced sporadically, for example, at weekends or on odd occasions. It does not affect family or school life, work or social relationships. The person can give it up at will.

• **Abuse.** The substance is used or the activity practiced regularly during the week. It affects school productivity and work, family and social relationships. Almost without realizing it, the person becomes an addict, increases her tolerance and suffers from abstinence syndrome. She must confront what is happening to her and seek help.

• **Addiction** or dependency. The substance is used or the activity practiced several times a day and every day. All relations with the family, school or work have deteriorated. The person obsessively and compulsively seeks out the drug or activity. It

is absolutely impossible for the person to abstain unless she receives help.

Female drug users often have self-esteem problems and low self-confidence and can feel powerless. Many female addicts do not seek treatment because, for example, they are afraid they will not be allowed to care for their children or keep them, or fear reprisals by their partner, punishment by the authorities, etc. Many state that their drug-taking sexual partners caused them to start taking drugs. Moreover, research indicates that drug-dependent women have great difficulty in abstaining when their partner's lifestyle relies on drug use. The woman must understand and know that it is possible to overcome the illness of drug addiction. Those women who have received support from their families and the health services have succeeded in overcoming the problem.

Addiction is not easy to diagnose and treat because it depends to a large extent on the affected person's accepting her situation and being prepared to do something to help herself, and that is not usual in addicts. Addiction produces a defense mechanism in them known as *denial*.

As they begin to suffer problems (at work, at home, socially), they start to deny that the drug or activity concerned constitutes a problem that they cannot control and that the negative effects on their lives are in any way connected with the use

Depression can affect a person at any stage of life, from infancy, adolescence or youth until old age. It can be of short duration or last for months or even years, and can appear episodically at different times of life. Some people make a full recovery, while others suffer from it all their lives. The degrees of severity are variable. When the condition is experienced slightly over the years, it is called *disthymia*.

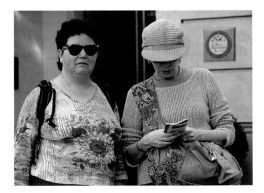

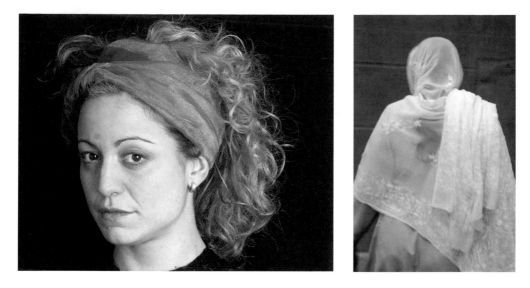

Women of all races and socioeconomic conditions suffer from the serious disorder of drug-dependency. They need treatment for drug addiction just as for any other problem that affects their physical or mental health. Many female drug-users have experienced other challenges to their health during their lives: research indicates that up to 70% of these women also report a history of physical and sexual ill-treatment.

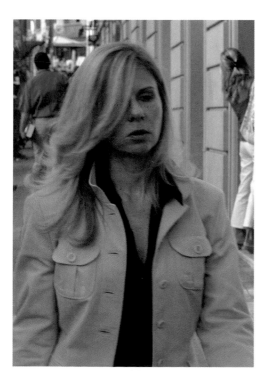

of the drug or the practice of the activity. Thus, they lose all contact with reality.

Moreover, there is the added difficulty of the false perception of self-control, typical of addicts. In this case, the person's will is insufficient when she tries to control the addiction. The substance or activity controls the person, but she thinks she can control the amount, dose, and frequency of the drug. This is naïve and forms the biggest obstacle to resolving the problem.

Toxicomania

The financially independent professional woman aged between 20 and 30, with low self-esteem, identity problems, and insecurities, has the profile predisposing her to potential addiction to tranquillizers, muscle-relaxants, and other medicines. Women self-prescribe more than men and usually take more sedatives and painkillers. The reasons seem to be the pressure they feel they are under regarding personal appearance (weight control), hormonal changes, and the physical and psychic overload with their multiple functions as productive workers and mothers.

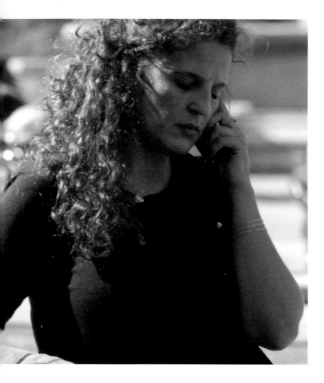

Addictive drugs constitute a group of substances that are very varied from the pharmacological or chemical point of view. Whichever drug is taken, all of them induce a pleasurable effect in their users that incites them to go on taking them.

Opium

Natural or semisynthetic opium derivatives create great physical and psychic dependency and cause all primary needs to disappear. Morphine is one of the semisynthetic derivatives of natural alkaloid opiates.

Heroin

The effects of heroin and morphine are similar. The principal difference is the greater power of heroin. There is no doubt at all that it is one of the most dangerous drugs and one of the most widely distributed. Its effects are felt within 10 minutes of taking it, peak after 60 minutes and cease after 3 to 4 hours.

Coca

Coca, the leaf of the shrub *Erythroxylon coca*, is a stimulant. Its effect on the central nervous system is not as strong as that of cocaine, because 160 coca leaves are needed to extract one gram of cocaine.

Cocaine

Cocaine is an alkaloid contained in the leaves of the coca shrub. It is an extremely powerful brain stimulant whose effects are similar to that of amp-

The excessive consumption of alcohol and tobacco and the use and abuse of other drugs prescribed as sedatives and tranquillizers is very widespread among women. This is a fact that is not admitted and is usually hidden.

The problem of addiction

- Addiction to substances that are harmful to health is sad and painful for the sufferer and for the family and friends.

- The problems created by drug dependency can become even greater when they affect particularly vulnerable people or lead to highly risky situations.

- Pregnancy is one of the situations in which the suffering of drug addicts becomes intolerable, as it demonstrates the harshness and harmfulness of drugs, not only to the person taking them but also to a defenseless being who is obliged to suffer the effects they cause.

- In the broad sense, it can be affirmed that the main effect of drug abuse in pregnancy is not only harm to the fetus, but the destruction of the mother's health, expressed as malnutrition, inadequate prenatal care, infectious diseases, psychosocial stress or poisoning from overdoses.

- All these factors contribute to the same or a greater extent to the complications of drug abuse during pregnancy than the effects of the drug itself.

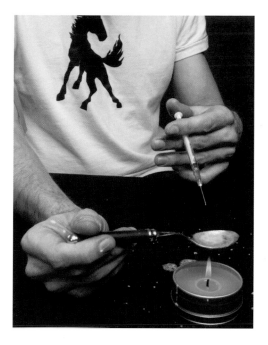

hetamines. It is also a vigorous blood vessel constrictor and a local anesthetic, being absorbed by the mucous membranes of the nose when it is drawn in.

Crack

Also called "the cocaine of the poor," it causes a serious social and health risk because of the dependency it induces and its harmful effects on the organism. It is obtained from macerating coca leaves in kerosene and sulfuretted compounds.

Amphetamines

The consumption of these stimulants is widespread in all social classes. Amphetamines are used by executives who claim to be overstressed, housewives seeking an appetite suppressant for their diets, and students preparing for exams..

MDMA

Methylendioximethamphetamine (MDMA), also known as XTC, Ecstasy, chalk, crystal, X, etc., is a synthetic psychoactive drug with emotively powerful and psychologically disturbing hallucinogenic properties and effects similar to those of amphetamines. Its duration varies from 3 to 6 hours after it is taken.

Cannabis sativa—Hashish—Marijuana

Its effect varies according to factors such as the speed at which it is smoked, the duration of inhalation, the amount inhaled, the length of time the smoker holds his breath after inhaling it, and his state of mind. The oral consumption of both marijuana and hashish has psychological effects similar to those experienced when it is smoked, but of greater intensity and longer duration, and it is more harmful. It affects the brain cells responsible for memory. This makes it difficult for the person to remember recent events (even what happened a few minutes ago) and to learn when under the influence of the drug. Recent studies show that marijuana creates mental dysfunctions and reduces intellectual capacity in people who smoke a lot of it over many years.

Barbiturates and sedatives

In small doses, these are used as tranquilizers, that is to say as a pharmaceutical to lessen anxiety and restlessness. In large quantities its effects are intoxicating, similar to those produced by alcohol. They are frequently taken at the same time as alcohol, increasing the effects of both drugs, characterized by psychomotor coordination problems and a reduced level of awareness. In large doses they can produce symptoms similar to the *delirium tremens* caused by alcohol.

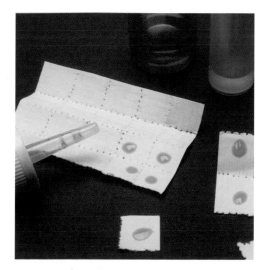

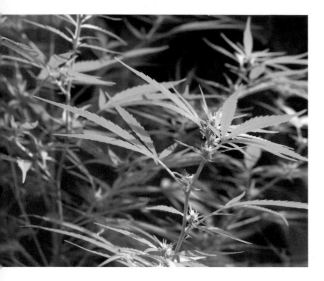

Hallucinogens

The term *hallucinogen* refers to substances that alter the senses, producing a distorted perception of sights and sounds and generating unreal sensations. LSD is a semisynthetic substance, a fungus extract derived from ergot. It is considered to be a psychedelic product that inhibits the ego's defense mechanisms and facilitates the distribution of sensitivity and the appearance of disconcerting images.

Alcoholism

Alcoholism in women requires separate consideration because, although it has characteristics in common with alcoholism in men, it is distinguished by sociocultural factors that determine the position of women in society. Society is less indulgent toward women, so alcoholism in women is more secret, solitary, and dominated by a sense of shame leading to self-blame. Alcoholism degrades women more rapidly and deeply in their social position and their feminine and maternal roles than men in their masculine and paternal roles. Social rejection and intolerance are more marked and occur earlier for women than for men.

The problem of alcoholism has probably become one of the most generalized social phenomena of recent decades. This has led to a great diversity of studies that attempt to establish its true dimensions. Many of these studies agree in pointing out the massive effect the consumption of alcoholic drinks has had in recent years on the health services, pointing out that the number of hospital beds assigned to drug addicts or alcoholics has doubled and that many of them are occupied by people with alcohol-related problems.

There is also a wide range of interrelated problems for which alcohol is directly or indirectly responsible. These include medical problems, both physical and psychological, family, work and social relations, domestic and traffic accidents and accidents at work, violence and self-inflicted injuries.

Years ago, alcohol addiction in women occurred mainly in two ways:

• In housewives, not leaving home and keeping it an unconfessable secret, making it difficult to seek medical assistance.

• As a social relationship, in which only women working in certain professions used to drink.

These days, women no longer devote themselves exclusively to domestic duties and are perma-

Ethyl alcohol is the psychoactive drug most used throughout the world. Alcohol abuse has now reached massive proportions in both developed and developing countries and is associated with a whole series of adverse consequences of which the disease of alcoholism constitutes only a small part.

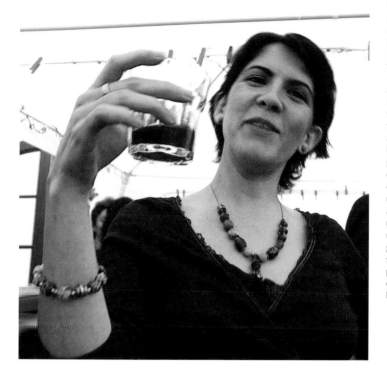

Alcoholism is a problem that has little to do with the type or exact amount of alcohol consumed or how long the person has been drinking. However, it has a lot to do with the person's uncontrollable need to drink. This definition of alcoholism helps explain why, for most alcoholics, a little willpower is not enough to stop themselves drinking. The alcoholic person often finds himself under the control of a powerful desire or necessity to drink alcohol, a necessity that can be felt as strongly as the necessity for water or food. Although some individuals can recover unaided, most alcoholics need outside help in order to get over this disease. With help, support, and treatment, many people are capable of stopping drinking and rebuilding their lives.

nently actively involved in the social and economic sectors. Their social role is no longer the same and their consumption patterns and behavior have adapted to that change. Women's behavior is now similar to that of men and, when addicted to alcohol, they match male consumption models, without the need to justify themselves to anyone, although they maintain a tendency to conceal or deny the problem. The age at which women start drinking alcohol has now become practically equal in both sexes, although the dependency pattern is still greater in males.

Treatment

The primary objective is to make the alcoholic person understand her illness and the necessity of taking adequate treatment. Then, the following stages will be alcoholic deintoxication, dropping the habit, and subsequent monitoring.

The effects of alcoholism

Alcoholism is an addictive disease characterized by the following effects:

- Insatiable need: the desire or strong and compulsive necessity for alcohol.

- Loss of control: the frequent inability to stop drinking alcohol once the person has started.

- Physical dependency: the appearance of symptoms after abstinence, such as vomiting, sweating, trembling, and anxiety when the person stops drinking after a period of consuming large amounts of alcohol. These symptoms are usually relieved when the person starts drinking alcohol again or some other sedative drug is taken.

- Tolerance: the necessity of increasing the amount of alcohol ingested in order to feel drugged or intoxicated.

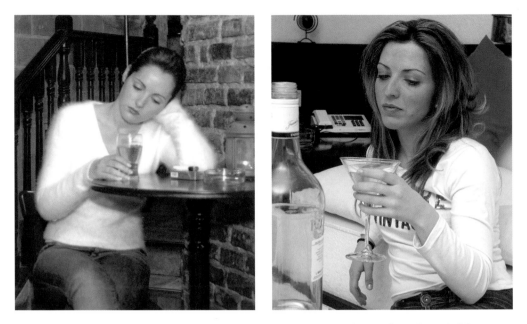

It has been established that many biological, psychological and social factors intervene in the genesis of alcoholism, and that the interaction between genetic and environmental factors contributes considerably to the development of problems.

For deintoxication, firstly the person must stop drinking alcohol and correct the nutritional deficit caused by its excessive consumption. Sedatives may be prescribed to confront the possibility, even minimal, that withdrawal symptoms may occur (anxiety, trembling, insomnia, abnormally fast heartbeat, sweating, nausea, vomiting, and diarrhea). Vitamin treatment is also advisable. In all cases, abstinence syndrome must be approached from the psychological point of view.

Another medication used is Disulfiram ("Antabuse"), which interferes with the metabolism

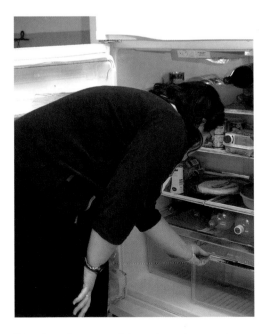

The most beneficial treatment for alcoholics is that provided through Alcoholics Anonymous. These groups put the sick person in touch with fellow abstainers who are always accessible in an environment where they can form social relationships outside the bar. This help can enable them to regain self-esteem and self-confidence and feel as they did before they came into contact with alcohol.

If the disease is not treated, depression and more serious anxiety attacks occur. Moreover, the patient gains weight and, consequently, heart and blood pressure problems may arise.

Symptomatology

- As a rule, alcoholics are over 40 years of age and have a history of drinking alcohol that dates back many years.

- Traditionally, their faces look red and swollen, the whites of their eyes look yellowish and their breath has a particular smell.

- Their speech is slurred and hurried, sometimes stammering, trembling round the mouth is observed immediately and they perspire easily.

- Psychic alterations start as character modifications: alcoholics are increasingly emotional, irritable and impulsive, jealous and moody and frequently have attacks of depression.

- At the same time, intellectual changes appear, with reduced productivity, difficulty in concentrating, attention deficiency, a certain confusion of the intellectual processes, a reduction in professional efficiency, absenteeism, behavioral regression and impaired social relations.

- They have memory lapses after drinking a certain amount of alcohol, whether excessive or not, in which they realize that they have forgotten what they were doing while they were drinking.

- The emotional results are fairly clear: egoistical tendencies, reduction in the sense of what is ethical and in the sense of responsibility, unconcern and indifference regarding the family, complaining of a lack of authority at home and the contempt in which they are held, especially by their children.

- Alcoholics often declare their repentance and vow that they will give up drinking.

- Digestive problems include frequent gastritis, abdominal pain, massive thirst, loss of appetite accompanied by nausea, as well as frequent and fetid diarrhea.

- The liver increases in size, with a feeling of heaviness in the right side of the abdomen and vomiting, finally leading to cirrhosis of the liver and the accumulation of liquid in the abdomen.

- Nervous system problems are characterized by minor rapid trembling of the hands and tongue, muscular cramp (especially in the calves), sudden jolts in the night, tingling sensations in the extremities and muscular atrophy.

- Fetal alcoholic syndrome can be observed in the children of alcoholic mothers, characterized by late development and growth, mental retardation and various congenital defects.

of alcohol by means of which intermediary products are accumulated. This causes symptoms of intoxication and intense problems such as facial redness, reddened eyes, throbbing headaches, abnormally fast heartbeat, and sweating. Thirty minutes to an hour after taking it, nausea and vomiting will occur and there may be reduced blood pressure, giddiness, and sometimes loss of consciousness. The effects are so intense that few patients risk drinking alcohol while they are taking Disulfiram. This medication should not be taken during pregnancy or by patients with heart disease.

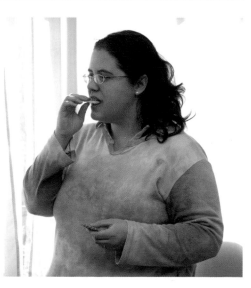

Almost all abnormal eating behavior occurs in adolescents and young people. However, this type of problem can also arise during menopause.

The principal characteristics of addictive behavior

1. A strong desire or feeling of compulsion to act in a particular way (especially when the opportunity of doing so is not available).

2. Reduced capacity to control the behavior (particularly when it starts, maintaining it or the level at which it occurs).

3. Feeling unwell and downhearted when the behavior is impeded or when the person stops it, with loss of interest in other activities.

4. Persisting with the behavior, in spite of clear evidence that it is seriously damaging the person's daily life.

Addictive behaviors

The idea that addictions exist in which no substance is involved is becoming increasingly widely accepted. This type of addiction is called addictive *behavior* or socioaddiction, as in the case of addictive gambling or compulsive shopping.

A central characteristic of addictive behavior is loss of control. People with addictive behavior have no control over that conduct, in addition to their dependency on it, tolerance, withdrawal symptoms, and a very considerable negative effect on their lives, which is in many cases why they seek treatment or are forced to seek it.

Eating-related addictions

Many women often suffer stress and anxiety caused by a multitude of situations and factors such as problems at work, with their partner or with the family. They channel this anxiety into an unstoppable impulse to eat. People with this kind of addiction to food or gorging can also suffer very serious problems such as depression, obesity, and heart and blood pressure complaints. This type of disturbance can become very severe and should be treated as early as possible. They are diseases that also require psychological support and pharmacological treatment to reduce anxiety.

Addiction to sex

This is an addiction in which the person feels the uncontrollable necessity for sex of all kinds, from sexual relations with other people to masturbation or the use of pornography. Female sex addiction is called *nymphomania*. It is important to differentiate addiction from high libido. All addictions are illnesses and, like almost all complaints, are characterized by feeling unwell, although the sufferer may not be aware of it or recognize it.

Kleptomania

Contrary to what is generally believed, kleptomaniacs do not steal everything they find indiscriminately, or enjoy doing it. Kleptomaniacs unexpectedly feel the impulse to steal something, often something of virtually no economic value or usefulness. It is an unexpected, unplanned, and unstoppable impulse for them and causes them great anxiety that turns into a feeling of satisfaction or relaxation once the theft has been committed.

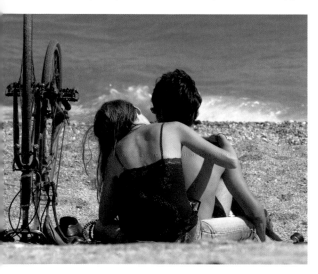

Addiction to sex is one of the least known and least visible dependencies, as its sufferers keep it secret and hide it, especially from people they know, but with whom they would feel embarrassed. It is estimated that up to 6% of the population suffers from it and that 2% of the people affected are women.

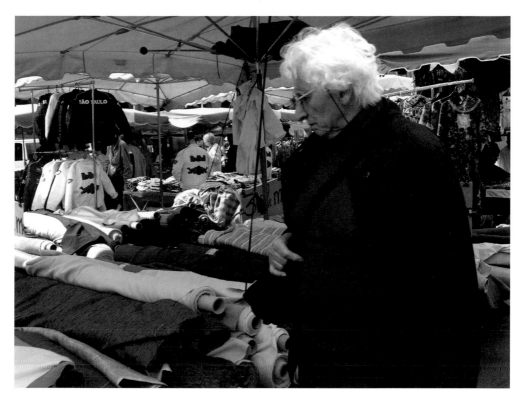

Kleptomania is a disorder of impulse control that mainly affects women and is usually associated with other pathologies.

But kleptomaniacs are at all times aware that stealing is an offense and that what they are doing is wrong, because the momentary euphoria rapidly disappears, giving way to guilt or anxiety and depressive states.

Addiction to gambling

This is an addiction to games of chance in their multiple varieties. The most widespread form concerns fruit machines or one-armed bandits, because they are so easily accessible. People are considered to be addicted to gambling when their condition causes personal, family, professional, and social problems, so that they think, live, and act in relation to the game. Having organized their lives around it, abandoning any other kind of activity, they thus become slaves to the game.

Emotional addiction

This does not concern immoderate love or pathological jealousy. Emotional addiction is a pathological attachment to the partner, an emotional dependency so exaggerated that it becomes an obsession, even leading to extreme situations such as those in which an abused woman will tolerate ill treatment for years because her emotional dependency makes her unable to break off the relationship.

Compulsive gambling

The most traditional profile of a pathological gambler is that of a capricious person with anxiety problems, social adaptation difficulties, and low frustration tolerance. Bingo, lotteries, casinos, and slot machines deserve special attention, if only because of their proliferation and immediate proximity.

Addiction to buying or compulsive shopping

Compulsive shoppers, like alcoholics and bulimics, suffer a breakdown in impulse control. Whenever they pass a shop they have to go in. The excitement of buying (often useless things, or the same things repeatedly) is followed by repentance and then depression, leading them finally to a state of anxiety about buying again. It should be pointed out that many compulsive shoppers are really depressives, and compulsive shopping is usually associated with bulimia and kleptomania.

Psychological ill-treatment and sexual aggression

Psychological ill-treatment is by no means a new phenomenon. What is new is that it is now denounced as a social problem. It is suffered by women of all ages, social and economic groups, cultures, and nationalities. The fact that it is so common, the seriousness of its consequences, its high social and economic cost, and especially the damage it causes to people's right to be treated with the respect deserved by all human beings, makes it a matter of great public relevance.

Psychological ill-treatment is based on deliberate behaviors carried out from a position of authority and aimed at devaluing, causing psychic harm, and destroying self-esteem and personal confidence. It leads to depersonalization and generates dependence in the person inflicting it. Its perpetrator uses insults, accusations, threats, destructive criticism, shouting, manipulation, silence, indifference, and sneering to inflict it.

Psychological ill-treatment is not as visible or obvious as physical abuse. Therefore, the victim is often not aware of it herself until she suffers a physical attack, but its consequences can be more serious and more lasting.

Continued attacks, both verbal and nonverbal (silence, indifference, gestures, etc.) create a harmful relationship of dependency between the perpetrator and the victim. In the end, they need one another. The victim, because on her own she feels she is nobody and fear and anguish paralyze her, and the perpetrator because he feels he is somebody through the domination he exercises. The dependency becomes so great that the victim ends by protecting and exonerating the person who is ill-treating her. This sets off a destructive process in which she starts losing confidence in herself and the capacity to respond, discounts herself and internalizes to the extent that she cannot escape and abandons all hope.

At the root of violence against women is the asymmetry of power caused by an overwhelmingly patriarchal and male-oriented system which has led to the abuse of the most disadvantaged person in it, woman. Therefore, experts prefer not to present it as a "women's problem," because, although women are the ones who suffer it, it is a problem of which men must be made aware and which they must work to overcome.

Physical symptoms and manifestations
- Back and joint pain.
- Irritability.
- Headaches.
- Insomnia.

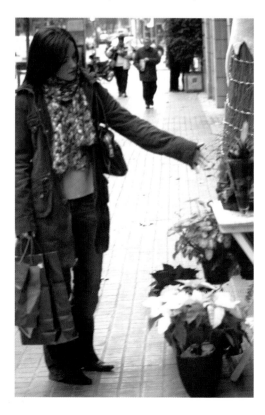

Women between the ages of 30 and 50 are usually the most inclined to be compulsive shoppers, but young people are increasingly exposed to it by the constant pressures of the consumer society.

- Permanent tiredness.
- Sadness, low spirits, feeling like crying for no apparent reason.
  - Anxiety and anguish.
  - Loss of sexual appetite.

Attitude
- Feeling of shame.
- Feeling of blame.
- Generalized fear.
- Averting the eyes.
- Social indifference and sparse communication: vague and confused explanations.

Alarm signals of behavior showing or deriving from psychological ill-treatment
- Ignoring his partner's feelings.
- Ridiculing or insulting women as a group.
- Ridiculing or insulting most of his partner's values, beliefs, religion, race, inheritance, or class.
- Using his approval, appreciation or affection as a punishment.
- Continually criticizing and insulting her or shouting at her.
- Humiliating her in private and/or in public.
- Refusing to maintain social relations in her company.
- Controlling money and all decisions.
- Refusing to share money or refusing to allow her to work.
- Not allowing her access to money, car keys or other goods.
- Frequently threatening to abandon her or saying he is leaving.
- Threatening to harm her or her family.
- Punishing or ill-treating the children when he is cross with her.
- Threatening to kidnap the children or take them away if she leaves him.
- Abusing, torturing, and killing domestic animals in order to hurt her.
- Accusing her of things he imagines her to be doing.
- Manipulating her with lies and contradictions.
- Destroying furniture, domestic appliances, or the home decor during arguments.
- Handling weapons in a threatening manner.

Sexual abuse

Sexual abuse means any act of a sexual nature performed without the consent of one of the people involved. It is an act of violence in which the human being is physically and emotionally outraged and his or her integrity and dignity is attacked. Violence against women is a serious offense. In the case of many victims, these acts of violence are reflected in depression or other mental health problems. In fact, a third of the victims of sexual abuse and attacks suffer posttraumatic stress, consisting of emotional states of anxiety and tension associated with remembering the violent incident.

There are several forms of sexual abuse:
- Rape. This is a sexual attack using force and intimidation against a person.
- Incest. This is a sexual act between people who are related in the first or second degree.
- Lewd acts. Any act of a sexual nature that does not include vaginal or anal penetration with the penis. These can involve kissing, touching, undressing the victim, anal or vaginal penetration with the fingers or some other object, penetration

What should the victim of sexual abuse do?

- Take refuge in a safe place.
- Contact someone who can help: family, friend, police, etc.
- She should not shower or change her clothes, drink or eat. All those actions could destroy important physical evidence if she wants to bring a charge against her attacker.
- Seek medical attention. She may have hidden injuries and also doctors will help her to prevent the possibility of a resulting pregnancy or contracting infectious diseases.
- Everything she remembers about the event should be written down, with all possible details. This may help the recovery process and will be of assistance in any legal action she takes.

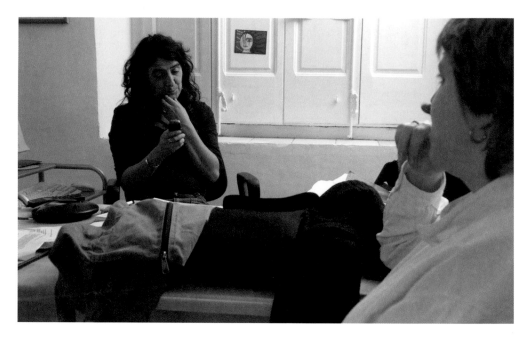

In the private sphere, although men also suffer sexual abuse, women are its usual victims. It also occurs in relations between parents and children, and an increase has been detected in the ill-treatment of children compared with their parents, as a consequence of increasingly permissive upbringing and the use of violence in disputes in the adult world. In the public sphere, psychological abuse in the form of bullying is present in the workplace and in school.

of the mouth by the penis, and obliging the victim to masturbate the attacker, among others.

• Sexual harassment. This consists of any kind of sexual approach or pressure, whether physical or verbal, not desired by the woman who suffers it, which arises in the workplace and results in a hostile working environment, prevents her carrying out her duties and/or affects her promotion or other professional opportunities.

• Obligation to undertake prostitution or exposure to pornography.

• Voyeurism. When someone is watched without knowing it.

Strategies for dealing with life after the attack:

• Obtain the support of friends and family members Try to identify trustworthy people to share your feelings with.

• Talk about the attack.

• Use relaxation techniques: physical exercise such as jogging, aerobics, etc. or relaxation techniques such as yoga, massage, hot baths, etc.

• Show affection. The body thus naturally releases analgesics against the pain.

• Remember that she is safe, even if she doesn't feel it. The attack is over now. She may think the unhappiness will last all her life, but in time she will feel better.

Addiction to tobacco

Tobacco addiction is a true epidemic that has spread over time through advertising and marketing and whose source of contagion is the tobacco industry. Many efforts are being made through government legislation and public opinion to reduce the opportunities to smoke and to discourage people, especially the young, from taking up the habit in the first place.

Tobacco addiction

The attitude to tobacco addiction has changed in recent decades. In the 1960s it was considered a habit, by the 1970s it was seen as a dependency, by the mid-1980s nicotine was considered a highly addictive substance, and in the 1990s the processes of diagnosis and therapy progressed. Nowadays, tobacco addiction must be considered as a drug addiction producing psychological dependence (factors in starting and continuing to smoke), tolerance of the addictive factor (nicotine), and withdrawal symptoms on giving it up. Like other euphoria-inducing substances (alcohol and cocaine), tobacco is capable of producing effects that affect the person's state of mind, and being deprived of it sets off the craving for the substance.

The addiction to byproducts of tobacco is the most widespread. Its cultural acceptance considers its use, firstly, as a source of pleasure and, secondly,

Tobacco is harmful

The link between the habit of smoking and the development of numerous serious illnesses is becoming increasingly clear. It has caused a rise in the number of consultations in the physical and mental health community. The WHO considers tobacco dependency to be an addiction. This type of dependency, like many others, must be properly treated, as nicotine can come to control important aspects of a person's behavior.

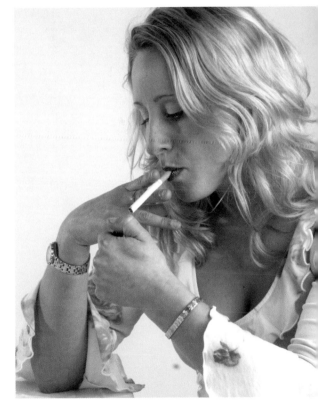

In recent decades, the tobacco industry has succeeded in making women into tobacco addicts, marked by an huge increase in the frequency of lung cancer in women compared with times past when smoking was not habitual among women.

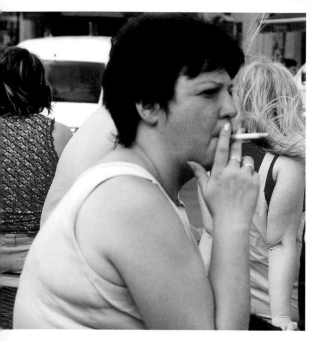

Female cigarette smokers have a considerably reduced life expectancy compared with the rest of the population. Some writers have estimated that they lose 5.5 minutes of life for each cigarette they have smoked. In a person aged between 30 and 35 who smokes two packets of cigarettes a day, life expectancy falls by between 8 and 9 years, compared with a nonsmoker of the same age.

as a simple vice or bad habit. It has been determined that cigarettes and other tobacco products, such as cigars, cheroots, pipe tobacco, or snuff (in powder form) are addictive, and that nicotine is the drug in tobacco that causes the addiction. Moreover, it is known that tobacco addiction is an important cause of heart attacks and strokes and is one of the leading factors in the development of cancer. In spite of that, millions of women use tobacco in its many forms.

Smoking is not only a habit, it is also a drug addiction, as the act of smoking tobacco fulfills all the criteria that define the consumption of such substances:

- Existence of tolerance.
- Dependency.
- Withdrawal symptoms in its absence.
- Compulsive behavior.

The substance most responsible for this dependency is nicotine, a highly addictive substance comparable to other drugs such as heroin or cocaine. Nicotine, one of the principal ingredients of tobacco, is a powerful stimulant. A few seconds after inhaling a mouthful of smoke, the smoker's brain receives a strong dose of this component, making the adrenal glands pour adrenalin into the blood, accelerating the heart rate, and increasing the blood pressure.

The consequences of using tobacco

In women, the damage to the lungs, heart, arteries, brain, and other organs caused by tobacco is similar to that suffered in men, but women suffer greater damage because of their special characteristics, not only during pregnancy but also to their systems or organs that are more predisposed to

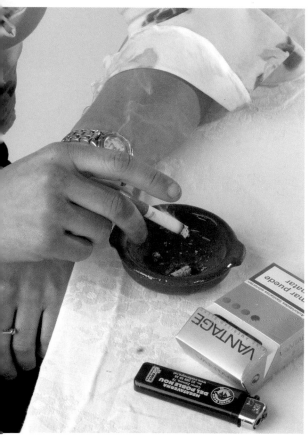

Tobacco is a legal, nonecological and toxic substance which creates addiction. The pressure against tobacco is increasing every day.

The effects of nicotine

• Nicotine acts on the body as both a stimulant and a depressive.

• It increases intestinal activity, saliva, and bronchial secretions.

• It stimulates the nervous system and can cause trembling in the inexperienced user, or even convulsions in high doses.

• This stimulation is followed by a phase that depresses the respiratory muscles.

• As a euphoria-inducing agent, nicotine causes stimulation and relaxation in stressful situations.

• On average, the use of tobacco increases the heart-rate by 10 to 20 beats a minute and raises blood-pressure readings by between 5 and 10 millimeters of mercury (because it contracts the blood vessels).

• Nicotine can also increase perspiration, nausea, and diarrhea. It raises the level of glucose (sugar) in the blood and increases insulin production.

• Nicotine also tends to increase blood platelet aggregation that can lead to the formation of blood clots.

• It temporarily stimulates memory and lucidity. Smokers often depend on it to help them do certain tasks at specific levels of performance.

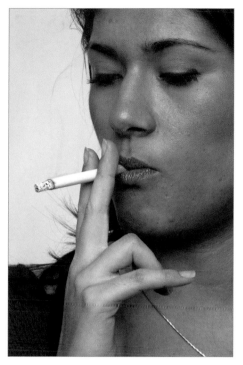

• It also tends to suppress the appetite which is why the fear of gaining weight also influences the some people's desire to stop smoking.

harm because of their delicacy and sensitivity, such as the skin, bones, and mouth.

The annual risk of death in women more than doubles in heavy smokers compared with those who have never smoked in the 45 to 74 year age group.

• The risk of contracting lung cancer increases according to the quantity, duration, and intensity of the habit. The risk of death from lung cancer is 20 times higher in women who smoke two or more

One of the reasons women continue the habit is stress due to tensions at work combined with domestic duties; cigarettes can be seen as a necessary recompense to help relax and deal with problems.

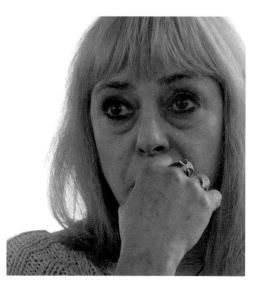

■ The effects of tobacco on the female skin

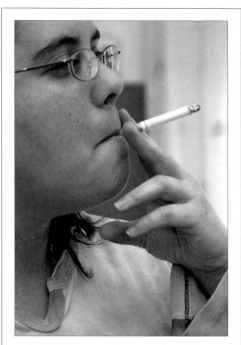

- The link between tobacco and wrinkles can be seen in people of both sexes aged over 30.

- Smokers aged between 40 and 50 are likely to have wrinkles identical to those of nonsmokers who are 20 to 30 years older.

- Women's skin is more affected by tobacco because of its delicacy, leading to premature aging.

- It suffices to observe the devastation nicotine causes in a woman smoker aged between 40 and 50 and compare it with a woman who doesn't smoke. The face of a woman who has been smoking for years shows the effect of aging skin and the accentuation of wrinkles round the lips and eyes. Her cheeks look deeply furrowed and many superficial lines can be seen in her cheeks and jaw.

- And her skin looks drab and gray as a consequence of cellular asphyxiation caused by damage to blood circulation in the dermis.

packets of cigarettes a day than in those who do not smoke.

- Women who smoke have a greater risk of suffering from strokes and subarachnoid hemorrhage.

- Addiction to tobacco is one of the main causes of coronary diseases in women. The risk increases according to the number of cigarettes smoked and the duration of the habit.

- Women who smoke increase their risk of dying from a ruptured abdominal aortic aneurysm. They also increase the risk of suffering from hardening of the arteries.

- Addiction to tobacco is one of the main causes of chronic obstructive lung diseases in women, the risk increasing according to the intensity and duration of the habit. In the United States, about 90 percent of deaths in women from these diseases can be attributed to using tobacco.

- Women who smoke increase the risk of difficulties in conceiving and primary and secondary infertility, and can suffer a slight increase in the risk of ectopic pregnancies and miscarriages. They experience the natural menopause at an earlier age than nonsmokers and, possibly, more menopausal symptoms.

- Postmenopausal women who smoke suffer osteoporosis (reduced bone-density) more often than nonsmoking women, as well as a greater risk of hip fractures.

- Exposure to tobacco smoke in the atmosphere, especially in an enclosed space, is believed to constitute one of the causes of lung cancer in women who have never smoked and is also associated with the increased risk of suffering coronary diseases.

The effects of tobacco in pregnancy

- Women who smoke more than 20 cigarettes a day reduce their fertility by 20 to 30 percent, and smokers have a 1.6 times greater risk of giving birth prematurely than nonsmokers.

- Women who smoke during pregnancy have babies with lower birth weights and a higher miscarriage rate compared with women who have never smoked.

- The prenatal mortality rate rises to 31.8 per 1,000 if the woman smokes a packet of cigarettes a day during pregnancy, whereas in nonsmokers the rate is 23.5 per 1,000.

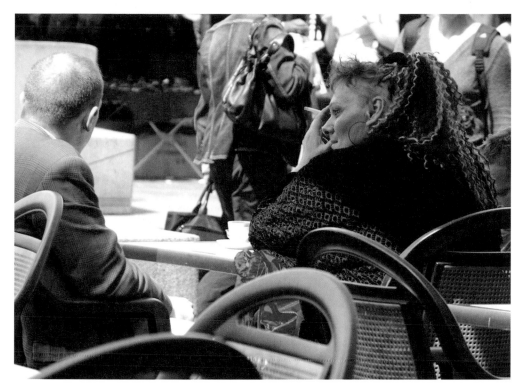

Tobacco addiction affects the bones due to its weakening effects, and reduced bone mass, leading to osteoporosis from antiestrogenic action, blood vessel dysfunction, and the inhibition of bone mass formation. The pernicious action of tobacco on the female skeleton is now becoming clear as, because of its antiestrogenic action, it aggravates the loss of bone mass after menopause.

• Tobacco use during pregnancy and tobacco smoke in the atmosphere after birth is believed to be a contributory factor to the sudden inexplicable death of a lactating infant under the age of 1 year.

• Sudden infant death syndrome is the sudden and unexpected death of an apparently healthy lactating infant. It represents the greatest cause of death in lactating infants under the age of one year, excluding the neonatal period, and is believed to be aggravated by the mother's addiction to tobacco.

There are many methods of giving up smoking and many ways of finding help. Family, friends, and co-workers can support or encourage the smoker, but the desire and commitment to give it up must be a personal decision.

Most women who have managed to stop smoking have made at least one unsuccessful attempt in the past. That is why it is recommended not to

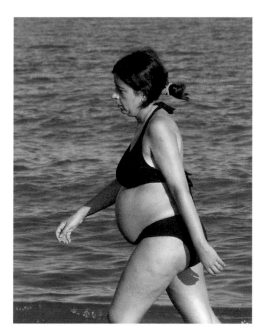

▪ The effects of tobacco on the mouth

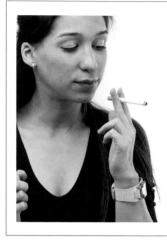

- Tobacco seriously affects the integrity of the mouth and the look of the face because of the injuries it can cause in visible areas.
- Stains on the teeth, bad breath, and a reduced sense of taste and smell appear in all cases and reduce the woman's self-esteem.
- Gum or periodontal disease or cancer of the lip and mouth can also occur.
- In themselves, oral diseases and complaints affect women's health and well-being throughout her life.
- Many of these conditions and their treatment can undermine the self-image and self-esteem, make normal social interaction more difficult and lead to chronic depression and stress, as well as costing a great deal of money.

view past attempts as failures but rather as learning experiences.

To stop smoking, a smoker has to pass through a series of temporary processes concerning her attitude to the habit, and those processes must be gone through in order to make the decision to stop.

Advice to women who feel ready to give up tobacco

- Write out a specific list of the reasons why you want to stop smoking, including the short and long-term benefits.
- Seek the assistance of a doctor who, if necessary, will advise you on nicotine patches and other methods to help you to conquer this addiction.
- Seek the support of family members, friends, and co-workers.
- Fix a date for stopping smoking.
- Get rid of all your cigarettes by that date—throw them away if necessary.
- Get it into your head that you're giving up smoking once and for all.

- Get exercise, as it will help alleviate the urgent desire to smoke.
- Learn self-hypnosis with a qualified doctor. Many find it helpful.
- Make plans for what you will do, instead of smoking, when you are stressed or at other times when you feel an urgent need for tobacco. Be as specific as possible.
- Avoid scenarios and situations where people smoke a lot and where you might feel more impelled to smoke.
- Like any other addiction, giving up tobacco is difficult, especially if you are acting alone. If the smoker joins programs designed for giving up smoking her likelihood of success will be greater.

Skin, hair and nails (I)

Much of the skin's appearance is the direct result of the amount of care it receives. This includes especially avoiding unprotected exposure to the sun, air conditioning, tobacco, environmental pollution or an inadequate lifestyle (poor nutrition, a sedentary life, emotional stress, etc.). Conversely, a balanced diet and lifestyle will go a long way to making skin look healthy. As well as water, the diet should include vitamins (such as A, B, C, and E) and minerals such as selenium, zinc and iron.

Skin, hair and nails

The skin

The skin is a surface organ that covers and protects the external surface of the body. Its total area is 5¼ to 6½ square feet (1.6–2 m²), it is 0.05 to 0.15 inches (1.5–4 mm) thick, and weighs about 11 lb (5 kg). It is a tissue with enormous vitality that acts as a barrier between the outside world and the organism and which needs more care than is sometimes realized. However, it is usually subjected to attacks that can damage it, make it sick, and age it prematurely.

The skin constantly renews itself at the rate of about 28 days. It is calculated that a person produces some 220 lb (100 kg) of epidermal cells throughout his or her life. This permanent renewal requires a constant supply of nutrients, as they are essential to the skin and their deficiency in the diet hinders its growth and damages its appearance. Therefore, a diet that provides the correct amount of all the necessary nutrients helps keep the skin in perfect health, prevents or considerably reduces lines, and maintains its freshness.

Hydration, which is so necessary for the skin, is achieved with the water in the food people eat and the water they drink. More than 90 percent of most green leaf vegetables and fruit is water, so it is worth including these in the diet, because much of the water needed is absorbed almost without

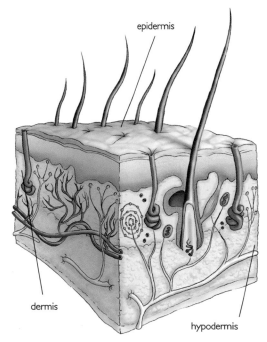

epidermis

dermis

hypodermis

The skin fulfills many functions. Above all, it is a barrier against the outside world and defends the body against environmental attack from heat and chemicals, radiation, and microorganisms. It forms an impermeable cover, reduces the impact of blows, regulates the body's temperature, enables us to feel numerous sensations, and plays an essential part in psychosocial communication, emotions, and pleasure. The appearance of the skin, especially the skin of the face, is a fundamental factor in assessing a person's age, emotional state, and character, but internal illnesses also manifest themselves in the skin.

▪ Fruit and green-leaf vegetables

What do they provide and where are they found?

• Provitamin A or beta carotene: It changes into vitamin A in the body as and when it is needed and is also an antioxidant. Green leaf, orange and yellowish vegetables contain large amounts of it (carrots, gourds, etc.) as well as certain fruits (apricots, cherries, melons, peaches, nectarines, etc.).

• Vitamin A: This is found only in foods of animal origin such as liver, dairy fats (cream and butter), egg yolk and full-fat dairy products. It plays an essential part in renewing the skin and mucous membranes.

• Lycopene: This is an antioxidant pigment that gives tomatoes their characteristic color and is also present in the flesh of apples, apricots, water melons, papayas, and pink grapefruit.

• Vitamin C: A powerful antioxidant related to the production of collagen, the protein that keeps the skin clear and wrinkle-free. The best way of ingesting this vitamin is from fresh fruit and green-leaf vegetables, in salads, for example. Pimentos, kiwi and citrus fruit, melons, strawberries, blackberries, tropical fruit, cabbages, and tomatoes contain large amounts of it.

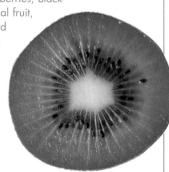

being noticed. It should be remembered that a person should drink about 2 quarts (2 liters) of water and other liquids to make up for losses and maintain the right level of hydration. Thus the skin will be kept perfectly hydrated and harmful toxins will be eliminated more easily.

What food does the skin need?

Fats

Fats supply nutrients that are essential to maintain a smooth, well-structured skin.

Where can they be found?

• *Monounsaturated fatty acids:* In olive oil and avocados.

• *Polyunsaturated fatty acids:* In seed oils, dried fruit, and fish (mainly oily fish).

Vitamin E: In vegetable oils and dried fruit, wheat germ, evening primrose oil, wholegrain wheat or cereals, and the leaves of some green vegetables. Vitamin E, an antioxidizing agent, neutralizes the harmful action of free radicals, which increase in summer due to the rays of the sun and are one of the causes of what are known as age spots.

Minerals

Which are the most important minerals?

• *Selenium:* An antioxidant mineral linked to a lower risk of the appearance of tumors, including skin tumors or melanoma. It is found in meat, fish, shellfish, cereals, eggs, fruit, and green-leaf vegetables.

• *Zinc:* It forms part of the epidermis and is present in meat, fish, eggs, whole-grain cereal, and pulses.

Green-leaf vegetables and foods of animal origin

These contain vitamins, minerals and proteins, among other nutrients, that are necessary to keep the skin healthy.

Group B vitamins: These play a part in the good condition of the skin and in cell-renewal. They are included in most foods of vegetable origin: greens, fresh fruit, dried fruit, cereals, pulses, beer yeast, and in foods of animal origin: meat and organ meats, fish and shellfish, eggs, dairy products.

Where can they be found?

- **Folic acid or vitamin B9:** This is related to cell renewal and is found mostly in green-leaf vegetables, green beans and peas, many fruits, enriched breakfast cereals, liver, and beer yeast.

- **Vitamin B2 or riboflavin:** This counteracts seborrhea. It is found in milk and its derivatives (yogurt, cheese, etc.), eggs, meat, fish, liver, pulses, and dried fruit (almonds, hazelnuts, etc.).

- **Vitamin B3 or niacin:** It participates in the synthesis of keratin. It is found in meat, fish, organ meats, whole-grain cereals, and dried fruit (peaches, apricots, figs, dates, etc.).

- **Vitamin B5 or pantothenic acid:** It plays an important part in the health of the skin. It is widely distributed in nature and a deficiency of it is very rare.

- **Vitamin B6 or pyridoxine:** It is linked to the correct metabolism of zinc, a mineral that forms part of the skin. It is abundant in oily fish, meat, eggs, dried fruit, whole-grain cereals, bananas, spinach, beer yeast, and wheat germ.

- *Iron:* An iron deficiency is the usual cause of pale skin resulting from a shortage of circulating hemoglobin (which transports oxygen and carbondioxide in the blood). It is found in organ meats, meat, fish, eggs, beer yeast, dried fruit, breakfast cereals, pulses, and green-leaf vegetables. In eggs and foods of vegetable origin it is found in its nonhemochemical form which is less easily absorbed by the body, although foods rich in vitamin C increase its absorption rate.

Proteins

These are the basic constituents of the skin. Where are they found?

Ingesting meat, fish, eggs and their derivatives, dairy products, legumes, cereals, and dried fruits according to the criteria for a balanced diet, is fundamental in maintaining healthy skin.

The number of individual hairs a person has is genetically determined. It is normal to have between 80,000 and 120,000 hairs, but fair-haired people have more and red-haired people fewer. Women usually have more hairs than men.

Hair grows at the rate of about ¹/₂ inch (12 mm) a month. It grows faster in summer and during sleep. If the hair is never cut it would grow to about 42 inches (107 cm) and then fall out. The average life of a hair is 7 years.

Between 50 and 100 hairs fall out every day. They are usually replaced by new ones, so the loss is not noticed.

Hair becomes dryer and more fragile with age. It changes color too, as the production of melanin diminishes and finally stops. As a result, the hair loses color and usually becomes gray or white.

It should be possible to stretch a healthy hair to 30 percent of its normal length before it breaks. It should also be capable of absorbing its own weight in water. A human hair is stronger than a copper wire of the same thickness.

◾ Skin care advice

- Always use soaps that do not alter the pH balance of the skin and do not remove oil. Don't use too much soap. Sometimes take a shower without soap—people use too much of it. Let the water flow over your body and then apply body oil while you are still wet. The water should not be hotter than 98–100°F (37–38°C).

- If you use degreasing agents, solvents, alcohol, or similar products at work, protect yourself with proper gloves or specific skin products. However dirty you may be, never use abrasives to wash yourself.

- Good hydration is essential—drink 3½ pints (2 liters) a day. Do moderately vigorous physical exercise to improve the blood and lymph circulation in the skin and make it look healthier, fresher, and smoother.

- Diet is important too. The vitamins and minerals in fruit and green-leaf and root vegetables help the skin maintain its youthful appearance. Vitamin A repairs the collagen and reduces wrinkles. Vitamin C seems to make the skin more elastic and flexible and also reduces wrinkles, and a derivative of vitamin A, retinoic acid, reduces abnormal pigmentation.

- If your life is stressful, practice relaxation. Stress causes constriction of the capillaries and reduces skin hydration.

- The repairing activity of sleep is crucial for the skin at night. The benefits of good rest are reflected in the skin.

- Wear cotton clothing if possible. Be careful about exposure to the sun. As well as increasing the risk of skin cancer, sunlight accelerates skin aging.

◾ The nails

Nail care requires a balanced diet and frequent cleaning, but there are certain products such as soap, detergents, and metal nail-files that damage them and make them more fragile and inclined to break. The foods that strengthen and improve the appearance of the nails are those with a high vitamin content—especially vitamin A and the group B vitamins, mineral salts—calcium, iodine, zinc—and proteins.
It is recommended to eat dairy products and seeds—sesame seeds for instance.

To achieve healthy nails and prevent breaking, certain points should be observed.

- Don't bite them.
- Protect the nails from soap and detergents.
- Cold water is better than hot for washing the hands.
- It is best to cut your nails after a bath.
- Filing the nails is better than cutting them.
- Using too much nail varnish (especially quick-drying varnish) dries the nails and makes them more fragile. Nail varnish remover (based on acetone) dries out the root of the nail.

Hair and nails

- The hair is one of the most visible and variable parts of the physical appearance, as well as having its own language of communication. Its condition affects not only the appearance but also the state of mind. The nails are also an important visiting card. Every detail counts.

- Hair loss and fragile hair are the problems that concern women most regarding their hair. The main causes of hair loss are usually reversible in women. Hormonal imbalance, using the wrong contraceptive, giving birth, the menopause, stress, and depression are the commonest causes. The solution in most cases is to take a complex of vitamins, amino acids, and trace minerals which help to renew the keratin in the hair, but it is best to visit a specialist to ascertain what treatment should be followed.

The hair is divided into three layers

Cuticle: The outermost layer, formed of flattened squamous cells. Its function is to provide a barrier against outside attacks and it serves as a support and anchorage inside the follicle. The hair's shine depends on the cohesion between these cells. If they are damaged, the hair will become dull and the ends will split.

Cortex: The middle layer composed of keratinized cells and variable amounts of pigment. It is responsible for elasticity and flexibility. It also gives the hair color and hydration. Permanent hair colorants act on this layer.

Medulla: The central part of the hair, formed by rounded cornified cells containing little pigment. It constitutes the link with the follicle.

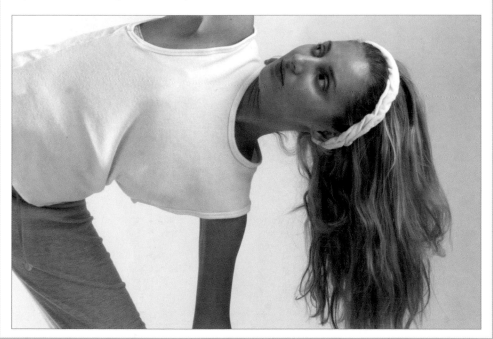

Factors that damage the hair

The principal factors that damage the hair over time are:

- **Chemicals:** Over-frequent use of temporary and permanent colorants.
- **Heat:** Hair-dryers, straighteners, and curlers.
- **Environmental factors:** Pollution, extremes of temperature, and ultraviolet rays.
- **Mechanical factors:** Setting, back combing, pulling, twisting, and ill-treating it with the hairbrush.
- **Emotional factors:** Some research has shown that people undergoing emotional stress play with their hair more—running their fingers through it, brushing and pulling it, which can cause increased mechanical damage and hence the loss of amino acids. When a person is anxious or stressed the scalp muscles contract, restricting the blood flow to the hair follicles.

All these factors contribute to the loss of amino acids and the hair has no internal structure to strengthen or regenerate itself.

The oil in the hair is its natural protector. Stress and illness, hormonal changes, and certain cosmetics or medicines can alter the activity of the sebaceous glands.

The color of the hair is determined by a pigment called *melanin*. The shape and number of melanin granules in the hair fiber determine its natural color. People with a large number of elongated granules have black hair, those with a smaller number of elongated granules have brown hair, and those with even fewer and smaller granules have blond hair. People with oval or spherical granules have red hair.

To achieve perfect nails

It is very important to care for your nails to prevent them looking unsightly. There are six fundamental steps to follow for perfect nails.

- Remove any remaining varnish with a good varnish remover. This will prevent your nails drying out.
- If your nails are very long, cut them with curved scissors. If they only need retouching, use an emery board to file them.
- The edges of the nails must be perfectly clean. To achieve this, dip your fingers in soapy water and then brush them. Another solution is to insert your fingers into a cut half-lemon.

- Surrounding bits of skin should be removed. To achieve this you can apply a moistening emulsion, massaging gently, and let it act for a few minutes, or a cuticle-removing product. Then, push the cuticles inward with a little orange stick. Don't cut them off.
- As there may still be some oily residue on your nails following the previous step, it is best to apply another layer of varnish remover, so that the nail varnish you are about to apply will adhere better.
- Apply a transparent hardening basecoat first, followed by two coats of varnish.

Skin, hair and nails (II)

Having healthy skin, hair, and nails is particularly important, not only for well-being but also because any problems with them cannot be hidden. In many cases these afflictions can cause a psychological complex suffering them, as regards both her self-esteem and the attitude of others.

Some skin, hair and nail complaints

An adult woman's 6½ square feet (2 square meters) ot skin not only protect her from infec tions and injuries and maintain bodily moisture and

 Acne

Acne, an eruptive skin disease, is caused by a change in the sebaceous glands in the skin of the face, neck, chest, and back. Common acne appears mainly in adolescence, but adults can also suffer from it. It is a consequence of hormonal changes that stimulate the production of sebum. Other factors are stress, some pharmaceuticals, large meals, and infections. Acne pimples do not indicate poor hygiene and can be prevented or, at least mitigated, with an adequate diet. Hygiene must be scrupulous to prevent additional infections.

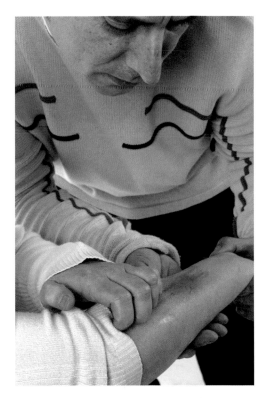

The word dermatitis describes an inflammatory response by the skin caused by contact with allergens or irritants, exposure to the sun, poor circulation or even stress. An example of atopic dermatitis is eczema, an itchy rash that causes reddening, blisters, and flaking. It should not be scratched. Scratching the rash can spread the inflammation, lead to infection, and even leave scars.

Urticaria

Urticaria is the allergic alteration of the skin characterized by the sudden or repeated appearance of skin blisters or eruptions accompanied by inflammation and itching. It is caused by a sudden allergic reaction after eating, inhaling, or injecting the specific antigen, or coming into contact with it. Many pharmaceuticals can cause it (penicillin, serums, insulin of animal origin), as well as insect stings or infections by parasites, various materials (wool, heavy metals, fur, silk), local infections (teeth, tonsils, etc.), exposure to ultraviolet rays or extreme temperatures. In many cases it is caused by emotional upsets.

temperature, but also the skin is the body's most evident way of showing various signs of illness.

The skin is likely to suffer diseases induced by both internal and external factors. Skin inflammation, or dermatitis, can occur after exposure to irritants, contact with poisons of vegetable origin or burns produced by excessive exposure to the sun's ultraviolet rays. Seborrheic dermatitis, an oily eruption on the scalp, face, and chest, and in the groin area, is due to excessive production of sebum by the sebaceous glands.

Bacterial skin complaints

The infection of the skin by certain bacteria produces rashes, and skin infections can spread all over the body (syphilis, smallpox, tuberculosis). General systemic diseases can cause skin symptoms, as in chicken pox and measles.

Other skin conditions include tumors, sebaceous cysts (wens), ulcers, pigmentations caused by congenital factors or changes in internal secretions (hormones) and melanomas (cancer).

▪ The hair

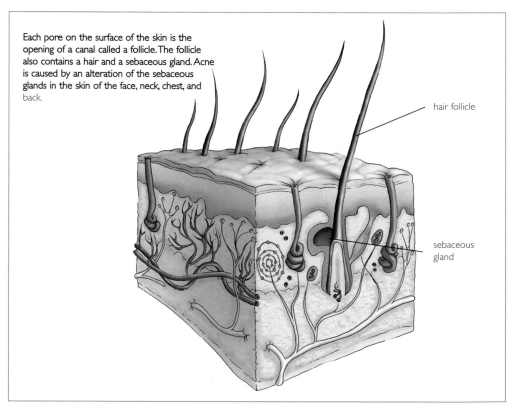

Each pore on the surface of the skin is the opening of a canal called a follicle. The follicle also contains a hair and a sebaceous gland. Acne is caused by an alteration of the sebaceous glands in the skin of the face, neck, chest, and back.

hair follicle

sebaceous gland

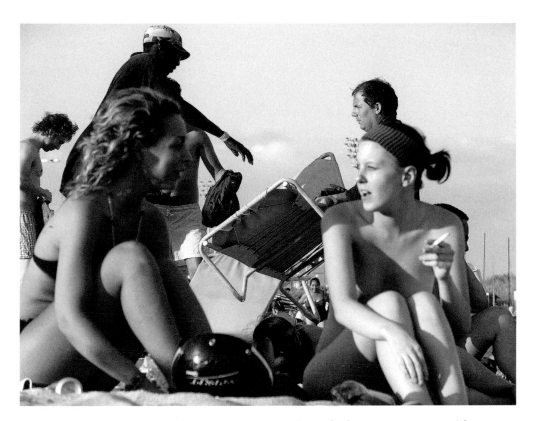

Young women with severe acne can benefit from treatment with contraceptives that contain antiandrogens. People with liver complaints should not take this type of pill.

Psoriasis, a chronic skin disease, is characterized by the appearance of inflamed scales on the surface of the skin ranging in color from red to brown. It mainly affects the elbows, knees, scalp, and chest, although it can extend all over the body.

Eczema is a noncontagious inflammatory and chronic skin disease. The word eczema is used to refer to a series of skin conditions that should really be called *dermatitis*. It is considered to be a symptom of a great variety of complaints, including local external irritations, blood changes, and allergies.

Marks on the skin

Marks on the skin are alterations in its color caused for various reasons. Many of them, such as moles or pregnancy spots, are no more than an esthetic problem. Sometimes, however, certain marks are caused by the malfunction of an organ, so their treatment, as well as being a question of personal appearance, means solving the health problem that caused them.

• **Freckles.** These are round accumulations of pigment that appear irregularly on the skin. They do not indicate any health problem. Sometimes they disappear as the person grows older. They are more abundant in fair-skinned than in brown-skinned people, and become more abundant with exposure to the sun.

• **Moles.** Their coloring ranges from brown to black and they can be flat or lumpy. Medically, a mole is called a *nevus*. They are caused by a surplus of pigmentation and the accumulation of small blood vessels. They are congenital. With age, they may disappear or grow bigger. They do not cause any physical problem, but are often an esthetic one. It is important to keep a careful eye on moles. They should not tickle, bleed or suddenly change color, size or shape. If they do, the person should consult their doctor or a dermatologist.

• **Some marks appear following excessive exposure to the sun due to an increase in melanin.** This type is very common in older people who have done a lot of sunbathing. These marks are more irregular and bigger than freckles.

• **Marks that appear during pregnancy (chloasma or melasma).** These are light brown marks. They are caused by a hormonal change during pregnancy, or as a result of taking contraceptives or hormones during menopause. They appear on certain parts of the face or cheeks and on the chest. Exposure to the sun makes them more likely to appear.

• **Blue spots on the skin.** They can appear as a consequence of a knock, but sometimes occur for no apparent reason. There could be various reasons, including medication based on anticoagulants, a kind of nutritional deficiency in which vitamins C, K or folic acid are lacking, infec-

Melasma, or pregnancy marks, are associated with high hormonal levels (estrogens and progesterone) and are most frequent in brown-skinned women (Hispano-Asian and Indo-Chinese). The marks often appear on the forehead, temples, cheeks, top lip, and nose, and can appear symmetrically (on both sides of the face). The marks are light or dark coffee colored.

Hormonal changes linked to the menstrual period and pregnancy can assist the development of acne, as can irritants in the environment, such as pollution, intense heat, humidity or cold.

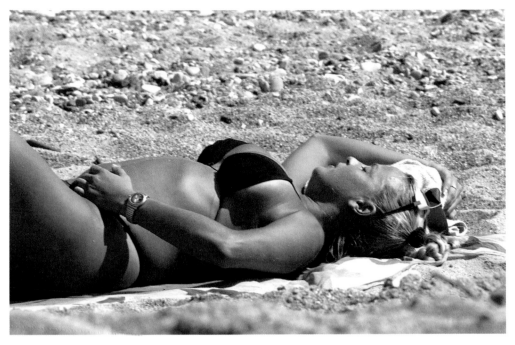

Marks can appear on the skin as a result of abnormal tanning in skins that are sensitive to sunlight (ultraviolet rays). This condition is called photosensitivity and can be caused by: contraceptive pills, cosmetics, a diet deficient in certain nutrients, heredity, antibiotics (sulfonamides, tetracyclins), nonsteroid anti-inflammatory medications, diuretics, painkillers, and some psychoactive pharmaceuticals.

tions of the blood or liver, or some types of cancer. If they appear and are not the result of a knock, it is best to consult a doctor.

• **Vitiligo.** This appears in the form of white patches, sometimes surrounded by a darker edge. They are caused by a loss of pigmentation in the skin for various reasons, including thyroid problems and autoimmune reactions by the skin itself.

• **Birthmarks.** These are reddish or brownish. People are born with them and they are of various shapes and sizes.

Depilation

People have always struggled against body hair. In Egypt, the pharaohs used stones or fire to eliminate the most unattractive looking body hair. Luckily, we have much more effective and less dangerous methods today.

Women have always wanted to eliminate their body hair as fast as it grows. In pictures of women from past centuries the face, legs, and arms are always represented free of body hair, and women used the most unexpected methods to achieve this.

Nowadays, nothing could be easier and, in many cases, the hair can take a long time to grow back again. Sometimes it grows less profusely than before, as the latest scientific discoveries used for hair removal (depilation) (using both chemicals and new laser technology) have definitely weakened or destroyed the hair, to the delight of women and, indeed men, who are increasingly using the depilatory methods available on the market.

❏ Tips for perfect hair removal

Before:
- Don't apply moisturizer before depilating with wax. The cream forms an oily film that makes the wax difficult to absorb.
- If bumps form because of ingrown hairs, rub them off in the shower using a luffa sponge (or similar) and apply cream to prevent subcutaneous hairs.

After:
- Once the hair has been removed from the armpits and groin area, a piece of cotton soaked in spirit should be applied to disinfect the area.
- Wipe an ice cube over the depilated area to prevent irritation.
- Keep out of the sun for at least 12 hours, and if you've used wax, wait a whole day, or dark marks may appear.

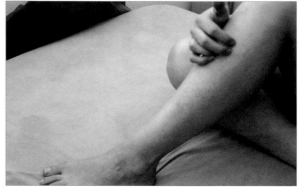

METHOD			
Cold, warm or hot wax	Eliminates hairs at the roots and is ideal for legs, groin, and armpits	May hurt a little. Don't use it for the breasts, navel or armpits.	2 to 3 weeks
Depilatory cream	Quick and easy to apply. Recommended for small areas.	May irritate the skin in very sensitive areas and cause allergies.	4 or 5 days
Depilatory foam	Quick and convenient to carry when traveling. Can be used on any area.	Hair grows again as fast as when using a razor.	4 or 5 days
Razor	The quickest and most convenient method. Ideal for armpits and legs.	Irritates sensitive skin. Doesn't hurt in delicate areas.	3 or 4 days
Lightening cream	Best for arms and tiny hairs round the navel.	Although they are lighter, the hairs can still be seen because they're still there.	1 month
Electric depilatory	Pulls the hairs out by the roots and is perfect for legs.	A slow and somewhat painful process if the person isn't used to it.	From 2 to 3 weeks
Laser hair removal (there are 3 types: diode, ruby, and Alexandrite)	Gel or anesthetic are not usually necessary, as a part of this laser is applied to the skin, chilling it. This avoids pain and possible burns. The diode method is 40% more effective than other light-depilation systems and ruby and Alexandrite lasers. Each laser shot (one per second) can destroy the hair follicles in an area 0.3 inch (9 mm), square so it is very quick.	The most expensive method. The price is fixed per session or per area to be depilated.	Permanent, but requires several sessions.

Sun and the skin

Sun damage is the principal cause of premature aging. It aggravates the appearance of brown marks and wrinkles and is also responsible for a more serious condition: skin cancer. Dermatologists stress the dangers of exposure to the sun and the serious long-term consequences it can have.

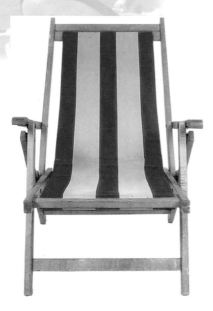

▪ Melanoma: cancer of the skin

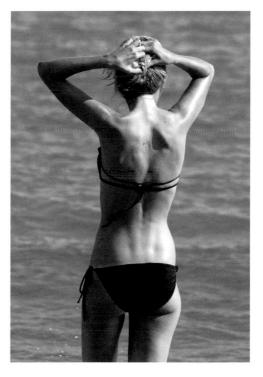

Melanoma is the most frequent skin cancer in women between the ages of 25 and 29 and the second most frequent in those between the ages of 30 and 34. Specialists affirm that, if detected in time, skin cancer is curable. Moreover, knowing what the risk factors are helps its prevention and treatment.

Although the sun affects fair skins more severely, too much sun always has to be paid for. In the end, exposure to ultraviolet rays is the most important external factor in aging of the skin due to light.

The fashion for looking tanned started in the 20th century with women's liberation and new social habits allowing both sexes to enjoy sport and the open air. This, combined with the fact that the sun ceased to be associated with the world of work, had a decisive effect. Very soon, tanned skin became synonymous with freedom, having the spare time to devote to leisure, and better health, looks, and vitality.

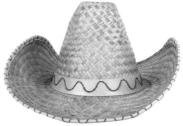

Sunlight

Sunlight is beneficial to the skin as it provides vitamin D, improves the blood circulation, protects the body against certain infections, and provides great vitality. Moreover, tanned skin looks attractive, but the price for displaying a golden tan is very high if the right recommendations are not followed.

However, there has been talk in recent years of the need to change some of these habits and of the damage caused by unlimited exposure to the sun. It has been demonstrated that the more a person is exposed to the sun the greater and quicker is premature aging in both men and women.

Specialists also warn that the sun should be taken in moderation. It should be avoided in the middle of the day—between noon and 4:00 pm—and it is best to use sun creams with a protection index to suit the skin of each individual.

The damage caused by the rays of the sun is cumulative. The amount of sun people can tolerate is limited and the time comes when they start to notice the changes in their own skin. This damage can range from abnormal reddening of the skin, speckled hyperpigmentations, loss of elasticity, dehydration, and deeper wrinkles to more harmful and dangerous effects, skin cancer, more cases of which are being diagnosed every year.

Whereas chronological aging is characterized by a soft, smooth skin with fine lines, light-aging presents thicker lines (furrows), rough, dry, leathery skin that is less elastic, with pigment changes (brown marks), broken capillaries and, in the most serious cases, precancerous skin tumors.

◾ Some advice

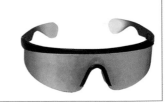

• When using a sunscreen, apply it at least half an hour before going into the sun and repeat the application every two to four hours, especially if you come into contact with water, and generally, don't use last year's creams. This is because solar protectors are very sensitive to temperature, materials that damage them often get into them, such as sand from the beach, and deteriorate fairly quickly, so it is not advisable to keep them for use next season once they have been opened.

• When sitting in the sun, always wear sunglasses with a high solar protection level to prevent eye damage. It is also advisable to wear a wide-brimmed hat, not just a peaked cap, and to use a high-factor protection cream to suit the photo-type of each person—the pharmacist will advise you—and apply it generously. It is crucial to avoid exposure to the sun between midday and 4:00 p.m.

• Children under the age of three should not be exposed to the midday sun and, whatever their age, should be protected with clothing and hats. Also, use creams with a high protection factor and make sure they drink water frequently.

• The recommended minimum protection factor is 15, but remember that protection cream should also be applied when you are in the shade, under a sunshade or on cloudy days and, even if your skin is already tanned, go on using sun-protection creams.

• The purpose of light protection products is not to enable you to spend longer in the sun but to provide adequate care during reasonable exposure and to enable you to tan without risk. These products prevent burning and help your tan to last longer.

What is your photo-type?

The photo-type refers to the capacity of each individual to withstand solar radiation. It is vital to know your photo-type so as to choose the right protection factor. It depends on the color of your skin, eyes and hair and how easily you tan.

• Red hair, light eyes, and white, sensitive skin. In these cases, the right protection will be a cream with a solar protection level of 40 to 60.

• Blond hair, light eyes, and sensitive skin that usually burns and hardly tans at all. The ideal protection will be a solar factor of at least 20.

• Brown hair, brown eyes, and light skin that goes red at first and then tans. It is recommended to use factor 20 solar protection at first, and factor 15 later.

• Dark skins that tan quickly and seldom burn nevertheless need to be protected with a factor 15 cream, that is to say the minimum recommended.

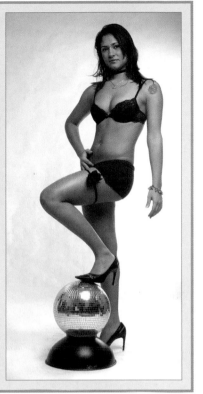

Dermatologists have noted the ever-increasing number of cases of skin tumors in which it has been demonstrated for certain that sunlight is the leading cause of the appearance of these cancerous lesions.

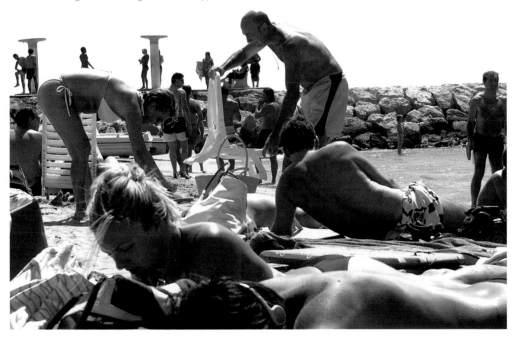

Changing the skin: tattoos and body piercing

Women have always been keen on personal adornment. Alongside progress as regards hair removal, the fashion for tattooing and body piercing has gained ground in the last decade, although it has a greater following among young women and adolescents.

Tattooing and piercing

It has become fashionable to decorate the body with elaborate and attractive designs. What is known as *body art*, has become a lifestyle and, for thousands of young people all over the world, a way of differentiating themselves. However, at the same time, tattooing constitutes an attack on the body and therefore the equipment and materials used must be hygienic to avoid infections trans-

mitted through the blood, such as the AIDS virus or hepatitis C. Before visiting a professional who applies these artistic techniques, it is best to be aware of some standards and the problems that can result from having tattooed skin.

Think hard before deciding to have a tattoo or a piercing because it is likely to last all your life. The design of the tattoo, its size, and the place where it is applied are of fundamental importance, and the same applies to a piercing. Basically, any part of the

From a medical point of view, there are three important points you should consider when having your skin tattooed: the risk that diseases may be transmitted, the possibility of allergies to certain tattoo ingredients, and the need to ascertain how the tattoo will be removed if one day you regret it.

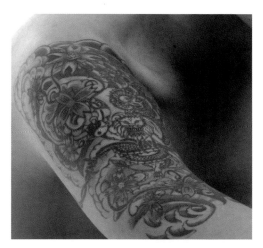

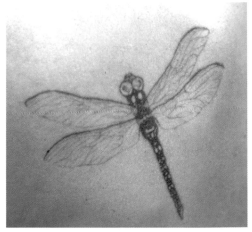

body can be tattooed or pierced, but remember that the pain you will have to endure depends to a large extent on the area you choose. Each individual's capacity for suffering will also influence the decision.

Before the tattooing session
• Make sure that the tattooing center is reliable and complies with all hygiene standards.
• Don't drink alcohol for at least 24 hours before the session.
• A pigment allergy test is necessary at least 24 hours beforehand.

During the tattooing session
• It is best, though not absolutely necessary, to have eaten something. An empty stomach can make you feel sick.
• If necessary, have the hair removed from the area to be tattooed by a specialist.
• The most important thing is to feel rested, and above all relaxed, when you attend the session. If the muscles are tense the pain will be greater. Stress can change the color of the tattoo and make its application more painful.

After the tattooing session
• The tattoo needs to be bathed three times a day for at least a week. Clean the area with damp towels.
• Apply antibiotic cream using a small spatula.
• Cover the tattooed area with a clean gauze held down with a plastic band-aid, as these cause the least irritation.
• Don't expose yourself to the sun or ultraviolet light for two months after the tattooing session.
• You can shower, but don't rub the area.
• A week later, apply moisturizing cream or body oil to the tattooed area to prevent it drying out or peeling.

People who must not tattoo themselves
• Hemophiliacs, because of their coagulation problems.
• People with a pacemaker. Due to the magnetic field the machine produces, tattooing could affect its operation.
• Epileptics.
• In temporary situations, people with herpes or fungal infections in the part to be tattooed.

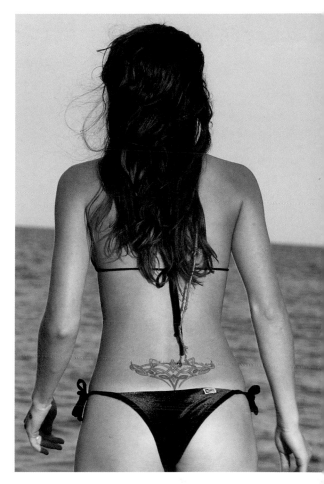

The risks of body piercing
• **Ear (lobe):** If the earrings are too tight they can cause keloids, recurring thick pink scars. They are also exposed to all kinds of infections.
• **Ear (cartilage):** As with all piercing, there is a risk of infection that increases if the perforation has been made with a piercing gun. This type of piercing is not recommended in summer, because it is the season of swimming pools and beaches, and the area will be wet much of the time, with the consequent risk of infection. As the cartilage of the ear is harder than the rest of it, it is a complicated area and, although certain intravenous antibiotics are used as a support, these perforations can ultimately deform the tissue.
• **Eyebrows:** Professionals recommend lateral piercing for this area rather than central piercing, as it is close to nerves and the supraorbital artery, and can also affect the behavior of the lachrymal gland.

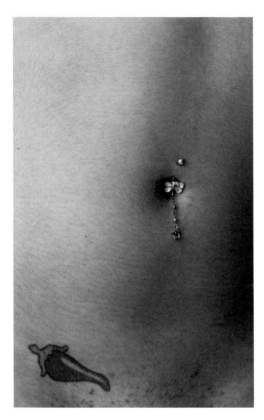

Before deciding to have a tattoo, always remember to take some precautionary measures. Otherwise, you run a serious risk.

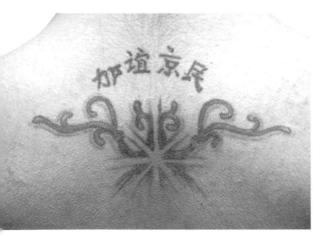

• **Lips:** If incorrectly positioned, this piercing can become infected, which can be very painful and cause dental irritation.

• **Navel:** If this part of the body is pierced, the risk of infection is caused by poor healing due to area being in permanent contact with clothing. Professionals recommend not having this piercing if the navel is prominent.

• **Nipple:** This area is very sensitive, so the risk of infection is high. It is also advisable not to wear the piercing ring or other adornment (in the case of an old piercing) if you are pregnant.

• **Tongue:** Because this part of the body is permanently wet it is slow to heal and piercing it can also cause irreversible damage to the artery and nerve underneath it. One of the secondary effects is swelling and engorgement of the tongue.

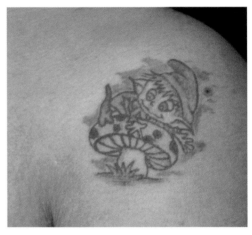

• **Female genitals:** This piercing can be rejected as a result of rubbing against underwear and can also cause reduced sensitivity in the area.

• **Nasal septum:** Although nose piercing was one of the original spots for piercing, that does not mean it is risk-free. It can seriously harm the cartilage.

• **Nose:** There is a high risk of infection.

Physical exercise and sport

Regular physical activity, combined with good dietary habits, can improve women's health and help prevent many of the diseases that constitute the main causes of death and disability that affect them worldwide.

The benefits of physical exercise

Specialists affirm that over 70 percent of the problems a woman suffers and feels throughout her life are directly or indirectly linked to being sedentary or not getting physical exercise. The accumulation of adipose tissue (fat) and fragile bones are among the problems that can be most effectively counteracted or prevented through a

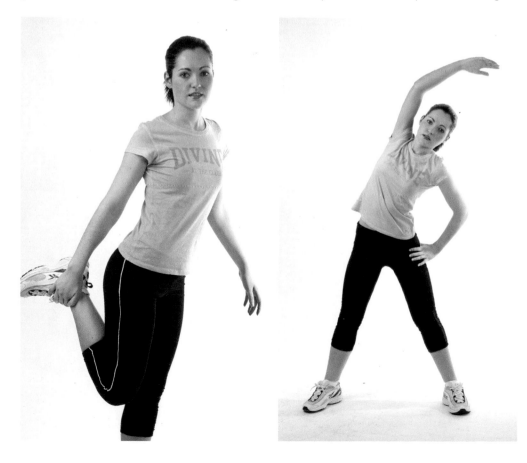

It has been amply proved that exercise helps prevent cardiovascular diseases. These diseases, which include heart disease, high blood pressure, and strokes, account for a third of female mortality throughout the world.

Cardiovascular diseases are responsible for 50% of deaths of women aged over 50 in developing countries.

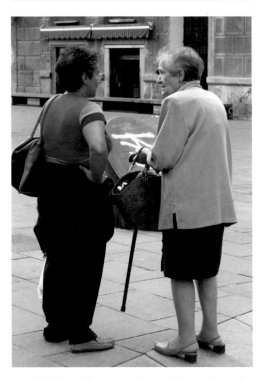

Physical activity can also enormously contribute to preventing and controlling osteoporosis. This is a disease in which the bones become weak and more likely to break. Women, especially after the menopause, run a greater risk of suffering from osteoporosis than men. This is due to a deficit in the production of the sex hormones which were essential to women for procreation and which they are no longer producing, but which also play a part in countless other female organic processes.

Weight-bearing activities, such as walking, dancing, and running, are essential for normal bone development in infancy and adolescence, and can help reduce bone loss. They also improve muscular strength and balance and reduce the risk of falling, thus helping to prevent fractures.

Arthritis is an important cause of reduced activity in adults and old people. Physical activity helps to control the inflammation and joint pain caused by arthritis, thus reducing its consequences and improving daily well-being in old age.

But exercise not only demonstrates its benefits at the bodily and organic level, it can also improve a woman's whole quality of life physically, psychically, and spiritually. Regular physical activity helps to relieve stress, anxiety, depression and the feeling of loneliness, which is particularly important for women, as their depression rate is twice that of

combination of good eating habits and regular physical exercise.

Diabetes affects more than 70 million women throughout the world. According to statistics, this figure will double by the year 2025. Diabetes, together with cardiovascular diseases, can lead to blindness, damage to the nervous system, kidney deficiency, ulcers, and amputation of the feet. According to a recent study, even moderate physical activity and some minor dietary changes can prevent more than half the cases of insulin-dependent diabetes.

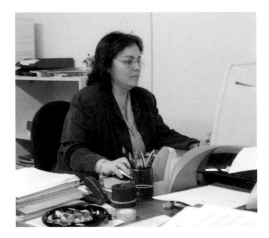

Physical exercise improves a woman's quality of life, as it offers emotional benefits, reducing stress, anxiety, and depression and helps improve self-esteem.

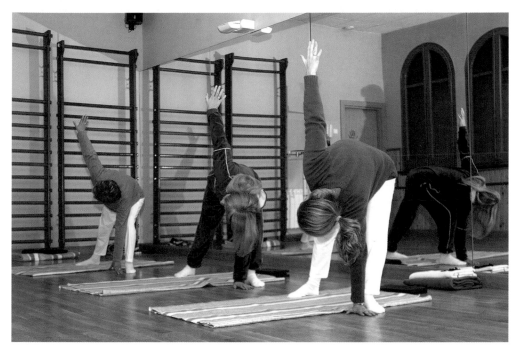

Increased physical activity can help to make people live longer, and improve their health. Exercise helps prevent heart disease and many other problems. What is more, exercise increases strength and energy and can help reduce tension. It is also a good way of limiting the appetite and burning calories.

▪▪ Sport and menstruation

Menstrual troubles are more frequent in women who practice sport intensively. This is because extreme exercise and a strict diet alter hormone production, which can delay the onset of the first period or make menstruation stop. Doctors believe that this factor is influenced by stress and the reduced percentage of fatty tissue in the body, because fatty tissue is necessary for the metabolism of female hormones. Consequently, the ovaries do not produce the estrogens necessary to enable the lining of the uterus (womb) to develop and menstruation to occur. But in any case, physical exercise produces beneficial effects before and during menstruation, as it stimulates the production of endorphins, the hormones responsible for inducing well-being and reducing unhappiness and, therefore, the symptoms of the premenstrual syndrome and period pains are themselves reduced.

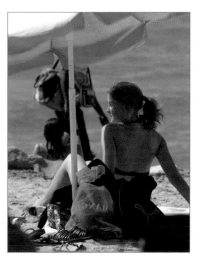

It may not be comfortable to exercise while menstruating because of abdominal pain and blood loss. Nevertheless, in spite of those symptoms, it is not inadvisable, but it is recommended only that the exercise should not be too strenuous (for example, walking, jogging, or cycling) and should be taken only when the effort does not cause additional troubles.

men in both developed and developing countries. Physical activity also helps develop self-esteem and confidence and promotes psychological well-being and social relations.

Increased physical activity can benefit almost all women. Most can start gradual and moderate exercise on their own. If a woman thinks she cannot exercise safely for any reason, she should consult a doctor before starting a program of activities. In particular, the doctor will check whether she has any problems with her heart, high blood pressure, and arthritis, and whether she feels nauseous, has chest pain or any other health problem before she embarks on it.

Physical exercise during pregnancy

Physical exercise improves the cardiovascular and muscular condition, encourages good posture and prevents excessive weight gain, improving the pregnant woman's general physical condition and enabling her to confront pregnancy and birth with fewer risks.

• Above all, a pregnant woman should not start or continue a physical training program before her obstetrician has examined her.

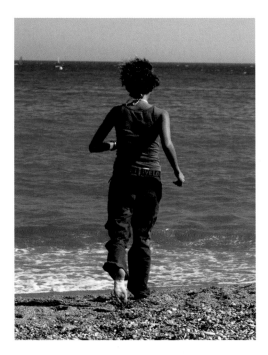

• Once she has been examined and if there are no obstetric or medical contraindications, she can do regular exercise during her pregnancy.

• Ideally, every pregnant woman should follow a personalized exercise program.

• This exercise should take account of the month of gestation, her physical condition at the time, and her experience, if any, of previous pregnancies.

Exercising or participating in an aerobic sport is very beneficial throughout pregnancy and after giving birth. There are many reasons why physical activity is especially recommendable during pregnancy.

• It prevents and reduces pregnancy problems. Physical activity is very beneficial because it helps prevent or reduce the appearance of stretch marks and varicose veins, prevents or alleviates constipation and hypertension, and reduces much of the pain felt in pregnancy, such as back pain.

• It prevents excessive weight gain. Gymnastics during pregnancy help burn up the calories the baby does not need.

• It increases self-esteem. Exercises improve the circulation and muscle tone, give greater flexibility and stamina and enable the woman to regain her figure more quickly after the baby is born. This enables her to feel more confident in herself.

• It prepares the woman for giving birth, which requires a great deal of energy and if the woman is fit she will be able to withstand it better. It will also enable her to recover much more quickly following the birth.

• It reduces stress and tension. In many cases, all the preoccupations, anxieties and changes of mood that pregnancy brings are responsible for the stress and tension a pregnant women suffers. These problems are harmful both to her and to the baby, as they cause muscular contractions, headaches, and backache. Physical activity is also very useful in these cases as it helps her to feel better.

• Another benefit of physical exercise is that it is tiring, enabling her to sleep better. As her preg-

Pregnancy is not an illness. It is a physiological state in which the typical recommendations for a healthy life can be followed perfectly. Physical activity is one of them.

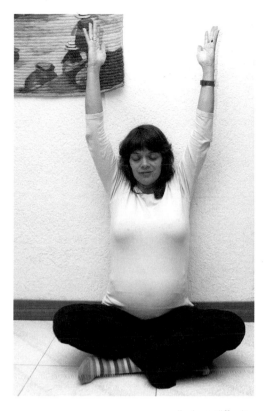

extra 300 kilocalories a day) and the calories needed for exercise have to be added to that figure. Thirst is not a good indicator of the degree of dehydration and a pregnant woman should drink before, during, and after the exercise session. Appetite and hunger can also be affected by the hormones of pregnancy and strict attention should be paid to nutrition with an adequate supply of minerals, especially iron, calcium, and vitamin supplements.

• Special attention should be paid to the practice of physical exercise according to the pregnant woman's symptoms, as less oxygen is available during pregnancy. If she feels tired she should stop once and for all, and avoid exhaustion (because of the risk of bradycardia or reduction in the fetal heart rate).

The benefits of sport

• It increases stamina, which declines considerably during pregnancy.
• It improves the circulation, enabling more oxygen to reach the baby's head.
• It stabilizes the blood pressure.
• It prevents osteoporosis.
• It exercises the birth muscles.
• It provides greater flexibility
• It produces physical and mental well-being.

Recommendations to pregnant women practicing sport

• Do exercises that increase stamina and coordination as these decline during pregnancy.
• Focus on strengthening the back and abdominal muscles as these are often highly sensitive and pregnant women can suffer back pain.
• It is much better to do your exercises gently and regularly (about three times a week) than to exercise intensely at longer intervals.

nancy progresses, a woman usually has difficulty sleeping because she feels uncomfortable and it is not easy to find a comfortable sleeping position. Physical exercise enables her to feel tired enough to fall into bed and sleep right through the night.

The ideal thing during pregnancy is for the woman to carry out the physical activities recommended to improve vitality and the sense of well-being. The most important thing is not to demand too much of the body, as excessive activity can cause uterine contractions and complicate the progress of the pregnancy. At the same time, it is important to follow a balanced diet during pregnancy, eating healthy food that will make the woman feel even better.

Health and diet recommendations before undertaking physical exercise

• Wear suitable and comfortable sports clothes.
• Do your exercises on suitable, nonslippery surfaces (surfaces that reduce impact on the feet: wooden floors, carpets, exercise mats, etc.).
• Drink plenty of liquids and eat adequately. More calories are required during pregnancy (an

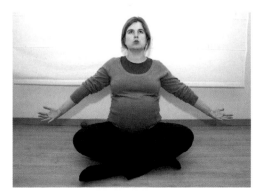

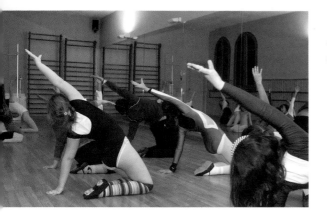

Contraindications concerning physical activity during pregnancy:

- High blood pressure induced by pregnancy.
- Premature breaking of the membranes.
- Premature birth pains.
- Inadequacy of the cervix or a history of miscarriages.
- Bleeding.
- Placenta previa.
- Delayed intrauterine growth.

Advice for pregnant women

If the woman is already used to doing gymnastics, she can continue provided her program does not include physical activities not recommended during pregnancy.

If the woman did not regularly get physical exercise before becoming pregnant, she should wait until the first three months of pregnancy are over before starting it, because during the first three months, typical symptoms such as drowsiness, digestive changes, nausea, tiredness, breast pain, and others, do not encourage her to find the energy needed for physical activity.

- Wear a special pregnancy bra to protect your breasts.
- Check your heart rate and don't let it exceed 140 beats a minute.
- Set yourself some limits if you are not used to practicing sport.
- Make sure that your exercises do not involve any risk of falling, fractures or bruising. Avoid sudden movements.
- There should be a warmup session before your sporting activity and a relaxation session after it.
- If any sign of weakness, raised heartbeat, breathlessness, giddiness, pain in the back, neck, or pubis, or any other anomaly occurs, stop the physical activity at once.

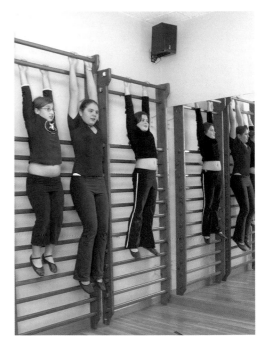

The importance of intimate hygiene in women

Bathing in public swimming-pools, keeping a wet bathing-suit on, sweat, menstruation, wearing tight underwear and poor ventilation of the genital area are some of the factors that can cause vaginal infection, a complaint that is easy to detect and treat, but is even easier to prevent with proper intimate hygiene.

It is generally accepted and well known that hygiene is necessary for health. Hygiene involves not only what a person eats and drinks but also the body itself and its most sensitive areas. And one of those sensitive areas in women is the genital area, which needs special attention and care to keep it constantly clean and dry, thus avoiding infections that could degenerate into more serious conditions and even, in the worst cases, lead to cancer. Hence the vital importance of proper intimate hygiene.

The vagina has an automatic self-purifying system—it cleans itself—which works by releasing a certain quantity of whitish fluid every day that cleans the vaginal walls. The acidity level of this fluid keeps the vaginal flora in balance and combats harmful bacteria, helping to prevent infections. This is why gynecologists advise against using products

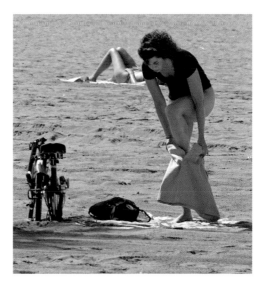

Vaginal hygiene

Although the vagina is self-cleaning, it is still necessary to maintain proper external hygiene, especially because, as the organ is almost constantly in contact with various liquids (urine, menstrual blood and/or sweat) and as the area receives little ventilation, the moisture generated by these secretions does not completely evaporate, making the vagina more vulnerable to attack by microorganisms. The genital area therefore requires washing—with just water, or water and a neutral soap.

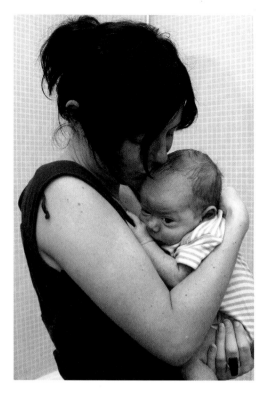

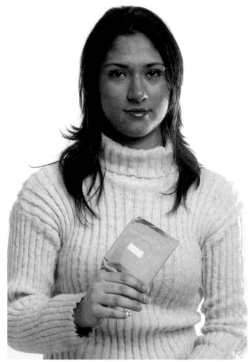

After giving birth, it is advisable to wash the whole genital area externally after urinating or defecating, especially if an episiotomy has been performed, as the stitches can become infected. If the woman is breastfeeding, the care and hygiene of her nipples should be meticulous. They should be cleaned with distilled water before and after each feed and protected from cold and knocks.

During menstruation, inadequate hygiene can give rise to most unpleasant odors. Many women nowadays use tampons, which, as they prevent the menstrual flow from emerging, avoid many unpleasant and embarrassing situations. But in spite of their convenience, women should use tampons correctly. The same tampon should not be left in the vagina for several hours.

marketed as vaginal douches for washing the vagina, as they neither prevent nor treat any infectious process. Moreover, the use of these chemical products can remove the vagina's natural flora or change its pH balance, giving rise to problems.

Basically, there are two risk factors that can give rise to vaginal infections: sexually transmitted infections and those caused by a process that encourages the proliferation of bacteria in the body.

Sexually transmitted infections can occur at any age and for various reasons. The most frequent of these infections is vaginitis—inflammation of the walls of the vagina—usually caused by bacteria from the anal area. This type of infection is very frequent in little girls who have just learned to use the toilet or in old women who cannot manage adequate intimate hygiene. But it is also normal in

women who, after urinating or defecating, clean their genital area by wiping the toilet paper from back to front, that is to say from the anal area toward the vulva. Thus, they move traces of excrement toward the vaginal area, and the repetition of this practice can encourage infection.

Another cause may be the excessive proliferation of fungi in the vaginal flora, the most frequent being *Candida albicans*. This is a fungus found naturally in the vagina and even in the skin. However,

Hygiene and healthy practices

The genitals are just one more part of a woman's body and, like any other, can easily be kept clean with a daily shower. As the genital area is delicate, it is always advisable to pay special, but not excessive, attention to cleaning it. It is perfectly normal and natural for the genital area to produce a certain odor specific to each person, which becomes an olfactory stimulus favoring the initiation of sexual relations.

In addition to washing with water and neutral soap, complete intimate hygiene should include the following care:

- After urinating or defecating, the genital area should be cleaned from front to back to avoid contaminating the vaginal area with fecal bacteria. Most people use only paper, but it is advisable to wash too because otherwise the area will remain dirty.

- Neither strong soaps nor any chemical product that could alter the vagina's pH balance should be used. It is not wise to apply intimate deodorants either, because they can cause irritation, inflammation, and even an allergy. What is more, they hinder the perception of any odors indicating conditions that could require medical treatment.

- Vaginal douches should not be used because they eliminate natural substances and microorganisms that protect the vagina.

- Cotton underwear is recommended, as nylon and other synthetic fibers impede perspiration, retain humidity and encourage the proliferation of germs.

- Very tight clothing should not be worn, to avoid scratching and encourage perspiration in the genital area.

- A sponge or synthetic gloves should not be used to wash the genital area, as germs accumulate in them.

- Tampons and sanitary pads should be changed at least every 4 or 6 hours. It is not advisable to use protective inserts every day because they impede adequate ventilation, increase the temperature of the area, cause the proliferation of germs, and facilitate the occurrence of complaints and infections.

- Before and after having sexual relations, it is advisable to wash the genital area, as well as the hands and mouth if you practice oral sex.

- Control the amount of medication you take. Antibiotics, for example, usually reduce the body's defense mechanism after curing the complaint for which they were prescribed. The result is that, after completing treatment with antibiotics, a woman is much more likely to contract vaginal infections.

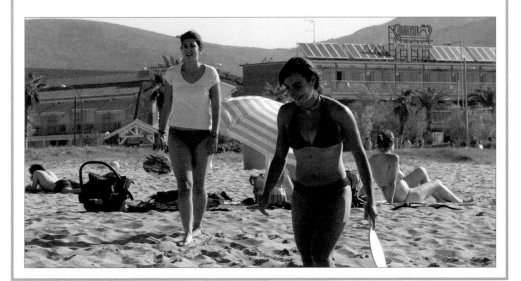

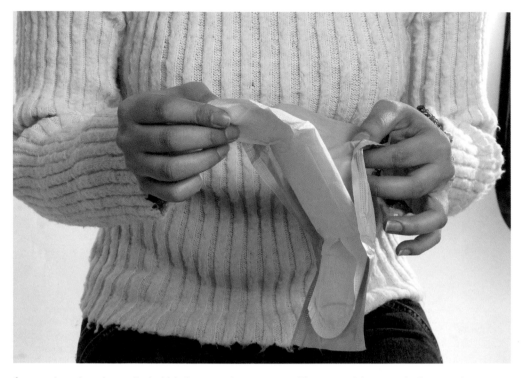

factors that alter the vaginal pH balance, such as wearing clothes that are very tight or made of synthetic fibers, using inadequately cleaned public swimming-pools or toilets, or keeping the genital area wet for a long time, can encourage it, with the consequence of infection.

As regards actual washing, it is recommended to wash the outside of the vulva, moving the fingers gently into the folds of the labia majora and minora and around the clitoris, as residues collect in this area too. The area should then be carefully dried to prevent its remaining damp. Unless the gynecologist prescribes otherwise in very specific situations, the inside of the vagina itself should not be washed as it has its own cleaning mechanism. To sum up, it is recommended to maintain adequate daily hygiene, practice safe sex, and visit the gynecologist at least once a year. Any small anomaly will be detected and treated easily during a routine examination and more serious problems will be avoided.

Factors that make intimate hygiene more difficult

To maintain proper intimate hygiene, the cleaning provided by a bath is not always enough, as certain external factors can alter it. These include:

• The natural hormonal changes that occur during puberty, pregnancy and the menopause.

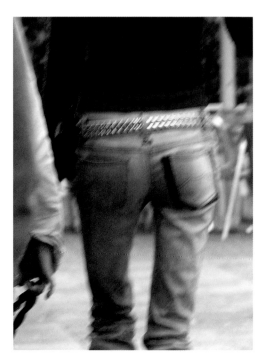

It is not true that older women have a special smell and need greater hygiene. They need the same dedication as a young woman and those who take a daily shower and wash themselves when necessary will have no fear of a body-odor problem. What is true, though, is that some women have a particular body odor all their lives and need to wash more often.

• Not changing tampons or sanitary pads often enough during menstruation. A tampon should never be kept in for longer than 6 hours.

• Perfumed soap and other products used to clean the genital area. These products can cause irritation, allergy and, ultimately, infection. It is therefore recommended to wash the area only with water, or with water and a neutral soap.

• Wearing underwear that is tight or made of synthetic materials. Slightly loose cotton underwear is preferable as it allows the area to perspire.

• The application of contraceptive sprays or spermicides, as they can upset the balance of the vaginal flora and cause problems. Some women also develop an allergy to such products.

• Sexual relations are the main factor that disturbs the balance of the vagina and can cause chemical changes. Sperm is alkaline and has a high protein content, which causes a change in the pH balance of the vagina and, as regards vaginal hygiene, remember that it is the channel that allows infections and sexually transmitted diseases to enter. Similarly, if oral sex is practiced without first washing the mouth, the genital area can be contaminated.

• The involuntary release of urine, or urinary incontinence, also represents a certain problem for female intimate hygiene, as both the genital area and the underwear remain damp, which can produce unpleasant odors and give rise to the production of microorganisms that cause infections.

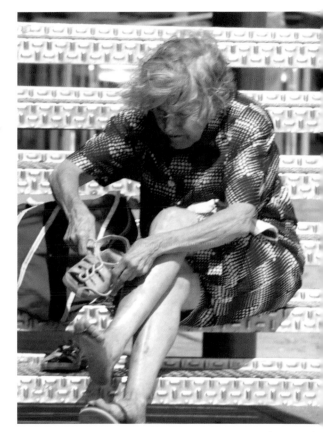

It is important to wash the genital area before and after coitus. Men are usually less scrupulous than women, so women are recommended to insist on this hygienic practice. Bathing or showering together can form part of loveplay or a pleasant ritual at the end of the day.

Deodorants and intimate hygiene products

As a result of the persistence of manufacturers of deodorants and intimate hygiene products, many people have become convinced that they should eliminate any trace of body odor, both the bad ones produced by sweat, and the sexual ones that are normal and healthy and do not need to be eliminated. These odors are caused by the sensitivity of the genital area. Intimate hygiene products usually cause irritation and allergies.

If your daily washing routine includes a shower, there is no reason why you should produce unpleasant odors. Men should pull back the foreskin and carefully clean the glans of the penis, which is the furrow formed where the foreskin joins it. This area produces a lubricating secretion called

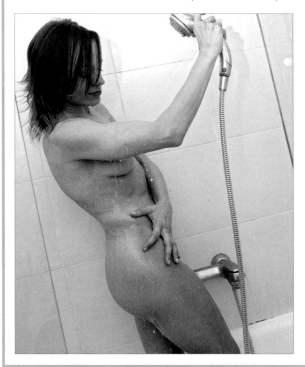

smegma which, if not carefully removed every day, can cause unpleasant odors and be the source of infections. Women should wash the vulva gently, using only water. The vagina has its own cleaning mechanism and any product can unbalance it and expose it to dangerous infections.

Bad odors, in both the sweat and apocrine glands, are caused by the accumulation of castoff salts and the action of bacteria that clear the skin of these salts. The best way of eliminating these salts is with water. Soap should be used only once a week, as it kills the bacteria, facilitating the proliferation of the fungi on which those bacteria feed. It is essential to protect the salts in order to keep the skin of this area in perfect condition.

Oral sex

Many people have the notion that oral sex is dirty, because the genitals are dirty, and think that using the mouth in this area must be very unpleasant. But, if hygiene is scrupulous, there is no reason not to practice it and enjoy it, just as deep kisses on the mouth are enjoyed, remembering that it is an area that produces its own fluid, saliva.

There are two types of vaginal secretion: the vaginal flow which is colorless and odorless, unless bacteria have acted on it because of inadequate hygiene or because the healthy practice of changing the underwear every day has not been observed, and a second secretion, the menstrual flow, which is bright red and usually lasts three or four days a month. Any variation in the quality or quantity of these fluids indicates that sexual health is not as it should be, in which case the woman should consult her medical center where someone will assess what is happening.

Work and health

Work is essential to the quality of a person's life and, at the same time, is an intrinsic part of it. There can be no quality of life without work: material needs and a large proportion of spiritual needs can be fulfilled only by work. Work cannot be viewed solely as a way of producing or rendering a service. It is much more than that: it helps a person to develop, mature, get to know people, and form relationships, and provides independence and autonomy. However, when work does not fulfill the appropriate conditions, it can have the opposite effect and become a health risk.

Work

Working conditions are a factor that directly affects health. The concept of health has evolved over time and does not refer exclusively to an absence of sickness but also to the environment, the work itself, and social relations—that is to say, to everything that physically or mentally affects a woman. When working conditions are analyzed, attention should be paid not only to matters of safety that prevent accidents at work—from using tools or machinery, fires, etc. It is also important to consider the environment in which the work is done—excessive noise, the lighting, temperature, humidity, etc. Some tasks require workers to handle chemical or biological substances that could be polluting or toxic.

Heavy tasks can cause physical damage that must be prevented. Not everyone is capable of carrying out the same tasks. As well as physical circumstances, there are other conditions that affect the worker, for example, mental pressure, the rate or quantity of the work, adequate training for the job. The stress a job can induce often constitutes a real danger to health. It is also essential to consider the way the work is organized, and factors such as monotony, autonomy, ability to communicate with other people, degree of participation in its organization, are highly influential.

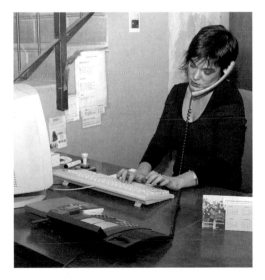

When work fulfils specific physical and psychological conditions it becomes an essential factor in human health and development.

Unlike what happened in the past, it is no longer possible to see the world of work and the world of the family as separate and divergent environments. Reality shows they are convergent and interdependent spheres that are essential for the formation of a full and satisfying life for human beings.

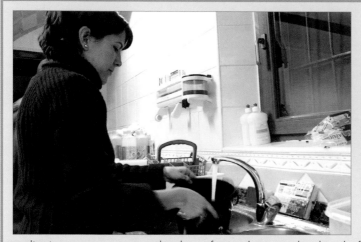

The double working day a woman is obliged to undertake, at work and at home, has prevented her from being available for work in the same way that men are. This has often stopped working women gaining access to responsible or managerial positions. The situation is changing and some women do succeed in gaining managerial posts, but normally it is at the price of losing family quality time or can even mean that the professional woman abandons the family altogether.

The world of work, working hours, and the way of relating are often still masculine and reproduce the traditional way in which men used to go out to work while women remained at home. The family is often still considered a woman's duty. Thus, for example, it is believed that a woman is absent from work much more often than a man. If that is so, it is because, while men are absent from work in order to carry out administrative duties, women are normally absent for family reasons, such as taking a child to the doctor, solving problems caused by the absence of the nanny or child carer.

Working women

Socialization is a process that starts in the early years of life. People learn to become involved in the world through the guidelines and patterns of behavior imposed on them by society. Normally, these guidelines and ways of behaving are not the same for men and women. Every person has a different role to play; a different way of behaving and feeling. This also considerably affects the world of work, which has traditionally been a sphere for male development, while women were relegated to the private or domestic sphere. It was assumed that the man was responsible for the financial maintenance of the home and he therefore had to devote himself to a career. Conversely, the woman devoted herself to the care of the family. Gradually, this division of labor has begun to change, but the burden of family life still weighs on the woman much more heavily than on the husband, who does not share in the domestic sphere and the duties it imposes to anything like the same extent. This has meant that the woman finds herself obliged to carry the double burden of work and home. What is more, she is still expected to adopt womanly attitudes, such as self-denial, pleasure in helping others,

availability, and an amiable disposition. This pigeonholes her into certain jobs in the labor market.

Society has accepted the female worker, but the image of her is false. Advertising shows a dynamic and determined woman who is capable of behaving like a man in the professional environment, but at the same time, her physical appearance is perfect and feminine, and without losing any of those attributes, she feels capable of caring for her family on her own.

The pressure on women nowadays to conform to the established image is changing, but no woman is capable of being perfect all the time, at work, with her husband, and with her children. This can be a considerable cause of frustration. The roles society fixes for men and women establish which jobs each sex can do. Some professions and trades have been considered masculine: electricians, truck drivers, mechanics, engineers, architects, pilots, etc., while women have been traditionally employed as teachers, telephonists, secretaries, nurses and so on.

Long-established attitudes to women and labor have disappeared in most progressive countries, although there are still matters such as equal pay to be resolved. The common belief that men

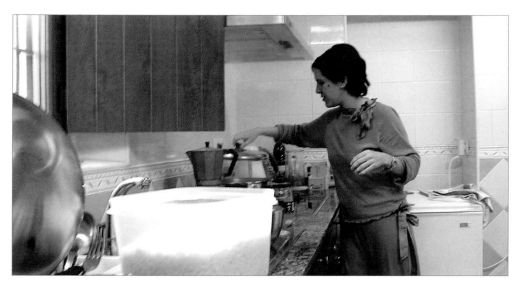

Mothers can develop a sense of guilt when she feels unable to combine her work with her family obligations.

need to work, while women only work because they want to is no longer valid. Current economic demands on the family have greatly increased the need for working mothers, while childless women also need to use the education and skills they have acquired to maintain their independent selves.

Domestic work

Women concern themselves not only with the material necessities of the home (washing, cooking, cleaning, etc.) but also act as the educator and nurse of their children, care for elderly parents, use psychology for all their family members, listening to them and supporting them when problems arise, and encourage the members of the family in all their projects.

This traditionally accepted attitude to domestic matters affects the woman's health, as her work is unpaid, no account is taken of the conditions in which she does it. There are no timetables for this work, no vacations, and virtually no leisure time. She works for hours on end, which can affect her physical and emotional health.

Domestic tasks can be hard, physical effort is required, and she also spends long hours on her feet. This can cause muscular pain and circulatory problems. The woman is isolated, loses her social life, and has no one to turn to when in need of help.

The people who live under the same roof as her take it for granted that it is the woman who will do everything.

Work and family

Combining work and family causes anxiety and stress in many women who work outside the home. This problem, which affects both parents and children, has become more marked since the mass incorporation of women into the labor market and because of the inadequate assistance provided by the institutions that facilitate the dual role of housewife and worker.

To help overcome the tensions that arise between work and the family, educationists and psychologists recommend following a series of guidelines:

• Be less demanding of yourself and accept that you can't do everything.

• Realize that the truly important thing is to find time for the most important matters—usually family and friends.

• Cleaning the house can wait, but never put off chatting with your children when they need the attention of their parents.

To make the best possible use of the time you spend with your children, it is best to accept that the quality of the time is more important than its amount. Therefore, your efforts should be concentrated on:

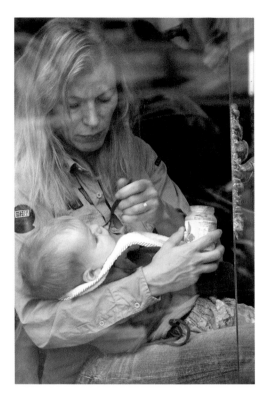

Work obligations often allow a woman little time to attend to her domestic duties. In this situation it is essential to pay more attention to the quality of the time you devote to your family than to its quantity.

• Making a great effort at weekends or on your days off. Use this time to do things together. It doesn't matter whether you play, talk about their concerns or enthusiasms, do homework, or get them to help with the household chores because, as well as teaching them the importance of working together as a team, it will help them become more responsible and self-confident.

• Trying not to overburden the child with extracurricular activities to keep him occupied while his parents haven't time to be with him.

• Reinforcing his understanding and the expression of his feelings.

• Monitoring the education he is receiving at school and from the people who look after him while his parents are busy. Also be vigilant about the influences he is receiving from all the educational agents to which he is exposed.

• Accepting his opinions, even if they differ from your own. This means not that you are giving in and complying with a child's will but that he will know that he can always count on your support even if his opinions differ from those of his parents.

• Cultivating patience and a sense of humor, qualities that will lighten any problem.

In addition to all this, there is one essential point: children need to be set clear limits and standards. Many parents try to make up for their lack of time by being permissive during the moments they

• Finding time to be with your children. If you don't have time, discipline yourself to make time, eat together, and help with homework, etc.

• Getting organized. Try to plan the time you have available as you would with any other obligation. The parents can take turns to go out before work to do the shopping, and to fetch the children from school. The obligatory items on your agenda must include being with them.

• Talking to them and giving them your full attention. You must stop and listen to everything your children want to say, which may be very important to them. If you don't have much time to be with them, the ideal is for them to feel really important at least during a moment's chat every day. This is the basis of communication and trust and, if you do not pay attention to a child during this time, he will stop spontaneously telling his parents everything and it will be very difficult to regain his trust in later years.

You have to do the impossible—find a moment every day to do things with your children. Communicating with them is a good basis for achieving trust both now and in the future.

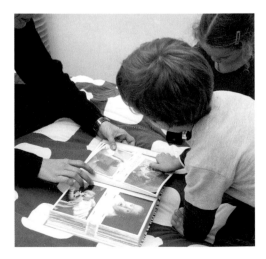

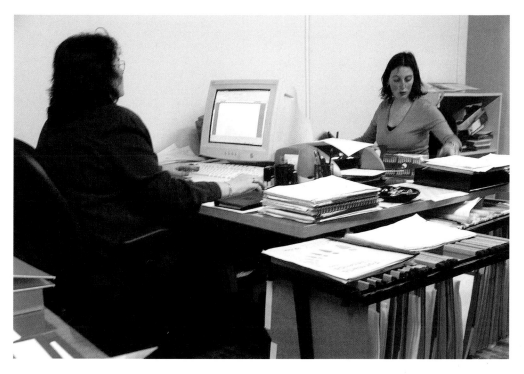

Although it is very important for a woman to be a professional in the world of work, she must establish a clear scale of priorities in her private life and know what is essential and what is ancillary.

spend with their children, but the purpose of those moments is not to make up for lost time with gifts, but to communicate with them, teach them principles, help them grow and develop, and show that we are coherent, understanding, and attentive, because an upbringing without any boundaries is the seed of many psychological problems and much future behavior.

Work-associated pain

Work, whether outside the home or within it, requires effort from the woman, and pain and complaints can arise as a result of it, secondary to the type of work and the character of each woman.

Mental and nervous complaints: stress and *burnout*

In the right amounts and circumstances, stress, like salt, is not a bad thing, but something that can add flavor, or even bring another dimension, to what is perhaps a rather mundane life. However, too much stress can be harmful and even biologically fatal to health.

Nowadays, in the sphere of teaching, there is much talk of stress and *burnout* (the syndrome of the exhausted professional), those terms being used indiscriminately and, at times, even being confusing. Although they are closely related in their meaning, being stressed and being burnt out are not the same thing.

Stress represents the accumulation of nonspecific changes in the body as its response to a stimulus. A positive stimulus does not usually cause problems, but a negative one does. The response to stress is automatic and with it the body prepares itself to face the new situation, activating all or part of the body. When the demands of the new situation have been resolved, the stress response ceases and the organism's balance is restored. When a great many extraordinary resources are activated the organism becomes exhausted if stress is repeated too often.

Burnout demonstrates its effect in exhaustion, debilitation, or psychological fatigue at work, generically as a form of affliction resulting from overexertion at work, and is manifested by severe losses of energy and a decline in the quality and quantity of performance. This brings with it emotional tiredness accompanied by a loss of motivation, usually progressing to frustration and failure. It also adds to feelings of despair and defenselessness, the loss of emotional resources, and the development of negative attitudes to work, life, and other people.

The consequences of stress and burnout

• Psychosomatic consequences: fatigue, headache, poor sleep, gastrointestinal disorders, high blood pressure, muscular pain, and menstrual troubles.

• Emotional upsets: emotional distancing, impatience and irritability, a sense of becoming despised, which can degenerate into distrust and defensive attitudes.

• Behavioral consequences: absenteeism, increasingly violent and risky behavior (dangerous games of chance, suicidal conduct, alcohol and drug abuse), family, and matrimonial quarrels.

Osteomuscular diseases

Most people have suffered an episode of intense back pain at one time or another. Some neurologists and traumatologists now call it "the disease of civilization." Not for nothing is back pain the commonest problem in industrialized societies.

It is so frequent that it is responsible for one in three resignations or dismissals in the world of work.

Everyone knows that the spinal column is the central axis of the human body. It is not a fixed and rigid structure, but allows considerable movement in all the activities of daily life. It enables the body to stand upright, bend or turn. It also covers and protects the spinal cord. The nerves branch out from the spinal column to the rest of the body.

Much back pain is caused by slight degenerative problems such as arthrosis. This pain can also be caused by diseases of the nervous system, traumatisms (such as fractures or sprains) or metabolic and decalcification processes, and by inflammatory diseases of the spine or joints.

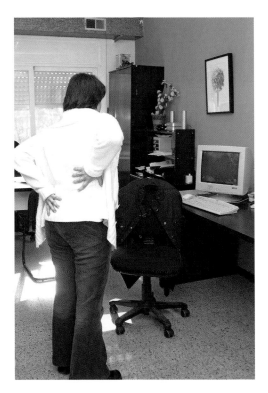

Back pain, resulting from the pace and stress of modern life and society, is one of the most frequent kinds of pain nowadays, and also affects women.

Restorative plastic surgery and cosmetic surgery

These days, having an operation to improve one's body image is considered a routine practice. However, a patient's eagerness to look great does not mean that she should ignore a series of fundamental precautions: a thorough knowledge of the possible risks and benefits, choosing the right professional service, and a genuine self-assessment of her reasons for seeking surgery.

The right to be informed

There is no reason for a person to undergo surgery, however noninvasive it may seem, without complete confidence in the specialist who will carry it out, and full knowledge of the procedures that will be used and their potential consequences.

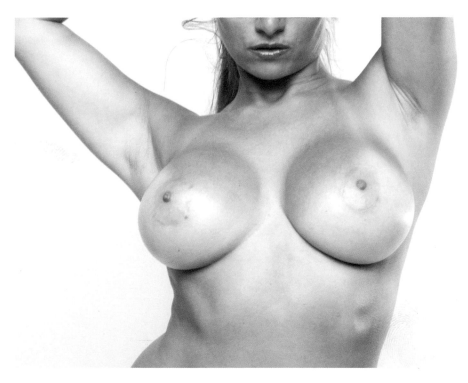

The aim of cosmetic surgery is not only to improve a woman's physical appearance, but also, and particularly, to give her a better and more positive image, improve her self-esteem and, hence, her quality of life.

Magazines and television programs often suggest that cosmetic surgery is frivolous.

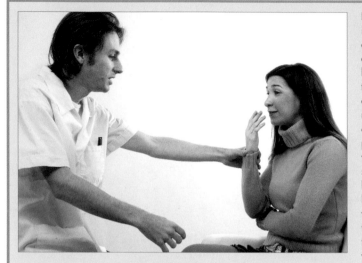

During the preliminary interview, the surgeon must ascertain any psychological aspects the patient may be hiding that could affect the successful outcome of a cosmetic surgical procedure. Thus, for example, the operation should not be performed on a woman whose husband has persuaded her to undergo it because he wants her to look younger, or on a woman who is seeking a facelift because she feels the need to compete with younger women, or thinks it will enable her to win back a partner. A patient suffering from depression should not undergo cosmetic surgery either. The surgeon is not a magician—he can only improve the woman's physical appearance, not solve her family or emotional problems.

When contemplating cosmetic surgery, it is important for the patient to have the consent of her family so they can support her adequately; otherwise they will not share the joy of a good result or support her if any problems arise.

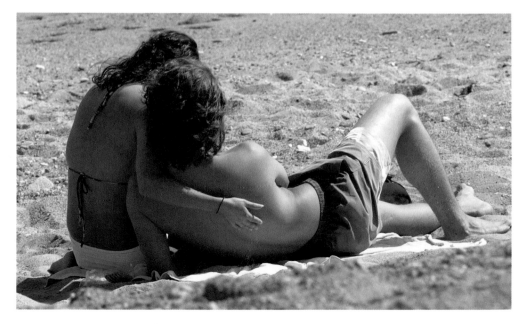

All patients are entitled to an explanation of the details of the procedure, the possible risks and complications, and the advantages and disadvantages of certain techniques, so that they can make their own cost-benefit analysis when taking the decision.

Firstly, the woman must be emotionally stable and calm, must not have false expectations of the operation (such as winning back a partner, or being more successful at work or in interpersonal relations), and must be prepared to confront her new image after the procedure.

This fundamental task demands time and good judgment so as not to make hasty decisions that may be regretted later. It is estimated that at least three independent specialists should be consulted so as to be able to make a comparison and choose the best.

It is best to consult a doctor who devotes himself exclusively to cosmetic surgery, although there may be other professionals who present themselves as capable of doing it—dermatologists, ophthalmologists, cosmetologists, and repairing surgeons—and who cover a wide field in this area.

The first visit to the doctor should never last less than 30 minutes. A good professional should take time to listen to the patient attentively, observe her, assess her expectations, and explain to her in detail the risks and benefits that can be expected from the procedure. The surgeon should never try to enthuse the patient, but should inform her as objectively as possible.

Professionals recommend that the patient should have no lingering doubts. The patient should ask for a description of the procedure, and about the risks she will be taking on, the type of anesthesia to be used, the duration of the operation, the postoperative period, etc. It is advisable that all the information the surgeon presents during the consultation, especially regarding possible risks and complications, should be given in writing, and that the patient should be given time to read it thoroughly so she can give what is known as *informed consent*. Good patient–doctor relations are also important if a successful operation is to be conducted.

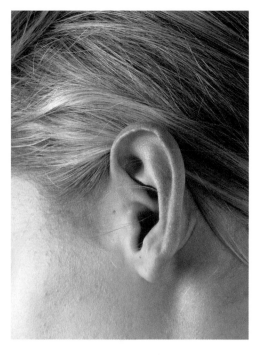

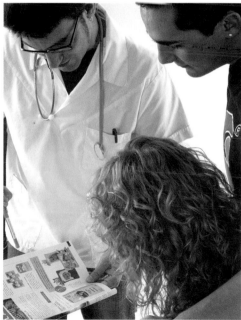

Cosmetic surgery, which is usually performed on healthy people who want to improve their appearance, requires a certain training and good judgment on the part of the medical team. The doctor must not agree to everything the patient wants. On the contrary, he must allow her to judge, acknowledge and accept the decision the plastic surgeon advises.

The most common cosmetic operations

Blepharoplasty

Eyelid surgery (technically known as blepharoplasty) is a procedure used to remove fat—and at the same time surplus skin—from the upper and lower eyelids.

Surgery can correct the separation of the upper eyelids and the bags that form under the lower eyelid that can disfigure the expression of the eyes and interfere with vision. However, this procedure does not eliminate the wrinkles known as *crows'* feet, and does little to mitigate dark circles under the eyes or lift fallen eyebrows. Although it can help increase the fold in the upper eyelid in Asian people, it cannot eliminate the signs of their ethnic or racial origins.

Blepharoplasty can be performed on its own or at the same time as other facial surgery such as, perhaps, facial skin stretching, or a facelift.

If the operation is performed on its own, the anesthetic used will always be local. The procedure will last about two hours if both the upper and lower eyelids are corrected. The scars appear as very fine lines which, on the upper eyelid, are hidden in its natural fold, while on the lower eyelid the scars are 1 mm below the point from which the eyelashes grow. The postoperative period is very brief and the stitches are removed within 4 to 5 days. The procedure is not painful, but it can cause slight conjunctivitis and watering eyes. This will clear up in a few days.

Before performing the surgery, the surgeon marks the incision points along the natural folds of the upper and lower eyelids.

The fat under the skin can be removed as well as the surplus skin and muscle.

In a transconjunctival blepharoplasty, a small incision is made in the lower eyelid and the fat is extracted using very fine forceps. No skin is removed and the incision is closed with self-dissolving sutures.

Rhinoplasty

Rhinoplasty, or surgery to change the shape of the nose, is one of the most common plastic surgery procedures. It can reduce or increase the size of the nose, change the shape of the tip or the bridge, reduce the size of the nostrils, or change the angle between the nose and the upper lip. It

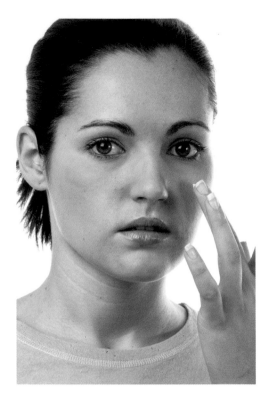

In a facelift, the tissue of the face and neck can be detached, as well as the muscles. The fat can be cut or sucked out and the internal muscle stretched. Once the internal muscles are stretched, the surplus skin is pulled back and cut off. Then the muscles are sutured back into place.

can also correct a birth defect or an injury, or help improve breathing problems.

The operation can be conducted under conscious sedation or a general anesthetic, and lasts between 1 and 3 hours depending on whether only the esthetic part or the functional part has to be corrected (nasal bone, turbinate bones, etc.). In both cases, the procedure ends with the insertion of a plaster rod and some tampons. The tampons are removed after 24 hours if the problem was only esthetic and after 4 days if the nasal bone or turbinate bones have been operated on.

The plaster rod is removed after a week and slips of paper are inserted and left in for a further 3 to 5 days. There is no pain, but there may be some discomfort because the patient will not be able to breathe through her nose. This problem will disappear with time.

Some advice

- Take time to choose your surgeon. Don't decide at the first consultation.
- Ask for a preliminary interview with the anesthetist, who is a key professional in the operating theater. You can also ask to meet the rest of the team beforehand and check their professional qualifications.
- All surgical operations should be performed in a fully equipped operating theater. Like the surgeon, the whole professional team should be specialists trained at recognized centers.
- Know the risks of any operation: infection, faulty healing, bleeding, unexpected complications, undesired esthetic effects, etc.
- Plan the operation, remembering that you'll need some time for recovery or to deal with any unexpected events. Avoid dates that are close to vacations, public holidays, or important events.
- Stay calm and, if you can't put the operation at the top of your agenda, postpone it until later.

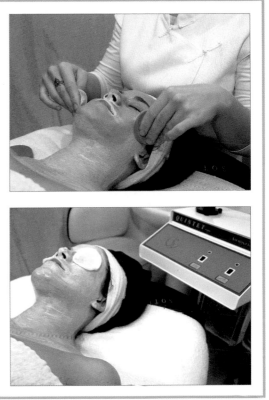

Otoplasty

Otoplasty is the procedure used to correct various ear defects. The commonest is the operation to reduce the size of the ears. In such cases, the natural folds of the outer ear are usually lacking and part of the ear is too big. The procedure is carried out under local anesthetic, unless the patient is very young. The incision is hidden in the fold behind the ear and is not visible. The result is very good, becomes apparent within 2 to 3 weeks, and definitive after 6 months.

Facelift

A facelift or stretching corrects the flabbiness produced by the passage of years and by certain circumstances such as weight changes, the action of the sun, external pollutants, etc. This procedure has two variants: for the upper part of the face and for the cheeks and neck. They can be performed separately or together (full facelift).

The procedure for improving the upper third of the face is called an endoscopic facelift. With three small incisions hidden in the hairline, the muscles of

the forehead are detached and pulled, so as to improve the appearance of the skin, eliminate forehead lines, and restore the eyebrows to their position, as they descend with time. The surplus skin is removed at the hairline, leaving no trace of the procedure performed.

The facial rhytidectomy is a method used to improve the flabbiness of the cheeks and neck that have the same causes as stated above (age, weight change, etc.). Incisions are made in front of and behind the ears, cutting out the surplus skin and returning the muscles and subcutaneous cellular tissue to their place. To improve the lower two thirds of the face, an inferior rhytidectomy or facelift is performed. The skin of the cheeks and neck are entirely detached and the skin and muscles pulled, to return the structures that have drooped with the passage of time to their place. The result is a scar that can barely be seen, because it is situated just in front of and just behind the ears.

In both cases, the postoperative period is easy. It should be explained that surgical procedures on the face are not painful, but they are visible. For

Botox

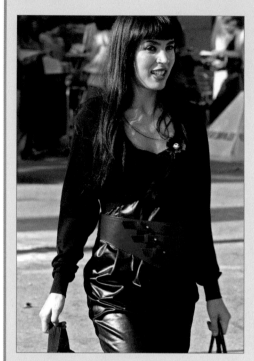

Botox is the trade name of the botulinum toxin. It can be injected into a specific muscle with the aim of weakening it and temporarily annulling its function. It has been used in medicine for over 20 years to treat various neurological and ophthalmic problems (tics, squints, etc.) and, although it was first used to lessen wrinkles in 1992, the treatment began to be widely used in plastic surgery from 2000. Botox acts by blocking the impulses originating from the nerve endings that contact the facial muscles, preventing those muscles from contracting. As the contraction does not take place, the skin on top of the muscles remains smooth.

What is Botox for?

- Correcting the furrows between the eyebrows that are produced by movement.
- Correcting crows' feet.
- Correcting forehead lines.
- Correcting the lines that appear on the neck during the contraction of the surface muscles (it does not correct the static lines that result from flabby skin).
- Correcting the unattractive expression lines of the nose.
- Chemically raising the eyebrows (it does not correct pronounced cases of fallen eyebrows).
- Reducing perspiration in the armpits and hands in cases that have resisted other forms of control.
- Botox treatment is said to have become popular in the United States to prevent the slipping caused by sweaty heels in wearers of high-heeled shoes.
- Its effectiveness has been described and proved in the treatment of certain headaches caused by muscular tension (each case of headaches should be medically assessed if their occurrence is frequent or intense, as they can have many causes).

this reason only, they require a postoperative recovery period of 15 to 20 days, after which the patient can resume her normal activities.

Liposuction

Together with breast enlargement, liposuction, lipoaspiration or liposculpture are the most frequently practiced procedures in cosmetic surgery. It is a surgical operation in which fat is sucked out using cannulas (small tubes) connected to a high-vacuum machine. Numerous tunnels are made with the cannulas, which are inserted under the skin through incisions measuring between 1/16th and ½ inch (2–10 mm). The incisions do not have to be made exactly where the fat will be extracted (this enables the small scar to be hidden in a place that is barely visible). As it is a surgical procedure, it must be carried out in a properly equipped operating theater. The areas to be treated are marked, focusing on those where a lot of fat needs to be extracted, and a small surrounding area is traced some ¾ to 1¼ inch (2–3 cm) outside the central treatment zone.

As with any intervention, a successful outcome depends on a thorough knowledge of the patient. The practitioner will ascertain her full history, including her previous illnesses, eating habits, whether or not she smokes, treatments of any kind, medication, etc. Her age, weight, and number of pregnancies are important. The patient's expectations should also be assessed because, in many cases, they are exaggerated, and she needs to realize that the surgeon is not a magician.

The period following a liposuction procedure

• Some bruising has occurred so the patient will feel a bit uncomfortable at first.

• After two or three days, the patient can lead a normal life, but she should wear a body belt for a while.

• Instead of traditional bandages that can create undulations in the tissue, the patient is usually fitted with a specially made elasticated bodystocking in the operating theater itself. This helps to remodel the areas operated on evenly, and promotes skin retraction. The belt should be worn for a period following the operation specified by the surgeon. A good outcome from the liposuction procedure depends on the patient adhering strictly to all of the surgeon's postoperative instructions.

• After that time, and only if the patient is not suffering any pain, she is advised to carry out a lymphatic drainage every other day. This drainage helps to reduce swelling and thus to eliminate possible irregularities caused by the hardening resulting from the healing process itself.

• Inflammation disappears some 15 days after the operation.

• It is recommended to practice gentle static cycling for 20 minutes a day to promote the elasticity of the internal scar.

• Hematomas can occur, although in ultrasonic liposculpture they are smaller than in traditional liposuction. The application of pharmaceuticals assists their reabsorption. For three weeks after the operation, it is wise to follow a low-salt, 1,300-calorie diet to avoid inflammation.

• No acute pain is caused, but minor aches are possible for the first two or three days, as if you had received a knock. They can be controlled with gentle tranquilizers and anti-inflammatory products.

Some preliposuction tests

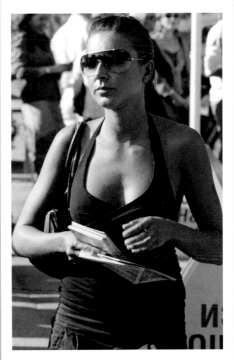

• Analysis of the deformity. The areas that are difficult and easy to treat are examined to ascertain whether there is enough fat to obtain a good result.

• Quality test. This consists of assessing the skin in the areas to be treated to ascertain the exact quantity of fat in each. It shows the elasticity of the skin and its capacity to retract.

• Pinching test. This enables the fat to be assessed exactly. The doctor can ascertain the type of fat in each area, so as to apply different and appropriate intensities or cannulas for each case. The areas to be treated must be discussed with the patient to inform her whether or not they will respond favorably to the operation. Once it has been decided which areas to treat and the preoperative procedure has been studied the procedure can begin.

Who can undergo liposuction?

As a general rule, everyone who is unhappy with their body and has accumulations of fat on their hips can undergo liposuction. However, the following are not considered suitable for this procedure:

- Seriously obese women, or women who are recommended to slim first.

- Moderately obese women, who are recommended to undergo sequential liposuction procedures and who, at the same time, are following an established diet corrected by an endocrine.

- Patients who are very flabby often do not realize that liposuction will not correct this problem.

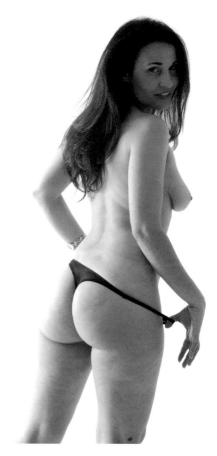

Cellulite is an condition found almost exclusively in women. Fourteen percent of cases of cellulite occur in puberty, 25% in the premenopausal period and many others during pregnancy or on starting to take the contraceptive pill.

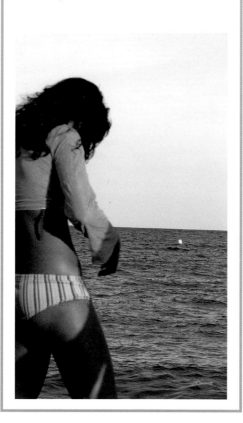

- Sun-bathing should be avoided at first. The skin, which suffers an internal wound, could become more pigmented than usual.

The consequences of liposuction

There are almost no contraindications regarding liposuction, but the commonest concern anesthesia. For this reason, patients with heart, circulation,

Is cellulite synonymous with obesity?

Not necessarily. Some thin people can have cellulite while heavier people may not suffer from it.

◼ Is cellulite the same as so-called orange-peel skin?

Not exactly.

Orange-peel skin refers to a number of irregularities that appear in certain areas of a woman's skin.

or coagulation problems should be treated with particular care.

Liposuction should be carried out in hospitals or clinics with adequate staff and teams who are prepared to overcome any kind of complication that could arise during the procedure.

Types of anesthesia

There are different types of anesthesia, depending on the size of the area to be treated, and on the surgeon.

• Ambulatory anesthesia, carried out by first applying ice and injecting a cold serum with a tumescent effect, is generally used for local liposuction procedures.

• Epidural anesthetic with sedation allows the patient to move during the operation but, as it dilates the blood vessels, it causes more hematomas.

• Local anesthesia using tumescence with sedation is employed for small areas where subsequent inflammation is less severe.

• General superficial and fairly shallow anesthesia can also be used, and is ideal for three-dimensional liposuction from the waist to the knee.

Cellulite

There are many theories on the origin of cellulite, but none is definitive. Studies have pointed out that the appearance of cellulite has little to do with a person's weight.

It is accumulations of fat that form in women because of the influence of hormones such as estrogen and progesterone. The fat appears crisscrossed by fibrous bridges leading from the skin to the subcutaneous cellular tissue giving the appearance of the peel of an orange.

• Does it appear only in certain areas?

The fat accumulation usually appears in typically feminine areas: on the hips, inner thighs, buttocks and sides of the abdomen. However, it can also appear on other extremities, including the arms.

• Are there different kinds of cellulite?

Yes, and some can even become painful to touch or pressure, especially those on the inside of the knee. The two most frequent types of cellulite are:

• **Hard cellulite.** This mainly affects young women and is localized on the thighs and pelvis.

• **Soft cellulite.** This is the most unattractive and difficult to treat. It frequently appears at around the age of 35 and its volume is usually much greater.

• What factors influence its appearance?

The factors are many and varied. Firstly, a natural predisposition to accumulate fat in certain areas, a sedentary lifestyle, smoking and alcohol habits, blood circulation deficiencies, and problems in puberty, pregnancy, or menopause. Secondly, there can be psychosomatic factors related to stress.

Food is also influential: eating a lot of fats, not drinking enough liquids, and an unhealthy diet directly affect appearance.

Breast surgery

In the modern world, the breasts are a symbol of femininity and play a very important role in a woman's sensuality. Nowadays, there are various ways of correcting the size and shape of the breasts, that is to say, their volume can be increased or reduced, making them firmer and reconstituting them in the case of breast removal.

Breast surgery

More and more women want to increase their bust size and are seeking surgery at an increasingly young age. It is quite usual to see women as young as 18 in the consulting room asking for breast enlargement or reduction surgery. The concept of the ideal size of the breasts has changed throughout history according to the tastes and fashions of each age.
However, the patient has the last word, and what matters is her assessment of beauty and proportion, refined by the concepts of the surgeon.

The female breast is composed mainly of fat mixed with connective and fibrous tissue. The circular region round the nipple is usually of a different color, that is to say that it is pigmented. This region is called the areola.

Mammoplasty for breast enlargement

By means of an incision in the furrow underneath the breast – round the areola or in the armpit – the tissue is raised in order to insert an implant between the breast and the pectoral muscle, or behind the muscle.

A silicone prosthesis filled with physiological serum or silicone gel is used (a kind of globe). These substances do not harm the body and are not associated with an increased risk of breast cancer. The implants do not affect fertility, pregnancy, or breastfeeding. The possibility of the implant's rupturing is very low and is usually caused by an accident, fall, etc. If this occurs, the patient will realize it because of the change in the appearance of the breast, and should visit a doctor to arrange for its replacement.

As a rule, breast enlargement surgery requires a general anesthetic, but it can be done under a local anesthetic with sedatives. It lasts about two hours and it is sometimes necessary to insert drainage tubes that are left in for one or two days. The skin is sutured and the stitches are removed after seven to ten days. The scar is red at first. After a few months it pales until it is almost imperceptible, but never disappears completely.

The patient can get up one or two days after the operation and return to work about 7 days later. During the first weeks, the breasts will be sensitive, so special underwear is recommended. The treating physician will give instructions on doing exercises and other activities.

This procedure is permanent, but age and gravity also affect it. The patient can have a mastopexy (breast-lift) after a few years if she wishes.

Like any surgery, this operation has its risks. A specific complication of enlargement mammoplasty is capsular contraction, in which the scar, or capsule, that the body develops round the implant shrinks. The breast feels hard to the patient in this case. The capsule can be removed or another implant can be inserted.

There can also be a change in the sensitivity of the nipples. Sensitivity can increase, diminish or cease completely. These symptoms usually disappear with time, but can be permanent. If an infection occurs, the implant will have to be temporarily removed.

When a mammography has to be carried out it is important to consult an experienced radiologist because it may be necessary to take more samples and other examinations may also be recommended, such as ultrasound and magnetic resonance tests. The idea is to check that the breast implant is not hiding a tumor that could delay its treatment.

Mammoplasty is a common surgical procedure designed to change the size of the breasts. Although we hear about breast enlargement more

A rare complication is permanent loss of sensitivity in the nipples and/or the breasts, or scars that do not heal well. If an injury occurs in the tissues of the areola or the breast, they can be reconstructed immediately with grafts.

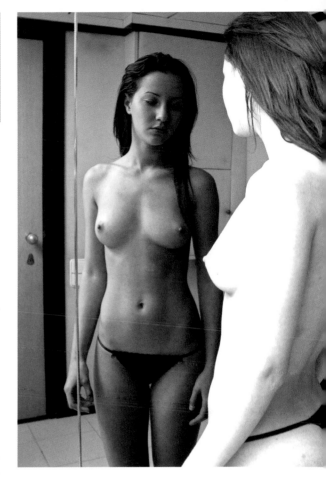

often, over half the mammoplasty procedures are carried out to reduce their size (breast reduction). Mammoplasty is also indicated when the breasts are markedly different in size.

Mammoplasty for breast reduction

This surgery helps to restore firmness and reduce the weight of the breasts on the shoulders, neck, and back, which in some cases can cause serious problems and prevent normal physical activity.

Three incisions are required, one round the areola, a vertical one from the areola to the furrow under the breast, and a horizontal one in the furrow itself. The lightest cases require only an incision round the areola.

In about three hours and under a general anesthetic, the plastic surgeon extracts mammary tissue and excess fat, relocates the areola and may also reduce its size. Sometimes, drainage tubes are inserted to eliminate fluids. Finally, the bust is wrapped in an elastic bandage.

During hospitalization, which lasts one or two days, postoperative pain is felt, but can be effectively treated with analgesics. The stitches are removed some 15 days after the operation. Scar healing is generally good. The marks do not disappear but become less noticeable with time. As a woman's breasts are naturally of different sizes, it is normal for that difference to persist after surgery. The important thing is that the difference should be small.

Depending on how quickly the patient recovers, she can return to her normal activity the day after leaving the clinic and should follow instructions such as sleeping on her back and avoiding sexual activity for at least a week. She is recommended to wear special underwear and not to practice sport

Mastopexy or bust-lifting

This surgery is especially effective for small or drooping breasts. Although it does not increase the capacity to breastfeed, it is recommended to postpone it if you are planning a pregnancy, because lactation distends the tissues, so part of the benefit would be lost. General anesthetic is customarily used for this procedure, which lasts about three hours. Three incisions are made in the shape of an anchor, one round the areola, another vertically from the areola to the furrow under the breast, and a horizontal one in the furrow itself. The skin is then pulled back and the areola is raised.

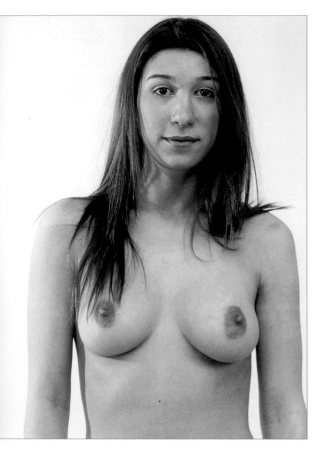

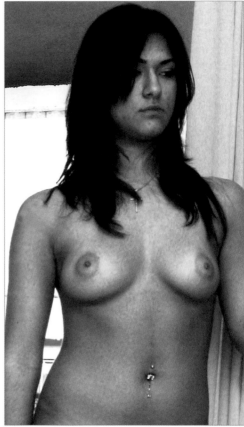

for three or four weeks. It is normal to feel some discomfort for a long time, but if severe pain occurs it is necessary to consult a doctor.

The results of this surgery are permanent, unless the woman gains a lot of weight or becomes pregnant, but the passage of time and gravity eventually leave their mark.

Breast reconstruction

One of the consequences that profoundly affects women who have suffered a breast tumor is mastectomy. It is now possible to remove the breast and reconstruct it in a single surgical procedure. In any case, it is preferable for the reconstruction to be done when the cancer appears to have been eliminated. Various techniques are used depending on the situation. Expansion and the insertion of a silicone prosthesis is one of them. An expander inflated with serum is inserted for several weeks. After the skin has stretched, the expander is removed and an implant is inserted. The areola and nipple are reconstructed in a separate procedure.

Sexuality and sexual relations

Human sexuality is not entirely focused on the genitals. Sex is of profound human significance with its own codes and signals; it is the supreme form of communication and expressing love through the body. It is not a question of understanding the female body only from the anatomical and physiological point of view. Both women and men are considerably more than just the sun of their parts. Sexuality affects psychic experience, interpersonal relations and social roles.

Sexual response

Human love has nothing to do with sex. People have feelings, attitudes, and convictions in sexual matters, but each person experiences sexuality differently, because it is viewed from a highly individualized perspective, one that emanates from both personal and private experiences and from public and social causes.

The action of the mind

The brain initiates the process of sexual arousal as a response to thoughts (sexual fantasies), visual stimuli (seeing the partner naked), audible stimulation (hearing the partner's voice), olfactory stimuli (the smell of the partner's body), and taste stimuli (the taste of the partner's body).

The body can initiate the process of arousal when the woman, or her partner, touch one another's genitals or breasts, the feeling of the air flowing over her naked skin, or her clothes stimulating her breasts or genitals. While the

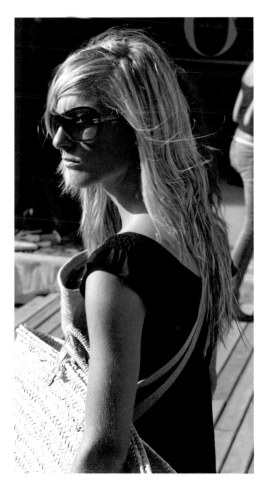

Having a healthy sex life is more than the right of every woman: it presupposes a positive way of communicating with others and with herself, sensing her own body, and developing her own capacity for pleasure.

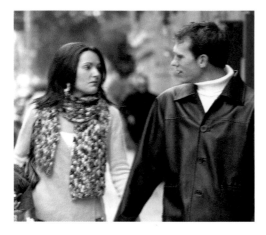

mind and the body can experience sexual arousal separately, they cannot experience orgasm at different moments. Orgasm requires the mind and the body to work together. Stimulation and arousal can originate in either, but orgasm occurs in both.

Both male and female sexual response are made up of five components which manifest themselves differently in each sex: sexual desire, arousal, the plateau phase, orgasm, and resolution. Sexual desire is influenced by a series of components that can be organic, psychological, cognitive, and environmental.

Sexual arousal

• Sexual arousal can be activated by a multitude of mechanisms that stimulate any of the senses and is intimately related to past experience. This sets off a physiological response in both men and women. In women, a component that can be compared to the erection of the penis is vaginal lubrication, which is the direct result of the increased flow of blood to the pelvic region, causing the blood vessels in the walls of the vagina to dilate and stimulating the vaginal secretion.

Motivation plays a very important part, as sexual arousal is not simply the need to satisfy a biological urge. There must also be a connection with the other person, the feeling of being in love, secure, and understood, a series of elements that lead the person to feel sexual desire for the partner. If sexual desire is absent, it should be remembered that many elements affect it and that they must be investigated to try and find a precise solution to the problem.

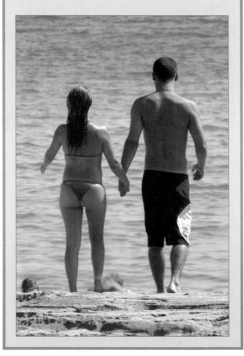

• In the external genitals, the outer and inner lips swell.

• A progressive erection occurs in the clitoris. The clitoris is a very excitable organ. However, it has been demonstrated that most women do not experience stimulation without some erotic foreplay. Vigorous stimulation of the clitoris can even cause pain, so indirect and gentle clitoral stimulation is recommended.

• There can be changes in the breasts. They can increase in size and the nipples can become erect.

• There is also an increase in the heart-rate, blood pressure, and general neuromuscular tone.

The plateau phase

• In this phase, the characteristic for both sexes is the presence of a high and sustained level of sexual tension, which is of short duration.

• In women, what is known as the orgasmic platform occurs, which, definitively, is an increase in the external volume of the vagina, secondary to the dilation of the blood vessels in that area. It produces a reduction in the interior of the

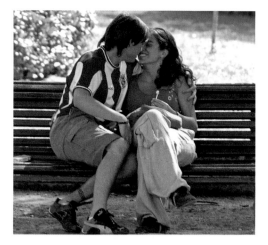

Sexual response is a complex process involving the whole woman, her mind and her body. The human mind receives sexual stimuli from the body, processes them and, based on what has been learnt previously, and on experience, makes the body respond to them.

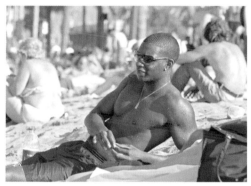

• The inner two thirds of the vagina swell. The woman may feel a strong desire to be filled, a vaginal ache.

• Vaginal lubrication may lessen during this stage, especially if it is prolonged.

• The clitoris remains constantly erect and its glans moves forward toward the pubic bone, hiding even further behind the clitoral cap.

• The swollen inner lips can open the outer lips, making the opening of the vagina more prominent.

• The color of the inner lips changes considerably, changing from pink to red in women who have not given birth, and from bright red to dark brown in those who have. The colors can vary, but the marked change does not.

• The areola, the pigmented area round the nipples, starts to swell.

• The breasts can increase in size by some

vagina and increased contact between the genitals, disregarding the myth concerning the thickness of the penis, as the cavity will adapt itself to its width.

• Vaginal lubrication increases, although if stimulation is too prolonged it can decline considerably and even stop. This would be equivalent to the loss of erection in the man and would be a completely normal response.

• The vagina increases in width and depth. Moreover, there are fewer nerve endings, so the depth of penetration does not increase the feeling of pleasure so a long penis can not necessarily produce greater sexual pleasure.

• The clitoris also increases in volume, as do the outer and inner labia and the breasts.

Effects of the plateau stage

• A marked increase in sexual tension.

• An increase in the congestion of the blood vessels of the vagina, causing the outer third of it to swell, so that the vaginal opening becomes smaller, sometimes by 30 percent.

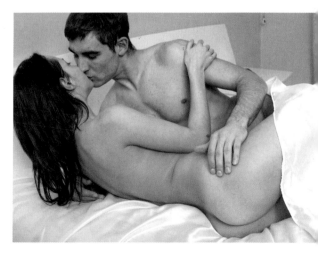

The sexual act must be considered as the ceremony of love and shared pleasure. Haste, the wrong mood, and inappropriate surroundings are not good conditions for complete enjoyment. Conversely, previous arousal, attention to all parts of the body, fantasy, everything that increases desire, are the best ingredients for reaching the orgasmic phase with great intensity.

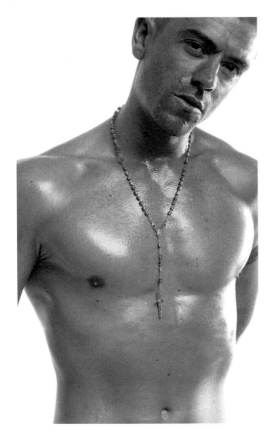

20 to 25 percent in women who have never breastfed, but in women who have, the increase is less marked, or does not occur at all.

• Some 50 to 70 percent of women experience sexual reddening in the chest and other parts of the body, resulting from an increased flow of blood to the surface of the skin.

• The heart-rate increases, sometimes with rapid palpitations.

• There is a marked increase in sexual tension in the thighs and buttocks.

• The woman's body is now completely prepared for coitus.

Orgasmic stage. Effects

• Rhythmic muscular contractions occur in the outer third of the vagina, the uterus (womb), and anus. The first muscular contractions are the most intense, occurring at a rate of a little under one per second.

• As the orgasm continues, the contractions become less intense and more sporadic. A moderate orgasm can generate 3 to 5 contractions, and an intense one, 10 to 15.

• Sexual reddening becomes even more intense and can cover a greater proportion of the body.

PHASES OF FEMALE SEXUAL RESPONSE

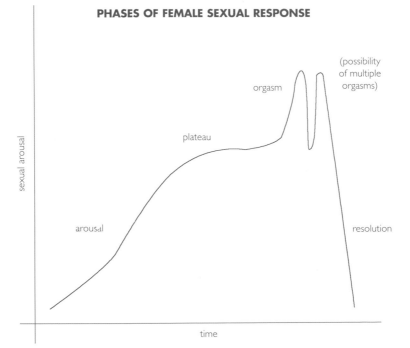

- The muscles of the whole body can contract during orgasm, not only those of the pelvic area.
- Orgasm also takes place in the brain, as shown by the brain waves monitored.
- Some women emit a little fluid from their urethra during orgasm. This is usually called female ejaculation. Although it has not been established whether the fluid expelled is urine or female ejaculate, the source of the fluid is not important; women often say they have had very intense orgasms when this has happened. That is all that should matter, the woman's pleasure, fluid or otherwise.
- Myotony (muscular tonus or tension) can be apparent all over the body, especially in the face, hands, and feet. The woman's facial expression can indicate that she is feeling pain, when she is really having a pleasurable orgasm.
- At the climax of the orgasm, the whole body becomes momentarily rigid.

Resolution phase

- If sexual stimulation continues, the woman may experience one or more additional orgasms.
- The vagina and vaginal opening return to their natural, relaxed state.
- The breasts, labia, clitoris, and uterus regain their normal size, position, and color.
- The clitoris and nipples may have become so sensitive that any stimulation can be uncomfortable.
- The sexual reddening disappears.
- The woman may perspire profusely and breathe deeply.
- The heart may beat rapidly.
- If orgasm does not occur, the woman experiences everything mentioned above, but to a much smaller extent. As it has not been dissipated by the muscular contractions of an orgasm, the blood trapped in the pelvic organs can produce a feeling of pelvic heaviness and discomfort.

Quality should always take precedence over quantity in everything to do with sexual pleasure, whatever its form. The greatest pleasure lies not in reaching a target, but in obtaining the highest degree of stimulation. This is the best guarantee of a fully satisfactory experience.

Response to sexual stimulation

As a rule, women react differently to sexual stimuli. The body has various sensitive, erogenous zones and each woman experiences different sensations when those zones are stimulated. The most important thing for the sexual act is good communication, which eliminates fears and anxieties, and gives free rein to enjoyment and pleasure. The woman should communicate with her partner so that he can stimulate the parts of her body that give her the greatest pleasure.

Sexual freedom: homosexuality, bisexuality and transsexuality

A human being is born male or female, and the sexual orientation of the individual is intimately linked to his or her own sex. Depending on their sexual orientation, people can be heterosexual, homosexual, or bisexual. Moreover, transsexuality includes people who were born biologically male or female, but who have a profound sense that they ought to have been born a member of the other sex.

The upbringing of most people is towards a heterosexual orientation, that is to say, it is assumed that girls will be attracted to boys and vice versa. This educative orientation is intimately liked to the belief that little boys and little girls will naturally behave in a typically masculine or typically feminine way, as if those patterns of

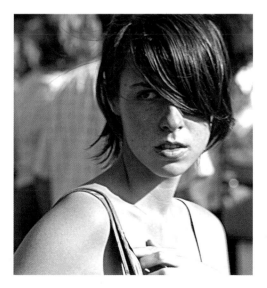

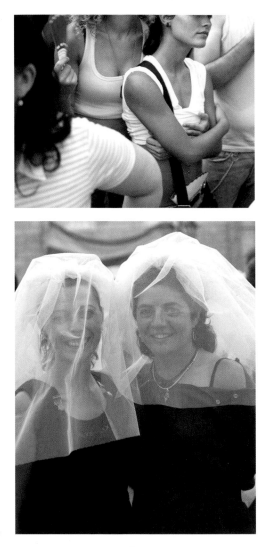

In recent years, the subject of homosexuality has been earning greater interest and respect from society, to the point that some countries have legalized the marriage of same-sex couples.

behavior were biologically determined by sex. Moreover, the family is the supreme social unit, and for a family to be created and have natural descendants, it is necessary to have a man and a woman. This has led to the determination of heterosexual union between a man and a woman as the normal one, sexually speaking, but people who feel other inclinations cannot be considered rare or abnormal.

Homosexuality can be defined as attraction or interaction between people of the same sex, and does not describe a uniform population, because men and women with that orientation constitute a group as diverse as heterosexuals from the point of view of their upbringing, occupation, lifestyle, personality, and physical appearance. There is great diversity in the definition of homosexuality in scientific literature.

Bisexuality

This is the orientation in which the person achieves sexual and emotional satisfaction with members of both sexes. Bisexuality is a permanent orientation, although the person's relations with both sexes may be limited to a particular period. Both men and women can be bisexual.

Transsexuality

A transsexual is a person who was born male or female biologically, but who has the profound sense that he or she should have been born a member of the other sex. Transsexuals are convinced that a biological error has been made concerning them and that they were born with a body that does not correspond to their feelings and desires. Many of them therefore seek medical help to change their physical identity and make it match their internal, emotional identity. The word transsexual can be used to define people with such feelings, regardless of whether or not they have undergone a sexchange operation. As soon as a *transsexual* male believes he is really a woman, it is logical for him to want to form a relationship with a heterosexual man. Transsexual men therefore have erotic, romantic, and emotional responses to men and sexual fantasies concerning them. Similarly, transsexual females think they are really men and so desire relationships with heterosexual women. They therefore have romantic, erotic, and emotional responses to women and erotic fantasies about them. These situations are difficult to confront, but transsexuals are not homosexual, and do not consider themselves or their relationships to be so. Conversely, most homosexuals are not transsexuals.

Safe sex

Regardless of each person's sexual choice, practicing unprotected sex makes the person vulnerable, as it leads to more infections by HIV and other sexually transmitted diseases throughout the world. The risk does not lie in sexual

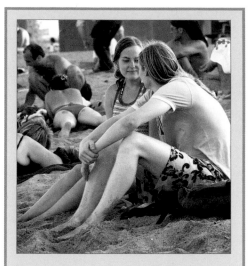

Homosexuality

Whatever their sexual orientation, most people include caresses, kisses, and embraces in their sexual repertoire. The great majority also include masturbation and oral sex. Gay women probably place more emphasis on rubbing their bodies against one another to achieve orgasm (which is called tribadism) than heterosexual couples, gay men probably place more emphasis on anal coitus, but none of these practices need be exclusively the sphere of gay men or women.

another's self-esteem, self-care, control, shared decisions and respect.

Masturbation

Between 70 and 80 percent of women have masturbated to orgasm at least once in their lives. Many women begin after the age of 20, or when they have already had sexual relations. Some may never masturbate.

Frequency tends to vary, depending on the circumstances of each person, but many women who maintain active sex lives masturbate as much as those whose sex lives are not active.

Masturbation is an excellent way of discovering ones own body and sexual responses, as well as satisfying ones own desires. It is a personal and private experience. Through masturbating, many women discover better ways of becoming aroused and reaching orgasm during coitus, and the practice can help some to experience multiple orgasms.

Some women lie down quietly to masturbate, using their hands only on their genitals. Others prefer to move vigorously and caress their breasts with their hands as well as their genitals. Lubricants can also be used to make the fingers more slippery so the friction on the genitals is gentler and more delicate, intensifying the pleasure derived from masturbating.

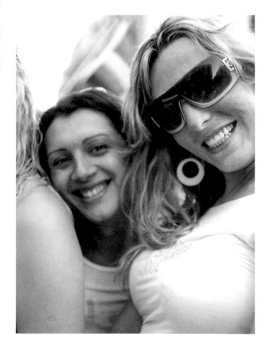

inclination, but in the lack of protection provided by using a condom.

Safe sex means taking precautions to avoid the risk and acquisition of sexually transmitted diseases (STDs) and AIDS from sexual relations. Safe sex should be practiced as a couple, meaning that both partners must share in carrying it out.

Couples should be prepared to reach an agreement about safe sex, considering one

The problems experienced by people who feel they have a body that does not belong to the sex with which they identify have received greater attention recently. Greater respect for the sexual condition of individuals has led to the search for adequate solutions for each case.

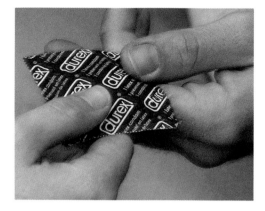

Regardless of each individual's sexual choice when embarking on active sex, whether they are heterosexual or homosexual, and regardless of the type of congress—vaginal, anal, oral—it is also very important to take appropriate measures to prevent what should be pleasurable from becoming a serious health problem. Sex should be satisfactory, but it should be safe too.

Solitary masturbation is 100% safe sex, as no sexually transmitted diseases are passed on and there is no risk of pregnancy. Moreover, by masturbating people learn to know their own body and explore their own sexuality. This helps them function better sexually with their partner and derive greater pleasure from sex.

Safe sex is more than the prevention of pregnancy. It means protecting oneself from sexually transmitted diseases, including those caused by the human immunodeficiency virus (HIV). Considering the seriousness of the consequences of some diseases contracted through sexual contact, the importance of always taking proper precautions cannot be over-emphasized.

The number of women who masturbate habitually is increasing all the time, progressively approaching the same proportion as men. As the role of women in society has become more highly valued and they have achieved greater independence, they have become increasingly interested in knowing their own bodies, their most erogenous zones, and how to achieve greater pleasure.

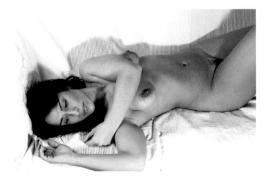

Female sexual dysfunction

Sexual pleasure, especially in women, is not something that happens automatically. A series of physical and psychological aspects must be appropriately fulfilled at the same time if it is to produce its effect. Many factors can prevent a woman from enjoying sex with her partner.

Origin

The origin of female sexual dysfunctions can be organic, particularly when other problems are also present, such as thyroid or hormonal troubles, diabetes, high blood pressure or high cho-

lesterol, as well as depression, anxiety, personality problems, sexual abuse, etc. Upbringing and cultural factors are also highly influential, as in many places it is still thought that women have no right

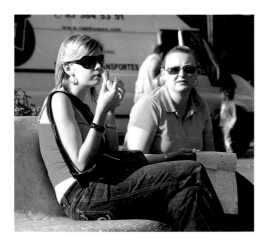

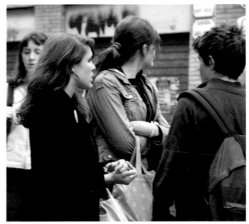

For a problem to become a sexual dysfunction, it must be:

- Of an erotic nature, that is to say it must be related to desire, arousal, and/or orgasm.

- It must be undesirable to the woman.

- It must be recurrent and persistent, as for many reasons the predisposition to sexual

pleasure and sexual relations may eventually be lost.

- There must be a combination of organic, emotional, and psychological symptoms.

to sexual pleasure and that feeling such pleasure casts doubt on her morality, so many women may feel guilty, ashamed, ignorant, and afraid.

Common causes

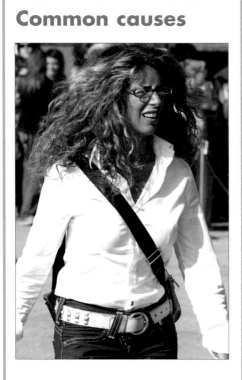

- Communication problems between the couple.

- Fear of pregnancy.

- Anxiety or depression.

- Feelings of guilt and shame about sex.
- Fear of pain or catching an infection.

- Lack of appropriate stimulation.

- Inadequate lubrication.

- Associated systemic disease.

- Menopausal changes.

- Damaged nerves due to surgery or injury.

- Medicines.

- Gynecological infection or disease.

- Previous sexual abuse.

The origin of a sexual dysfunction usually lies in several factors at once, so clearly identifying the causes is vital to treat it adequately and enable all women to understand and make the most of their sexual rights. Since it is an integral part of her health and development, it can affect a couple's life together and can even lead to severe depression and marital and family problems.

Classification

There are four main types of female sexual dysfunction, related to: desire, arousal, orgasm, and others that generally affect sexual expression. They can occur when the woman's sex life begins (*primary*) or may appear after a person has experienced her sexuality and soon has problems with one or more of the aspects mentioned (*secondary*). Female sexual dysfunctions can be classified by their origin into:

- Desire-related dysfunctions or upsets, which include hypoactive sexual desire, hyperactive sexual desire, or an aversion to sex.
- Arousal dysfunctions or upsets.
- Orgasm-related dysfunctions or upsets, such as female anorgasmia.
- Pain-related sexual dysfunctions, such as dyspareunia or vaginismus.
- Sexual dysfunctions due to disease, caused by medicines or taking drugs.
- Psychological sexual dysfunctions.

Sexual dysfunctions impede and damage the woman's sexual and social life and life as a couple.

- As a whole, whether it occurs when the woman touches her own body or when her partner touches her.

- Partially, when the problem occurs only in the partner's company, although individually they can achieve pleasure, or selectively, when the problems arise only with a particular person, behavior, attitudes and effects being very different with someone else.

It is wise to consult a doctor whenever this problem arises. The doctor will make a physical examination that can include a pelvic examination, and can ask about the couple's sexual relations, customary sexual practices, attitudes to sex, any medication being taken, and other possible symptoms. The treatment of the sexual dysfunction will depend on its cause and can invol-

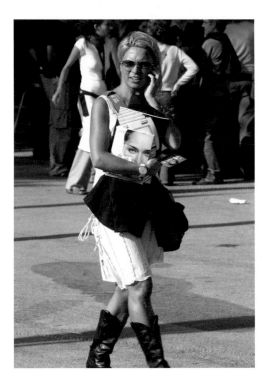

It should be remembered that in most cases, while the woman is starting menopause, her partner is very probably also experiencing biological and psychological changes that will alter his own sexual response. An alternative way specialists have found for treating loss of sexual appetite in some women during menopause is the use of hormone replacement therapy, as it has been demonstrated that it helps repair vaginal weakness and elasticity and alleviates vaginal dryness. However, it is important for every woman to consult her gynecologist to obtain the right treatment for each case.

cal reasons such as lack of arousal, tiredness, tension, uncomfortable sexual positions, anal coitus.

• **Anaphrodisia.** This is inhibited sexual desire, either because the women who suffer from it do not want to have sex, or because they deny themselves pleasure, are afraid of rejection, have difficulty in demonstrating sexual desires, fear previous traumatic experiences, or have other psychological problems.

ve changes in current sexual activities, suspending or changing medication as far as possible, adding a new medication, or surgery.

It may be necessary to consult a specialist in the treatment of sexual dysfunction. A psychological assessment may also be recommended.

Various dysfunctions

Female sexual dysfunctions concern arousal, penetration (or coitus), or orgasm, and can originate from an organic or psychological cause.

• **Anorgasmia.** This is a blockage of the orgasm, although not of arousal. As in men, its origin is psychological. Its causes are physical only in a tiny percentage of cases. The principal causes are: having previous experience of rape or sexual abuse, worry, fear, stress, depression, or problems resulting from a sexual upbringing emphasizing that women should not enjoy sex.

• **Dyspareunia.** This is pain that can occur during or after coitus. It can be experienced as vaginal pain or irritation. Its causes include: infections, genitourinary diseases, rejection of barrier contraceptive devices such as the diaphragm, IUD, condom, or spermicides, or for psychologi-

Important psychological aspects

- Understanding changes in sexuality.
- The processes at the root of the woman's sexual response.
- The emotional state.
- The level of available energy.
- The woman's own attitude to herself, including her body image and her self-esteem.
- The memory of past experiences.
- Her imaginative capacity, that is to say the facility of evoking pleasant past experiences for the development of sexual fantasies.
- Beliefs and expectations.
- The relationship with the partner.
- The partner's functional skill.

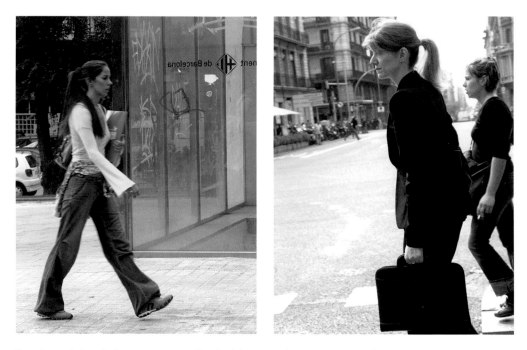

Every human being, whether man or woman, has the right to experience sexual pleasure. This experience can be made more difficult by many factors, most of which can be completely overcome.

• **Hypoactive sexual desire.** This is characterized by never or almost never wanting to have sex, nor having sexual or erotic thoughts or fantasies. When the woman thinks about her behavior, she realizes that having sex matters to her less and less, with the result that she not only avoids them but seldom or never initiates them with her partner.

• **Hyperactive sexual desire.** This is a problem reflected in the woman's constant desi-

VAGINAL INJURIES OR DISEASES CAN MAKE THE SEXUAL ACT PAINFUL

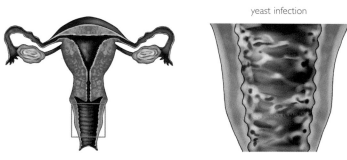

yeast infection

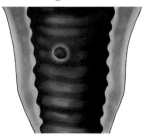

vaginal ulcer

Painful coitus, or dyspareunia, is the name given to the problems that arise in the pelvic area during or after active sex and can affect both the man and the woman. In addition to possible physical causes, the pain can be associated with psychological factors such as previous sexual trauma or a very restrictive upbringing.

How to improve sexual relations

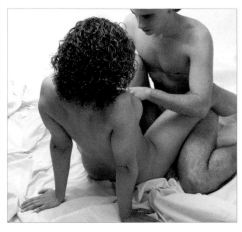

At some time in their lives, almost 50% of women experience a reduction in sexual appetite. The fact is that present-day society, in which home has to be combined with her work and family, in addition to sex and her partner, generates stress that can make even the most ardent couples sometimes suffer what experts call *inhibited sexual desire syndrome*.

But giving up the most animal side of our nature directly harms physical and mental health. The absence of pleasure can cause an increase in headaches, bouts of depression, low self-esteem, unhappiness, and even the separation of the couple. The lack of physical contact between the couple is one of the main causes of family breakdown.

The lack of sexual desire can be set off by many factors, including physical problems, such as hormonal deficiency, diabetes, vaginal infections, high blood pressure, recently giving birth, or the menopause, which can cause painful coitus, inflammation, an absence of vaginal lubrication, and hence, aversion, and taking drugs, pharmaceuticals or alcohol, which induce low libido.

Other frequent causes are psychological. Traumatic events such as rape, abandonment, and disappointed love, can cause a decline in sexual desire. Similarly, very low self-esteem, anxiety, worry, or depression can banish pleasure.

Lastly, the enemy of sex in the new millennium has appeared in the form of stress. Home, work, credit card debt, and children are totally incompatible with libido. The tiredness generated by so much daily activity prevents people from thinking about anything other than sleep when night falls.

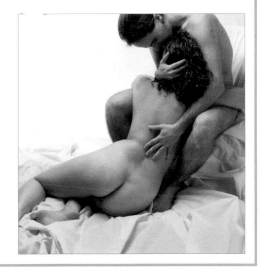

re to have sex. It is also known as compulsive sexual behavior, and as a rule the frequency or intensity of active sex or the desire to have them interferes with her daily life. This dysfunction is of psychological origin and can be motivated, among other causes, by an enormous hunger for affection and caresses, however artificial they may be.

• **Arousal dysfunctions.** Conditions in which the woman has great difficulty in becoming aroused and hence failing to achieve vaginal lubrication before penetration, making coitus difficult and painful.

• **Inhibited sexual arousal.** This occurs during sexual activity when vaginal lubrication is inadequate or nonexistent, or when the woman does not feel aroused during it and feels disconnected from her body.

• **Inhibited orgasm.** This occurs when the woman experiences difficulty in achieving orgasm, both on her own and with her partner. It is the most frequent dysfunction in women

Training the senses

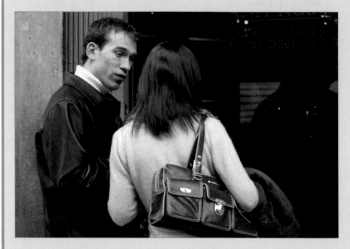

- This technique is often recommended by sex therapists to reduce anxiety about the sexual act, focusing on the stimulation of the senses.

- Directed by the therapist, the couple will practice these exercises for an hour every week, in a comfortable well-lit place.

- The couple will take it in turns to play the active role.

- They undress, lie down and explore the pleasures of the senses (embracing, kissing, caressing, etc.), but without at any time performing the sexual act (if one of them becomes excessively aroused, he or she will masturbate, and then continue the experiment).

- The method can include taking a pleasant shower together.

- If one of them wants to stop the session, it will be suspended.

- The couple will report their experiences to the therapist, who will usually give them further instructions and introduce sexual games. When the therapist considers the moment is right, he or she will advise the couple to have full active sex at the end of their sessions.

- This technique will therefore revive and refresh the sexual life of couples who are prepared for it.

worldwide and has much to do with their sexual upbringing.

- **Orgasmic insensitivity.** When the woman does not feel the contractions produced during orgasm, although she has achieved it.
- **Other problems.** The problems that prevent sexual enjoyment include vaginismus, that is to say involuntary movements of the vaginal muscles which make it impossible for the penis to penetrate, dyspareunia, or painful coitus, and phobic avoidance—fear of a sexual relationship.

Some ways of overcoming apathy

- **Yoga.** Although physical activity may seem the opposite of relaxation and rest, keeping the body moving releases tension and activates the circulation.
- **A healthy, balanced diet.** If the body has enough energy it will be able actively to tac-

kle all the challenges of the day and the night. It is recommended to opt for a Mediterranean diet and avoid stimulants which, although they can reawaken desire, cause poor sexual performance (alcohol, coffee, tea, cigarettes, drugs).

- **Relaxation with music.** If the nerves are on edge, music can be an excellent ally.
- **Empowering self-esteem.** Libido will depend to a large extent on a healthy level of self-esteem and a good self-image. Insecurity generates tension and tension inhibits sexual desire.
- **Masturbation.** It is useful to masturbate on your own terrain, alone, only in the company of your own body and with the help of your imagination. It is good to lose your inhibitions, release yourself, and enjoy your own body without any embarrassment or psychological
- **Burdens.** Masturbation is the best way of discovering the physical and mental stimuli that awaken your desire and sexual responses.

▪▪ Learning to communicate again

Sexual relations are a reflection of the existing relationship between the couple. Respect, tenderness, details, suggestions, and preliminaries are fundamental to maintaining a satisfactory sex life.

One of the basic rules for maintaining a satisfactory sexual relationship with a partner is to talk sincerely, that is to say, always to show the other person what you want and feel. It can be affirmed that frankness is the key to the door of sexual satisfaction. The following advice will probably be very helpful.

- Take the trouble to ascertain the preferences of your partner and find out how to satisfy them.

- During the sexual act, specify what you want or like: frequency, method, speed, intensity, etc.

- Never be afraid to express everything that worries you, especially if it concerns an aspect of your own sexual satisfaction, such as, anorgasmia, for example (difficulty in reaching orgasm).

- Problems must not be evaded: you should discuss them sincerely and try to resolve them together.

- When a couple has problems, they directly affect their sex life. That is why it is so important to maintain a good communication system and so overcome any obstacle that may be hindering the relationship, otherwise they can end by reducing the sexual appetite.

Moreover, disappointment with sex as a couple often derives from the inability to reach orgasm in coitus. Masturbating in private helps discover the best ways of reaching climax, and even multiple orgasms, as the vast majority of women easily reach climax while pleasuring themselves.

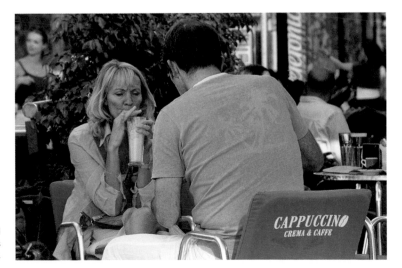

The basis of any good sexual relationsip is confidence.

Some myths

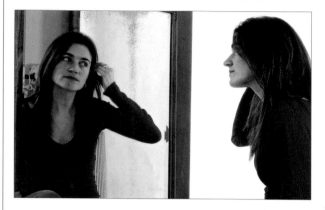

• **Women don't have wet dreams**. Nocturnal orgasms are the female version of male wet dreams. The fact that female arousal during deep REM sleep is not externally visible does not mean that it does not occur.

• **Simultaneous orgasms give greater pleasure than orgasms experienced separately.** The idea is romantic and there is no doubt that achieving orgasm together produces a very special feeling. The problem arises when the idea becomes an obsession. Mutual satisfaction should be sought, regardless of when each person experiences pleasure.

• **Impotence in old age has physical causes. Sexual desire and capacity diminish after the age of 50.** It is difficult to determine whether the decline in active sex observed in studies of people after a certain age is due to purely physical causes, or whether cultural conditioning plays a part in it. The passage of the years does not have to affect sexual desire or cause impotence, but external causes have to be considered, such as illness or the family situation.

• **Vaginal orgasm and clitoral orgasm are different things.** The clitoris is a fairly long organ, and much of it is internal, just above the entrance to the vagina. It is therefore impossible to have a vaginal orgasm without the participation of the clitoris.

• **Coitus should be avoided during pregnancy.** This myth is still alive because of the fear of affecting the progress of the pregnancy and the lack of available information. Although during the first three months the woman may suffer reduced sexual desire due to the physical changes caused by the start of gestation, in the second three months it usually reappears, together with arousal and the capacity to increase the quality of the orgasm.

• **Alcohol and marijuana are sexual stimulants**. The fact that alcohol and marijuana remove inhibitions makes many people believe it helps improve their sexual performance. However, the fact is that in many cases two or three drinks are enough to eliminate erection in men and make orgasmic response more difficult in women, because alcohol is a powerful depressant of the nervous system. Marijuana works very similarly and, as with alcohol, if it is smoked regularly it can lead to a loss of interest in sex in both men and women. In women, vaginal lubrication is reduced, which can make coitus painful. Men can find their sperm production reduced and weakened.

• **Anal sex indicates homosexual tendencies.** The desire to experiment with anal sex has nothing to do with homosexuality, as the practice is not confined to homosexuals. Forty percent of heterosexual couples acknowledge that they have tried it at least once.

• **Oral sex is perverted.** We may like it or not, but not only is oral sex not a perversion, it is one of the most gratifying ways of enjoying sexuality and a way of activating and intensifying arousal.

• **Masturbation is a habit indulged in by young and immature people.** Although masturbation is usually started in puberty, many people never give it up, as it helps them discover their own body and enjoy it. It makes it easier to explain to the partner which are the most excitable zones, the actions a person desires at any moment, and what will cause the greatest pleasure.

Family planning and contraceptive methods

It is every woman's right to plan her family. To decide freely, responsibly, and in an informed manner about the number and spacing of her children is fundamental, although of course her partner should also share in the decision.

What is family planning?

Family planning is the use of natural or artificial procedures to prevent pregnancy, giving couples the opportunity of deciding both the number of children they will have and the intervals between births completely voluntarily. These procedures can be temporary or permanent.

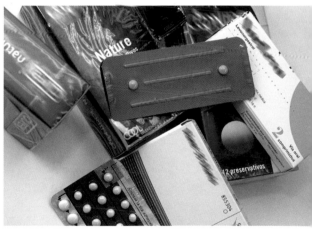

It is important to know and follow the instructions for use of each contraceptive method, as the correct use of the method chosen is the best guarantee of avoiding the risks of sexual relations (unplanned pregnancies and, in some cases, sexually transmitted diseases).

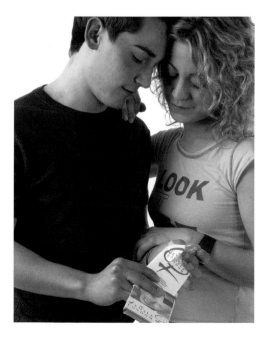

Contraceptive methods are defined as all actions designed to enjoy the erotic sexual function, exercising voluntary and responsible control over reproduction. There are methods of regulating fertility that differ in their characteristics, level of effectiveness, side effects, and functionality. The principal function of these methods is to facilitate

EFFECTIVE, EASY TO USE CONTRACEPTIVE	
Once a day	• Combined pills
Once a week	• Gestagen pills
Once a month	• Intravaginal contraceptive ring • Intramuscular progestagen injection

EFFECTIVE LONG-TERM OR PERMANENT CONTRACEPTIVE	
Temporary	• IUD (intra-uterine device) • Hormonal implant
Permanent	• Tying the fallopian tubes • Intratubal devices • Vasectomy (for the man)

responsible sexuality, which is considered a sexual and reproductive right of men and women.

Other less effective contraceptive methods

The rhythm method confines protected sex to the part of the menstrual cycle when a pregnancy could occur, between its 10th and 18th days.

It is a very unreliable method.

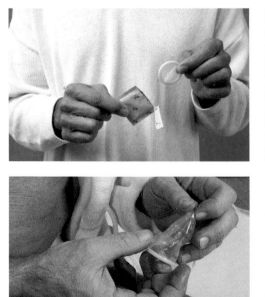

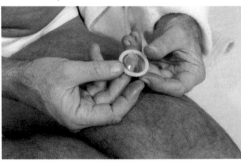

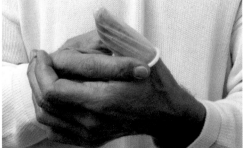

EFFECTIVE, EASY TO USE CONTRACEPTION

ONCE A DAY	ONCE A WEEK	ONCE A MONTH

Combined pill

Contains contraceptive hormones (estrogen and gestagen) that impede ovulation and, depending on the type of pill the doctor prescribes, a different pattern is followed.

Advantages:

• Easy to use.

• Reduces/eliminates menstrual pain.

• Regulates the menstrual cycle.

• Reduces acne and unwanted body hair.

Disadvantages:

• Becomes less effective in the case of vomiting or taking certain medication, some antibiotics, for example.

• Must be taken correctly. No pill must be missed.

• There are certain medical contraindications with this method, so it must be prescribed by a qualified person.

Mini-pill

Contains only gestagen, also spelled progestagens, (progesterone), which impedes ovulation and so is as effective as the combined pill. It is taken daily without any break. These pills are especially indicated for women during breastfeeding, or for those who are intolerant or present certain contraindications for estrogens.

Advantages:

• Easy to remember, as it is taken without a break.

• Useful for estrogen-intolerant women.

• Indicated during breastfeeding.

Disadvantages:

• No pill must be forgotten.

• Bleeding pattern variable and unpredictable in each woman.

Contraceptive patch

Releases contraceptive hormones that are absorbed through the skin. Can be placed anywhere on the body when the skin is clean, dry, and hairless. It is pressed on firmly for 10 seconds to ensure it has stuck properly. The patch is used weekly. It is changed every week for the 1st three weeks followed by a patch-free week. The wearer must ensure that the patch is firmly stuck.

Advantages:

• Very effective, just like the pill.

• Avoids having to take a pill every day.

• Less likelihood of forgetting.

• Easy to use.

Disadvantages:

• Not very discreet.

• You have to make sure it is firmly stuck, as it can come off and cease to be effective.

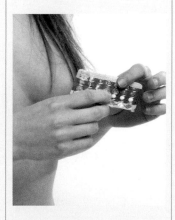

As a rule, any healthy woman can take the pill. However, it is not recommended to take it before the age of 16, to allow sexual maturation to take place naturally, or after the age of 45. At that age, the risk of heart or blood vessel problems increases. Between those two ages, and if there is no disease and no history to contraindicate its use, the pill is a safe and effecttive alternative. It is also not recommended to smoke while taking the pill. This warning becomes more important as the woman approaches the age of 35.

Vaginal contraceptive ring

A flexible plastic ring which the woman places in her vagina like a tampon. The ring has to remain in place for the next 3 weeks. It is removed after the 3rd week, when the period will occur. This ring releases contraceptive hormones in very low, regular doses, which pass into the blood through the vaginal walls, preventing ovulation.

Advantages:

• As effective as the pill.

• Monthly method.

• Little likelihood of forgetting.

• Easy to use.

• Comfortable, imperceptible, invisible, does not fall out.

Disadvantages:

• Some women find it hard to get used to handling and inserting the ring into the vagina.

• Must not remain out of the vagina for more than three hours.

• Must be prescribed by qualified staff.

Intramuscular progesterone injection

This is an intramuscular injection of progesterone that impedes ovulation.

Advantages:

• Can be administered monthly or 3-monthly.

• Is very effective.

• Less likelihood of forgetting.

Disadvantages:

• During the first months, there can be irregularities in menstrual bleeding.

• The periods can cease.

• There is a risk of weight gain.

• It must be prescribed by qualified staff.

TEMPORARY	PERMANENT	BARRIER CONTRACEPTION: EFFECTIVE AND PROTECTS AGAINST SEXUALLY TRANSMITTED DISEASES

Intrauterine device (IUD)

Made of copper, it prevents the passage of sperm into the uterus (womb) and avoids fertilization of the egg and its implantation into the wall of the uterus. It lasts three to five years. IUDs with hormones combine the effects already described with the hormonal effects of progestogens. Combined IUDs are effective for longer, up to 5 years.

Advantages:

• Easy to use.

• No risk of forgetting.

• Very effective.

Disadvantages:

• Some women have copious and painful periods.

• Can be spontaneously expelled.

• Intolerance and secondary effects can occur.

• Relative contraindication for women who have never been pregnant.

Hormonal implant

A hormonal implant is a small rod inserted under the skin of the arm that releases hormones. It is especially appropriate for women seeking long-term contraception for whom estrogens are counter-indicated or who want an alternative to having their fallopian tubes tied.

Advantages

• It reduces menstrual pain

• There is no risk of forgetting

• It is easy to insert

• It is very effective

Disadvantages

• It must be inserted and removed by a trained doctor

• Menstrual bleeding can be variable and unpredictable.

Tying the tubes

During a surgical procedure, the uterine or fallopian tubes are cut and tied off, thus preventing the fertilized egg reaching the uterus, permanently preventing fertilization.

Intratubal devices

In a single operation, an intratubal device is inserted into each tube, causing an inflammation that obstructs them. An alternative method (e.g. condom or contraceptive pills) must be used for 3 months after the operation, until the doctor has checked that the tubes are totally blocked.

• In men, the surgical method equivalent to tubetying is vasectomy. This is a very simple operation in which the tubes that carry the sperm are cut and tied, thus preventing their inclusion in the ejaculate. Only a few weeks afterwards, it is safe and permanent. An alternative method must be used (e.g. condom or pills) until a check has been carried out to confirm the absence of sperm.

Condom for men

A latex sheath that covers the erect penis during coitus and retains the semen. Press the end of the condom (deposit), remove any air remaining in the chamber and roll the condom along the erect penis to its base. Once coitus is over, remove the condom before the penis loses its erection, squeezing it by the base to prevent it staying inside the vagina.

Condoms for women

A transparent plastic sheath with two rings at the ends that adjust to the walls of the vagina and retain the semen.

• It is inserted into the vagina, grasping the ring at the closed end, from the end of the condom.

• IThen a finger is inserted into the condom to locate it deep inside the vagina, leaving the external ring outside to prevent the penis contacting the vagina.

• IAfter coitus, the external ring is given a couple of turns to prevent the semen coming out, and the condom is removed.

Advantages:

• Both types of condom are easy to obtain and fit, and offer protection against sexually transmitted diseases.

Disadvantages:

• They can break.

• The penis must be withdrawn immediately after ejaculation.

• Although the condom for women enables the woman to deal with her own contraception, it does make some noise and is not very esthetically pleasing.

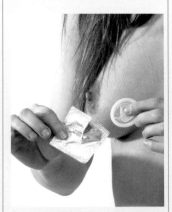

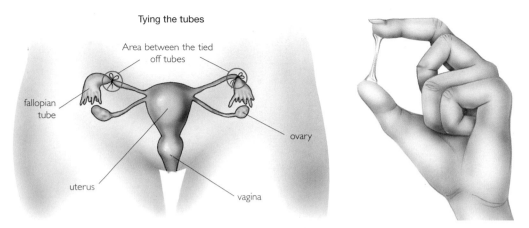

Tying the tubes

Area between the tied off tubes

fallopian tube

ovary

uterus

vagina

The elasticity of the mucous in the vaginal fluid varies during ovulation, and can be detected with careful observation.

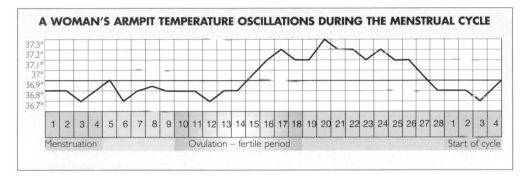

A WOMAN'S ARMPIT TEMPERATURE OSCILLATIONS DURING THE MENSTRUAL CYCLE

37,3°
37,2°
37,1°
37°
36,9°
36,8°
36,7°

1 2 3 4 5 6 7 8 9 10 11 12 13 14 15 16 17 18 19 20 21 22 23 24 25 26 27 28 1 2 3 4

Menstruation   Ovulation – fertile period   Start of cycle

◢ Which contraceptive method to choose?

- No method of contraception is perfect. The choice of method is a decision which the couple, or in this case the woman, must take freely, bearing in mind a series of factors such as, for example, the type of relationships she maintains, their frequency, her age and state of health, her partner's situation, the doctor's recommendation, etc.

- To make the right choice, she needs to know the different methods, their advantages and disadvantages, their effectiveness and price, how to obtain them, etc.

- Before choosing a contraceptive method, she should consult a gynecologist about their characteristics, use, advantages, disadvantages, effectiveness, etc.

- Coitus interruptus (withdrawal)

The man withdraws his penis from the vagina before ejaculation. There is a risk that some sperm may escape from the penis. It is a very unreliable method.

- Basal temperature method

The temperature must be taken (under the arm, under the tongue or anally) every morning before getting up and before taking physical exercise. Ovulation is determined by a slight rise in the temperature—less than 2°F (0.5°C). During this time the couple should abstain from having sex until the temperature falls to its initial level. Because many factors can affect the basal temperature and the temperature rise is not clear, it is a very unreliable contraceptive method.

- Cervical mucous method

The woman has to put a finger into her vagina, remove a little cervical mucous and check its viscosity. During ovulation it takes on a viscous appearance similar to egg white. A very unreliable method.

EFFECTIVE CONTRACEPTIVE THAT PROTECTS AGAINST SEXUALLY TRANSMITTED DISEASES (STDS)
• Condom for men • Condom for women

PACKET CONTAINING	TAKING THE PILL	REST PERIOD
21 pills	One pill a day for 21 days	7 days
22 pills	One pill a day for 22 days	6 days
28 pills	One pill every day for 28 days	No break

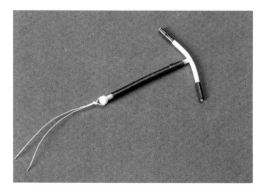

• Spermicide

This is a cream which is applied inside the vagina and supposedly deactivates sperm. It is an unreliable method, but one which can be very useful for avoiding pregnancy when used together with a condom.

• Diaphragm

This is a barrier contraceptive method consisting of a flexible circular rubber cap that covers the neck of the uterus, preventing sperm from entering the cervical channel. It is important to combine it with a spermicide. It is not a very safe method.

The diaphragm is a rubber disk or cap that the woman places inside her vagina before starting the sexual act. The woman needs previously to have been taught how to insert it and locate it over the neck of the uterus with her fingers.

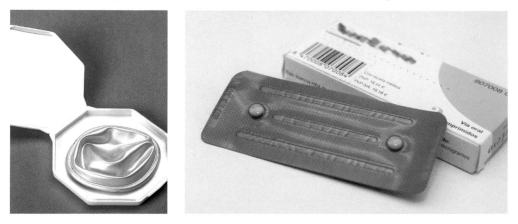

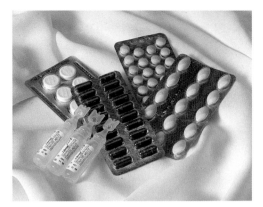

Hormonal methods. These are based on the administration of medication containing synthetic hormones, similar to female hormones, that prevent the ovary from ovulating. They can be used in the form of pills that are taken every day for 21 days following the first day of menstruation, never forgetting to take one. During the 7 days following the last dose, a period will occur and a new cycle will begin. Nowadays, this method can take the form of a single monthly injection or of implants placed under the skin that release hormones progressively. In certain cases, hormonal treatment gives rise to complications, so women should consult a gynecologist before adopting this method.

■ Other, less effective, contraceptive methods

- Rhythm method
- Coitus interruptus
- Basal temperature method
- Cervical mucous method
- Spermicides
- Diaphragm

RHYTHM METHOD

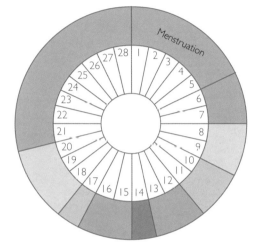

- Low risk days
- High risk days
- Ovulation (high risk day)
- Moderate risk days for regular cycles
- Moderate risk days for irregular cycles

- The "morning after" pill

The postcoital pill is not a contraceptive method but an emergency remedy. It is a combination of hormones that alters the female reproductive cycle, preventing a pregnancy from going to term if one has started. The morning after pill acts by inhibiting ovulation and preventing fertilization. It is almost 100 percent effective when taken within 24 to 72 hours of unprotected coitus.

This product does not have the undesirable side effects of the contraceptives usually taken to avoid pregnancy. Emergency contraception must be administered within 72 hours of the act of unprotected coitus (that is to say, sexual relations without any kind of protection). It can be administered only on a doctor's prescription.

It is not recommended as a customary contraceptive method, but should be considered only as an emergency method, that is to say, for use in exceptionally unforeseen situations.

The perfect age at which young people should start to have full active sex cannot be established, because it depends on each individual's personal circumstances. However, the time when they should start using contraceptive methods to avoid pregnancy can indeed be clearly determined—from the first moment when they have sex involving penetration.

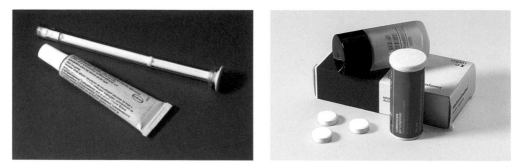

Spermicides are creams or gels containing substances that destroy sperm and should be used in combination with the diaphragm.

Starting to use contraception

A person's first sexual relationship is a vital experience requiring a series of precautions that few adolescents take into account. Losing one's virginity should not be viewed as a challenge, achievement, or escape, or be done to avoid ridicule from friends. It is essential to feel loved in return and to take the time necessary for the sexual act not to be experienced under pressure or with feelings of guilt. Using your head before going to bed with someone should be an obligation shared by the couple embarking on sexual love, so as not to run unnecessary risks such as premature pregnancy, venereal diseases, or big disappointments.

Young people should not rely on the contraceptive information given by friends and companions of their own age, but should seek information from family planning centers dedicated to that function.

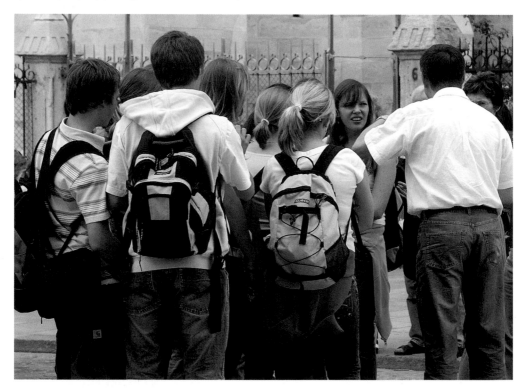

The most reliable information on contraceptive methods is available to all, although many prefer to ignore it, by believing in some old wife's tale or remembering the date of the girl's period that they will not be in any danger, but that is not true.

Most adolescent pregnancies could have been avoided if adequate methods had been used.

Contraception is the way to avoid pregnancy using methods or products which interfere with the mechanisms that make it possible. It is wise to remember that if a person has sex quite regularly and does not use any method of contraception, the probability of pregnancy is very high: about 80 percent in a year. It is most important to understand all the existing contraceptive methods so as to be able to choose the right one for each case. The choice of one method or another will depend on many factors, such as the frequency of sex, the person's age, personal preferences, etc. In any case, if no method is to hand, petting is the most reasonable practice.

When young people ask what is the best contraceptive method, specialists usually reply that no ideal method exists that suits everyone, but what they will say is that the best contraceptive must possess the following characteristics: it must be reliable, innocuous, and readily accepted by the couple.

EFFECTIVENESS OF CONTRACEPTION	
Method	Percentage of women who become pregnant during the first year of using it
Hormonal implants	Less than 0.1
Oral contraceptives: • Estrogen-progesterone combination pills • Progestagen pills	0.1-3 0.5-3
Injectable medroxiprogesterone	0.3
Intrauterine device	0.6-2
Condoms • For men • For women	3-12 5-21
Diaphragm with spermicide	6-18
Cervical diaphragm with spermicide	11.5-18
Rhythm method	20

THE MOST WIDELY USED CONTRACEPTIVE METHODS

Oral contraceptives
Disadvantages and risks
- Gives no protection against sexually transmitted diseases (STDs) and AIDS.
- Must be taken every day.
- Can cause side-effects such as nausea, painful breasts, weight gain, fluid retention, increased blood pressure, mood changes, and migraines.

Effectiveness: 98%
Comments
- Not recommended for women aged over 35 who smoke or have suffered heart attacks, embolisms, or severe circulatory problems, cancer, liver troubles or high blood pressure.
- The periods will be more regular.
- Helps prevent cancer of the ovaries and uterus.
- Reduces menstrual pain.

Implant
Disadvantages and risks
- Gives no protection against STDs and AIDS.
- Irregular periods and bleeding during the first year.
- Possibility of painful breasts, weight gain, and pain in the implant area.
- Small incision necessary to implant it which must be done in a medical center.
- The surgery to extract it can be complex.
- The wounds it causes can leave bruising or scars.

Effectiveness: 98%
Comments
- Not recommended for women suffering breast cancer, phlebitis of the tubes, or serious liver diseases, or women taking medication against convulsions.
- A good option for women who forget to take the contraceptive pill.

Injection
Disadvantages and risks
- Gives no protection against STDs and AIDS.
- Changes in menstruation.
- Weight gain.
- Infertility can last up to 18 months after the last injection.
- Increases the possibility of breast cancer.
- Bone density may decrease after about 10 years and cause osteoporosis in the long term.
- Nervous problems, headaches, apathy, mood changes, and depression.

Effectiveness: 97%
Comments
- Almost all women suffer menstrual changes.
- Requires four visits to the gynecologist per year.
- The injection is better than the pill for women who smoke, because it does not contain estrogen.
- It can be used when breastfeeding, after giving birth.

IUD – Intrauterine device
Disadvantages and risks
- Gives no protection against STDs and AIDS.
- The periods may be heavier.
- There is a possibility of contracting a womb infection, especially if the woman has sex with different partners.
- In some cases the womb may be perforated, leading to hemorrhage or infection, and resulting in infertility.
- The body may expel the IUD.
- The man may feel the thread.

Effectiveness: 95%
Comments
- A mutually monogamous relationship is recommended

Cervical cap
Disadvantages and risks
- Without a condom, it does not prevent the propagation of STDs and AIDS.
- It may interrupt foreplay if it is not been inserted beforehand.
- Some women find it difficult to insert and remove.
- There is a risk of cervical irritation or allergy.
- It may come loose during the sexual act.

Effectiveness: 70%
Comments
- Infection is less likely than with a diaphragm.
- Not recommended if the user has suffered toxic shock syndrome or pelvic inflammation, or any cervical or vaginal infection.
- Helps a woman to become more familiar with her body.
- Needs to be adjusted after giving birth.

Diaphragm
Disadvantages and risks
- Without a condom, it does not stop the spread of STDs and AIDS.
- It may interrupt foreplay if it has not been inserted beforehand.
- Some women find it difficult to insert and remove.
- Increases the possibility of suffering infections.
- Possibility of allergic reaction.
- If the woman's weight varies, the size of the diaphragm needs to be adjusted.

Effectiveness: 75-80% and higher if used with spermicides.
Comments
- A good option for women who are breastfeeding and don't want to take hormones.
- Should not be used if the woman has suffered toxic shock syndrome.

Spermicides
Disadvantages and risks
- Are not very hygienic.
- Can interrupt foreplay.

- Risk of vaginal infections.
- Possibility of allergic reaction.
- The smell and taste of the chemicals could reduce oral sexual enjoyment.

Effectiveness: 35-50%
Comments
- Should not be used if the woman has suffered toxic shock syndrome.

Condom for men
Disadvantages and risks
- Has to be put on before active sex.
- Can reduce sensation in the man.
- Possibility of allergy to latex.
- There may be leakage, or it may break.
- The erection may fail due to the interruption of foreplay.

Effectiveness: 80-90%
Comments
- Should not be used with lubricants such as Vaseline or baby oil.
- Two condoms at once, or the condom for men and the condom for women, should not be used together.
- To facilitate putting it on, it can become part of foreplay.

Condom for women
Disadvantages and risks
- Can reduce the sensitivity of the partner, and even of the woman herself.
- Possibility of allergy to latex.
- Can become dislodged or break.
- Can be uncomfortable for the outer part of the vulva.

Effectiveness: 80-90%
Comments
- Should not be used at the same time as the condom for men.

The morning after pill
(emergency contraceptive)
Disadvantages and risks
- Can cause nausea or discomfort associated with the high hormonal level.
- Works only up to 72 hours after having unprotected sex.

Effectiveness: 80-90%
Comments
- Is not a contraceptive.
- Was not created for continuous or regular use.

Tube tying
Disadvantages and risks
- Requires medical supervision before, during, and after the operation.
- Anesthesia brings risks.
- Possibility of regretting having it done.
Effectiveness: 98-99%
Comments
- This is the best option, if the woman is sure she never wants to become pregnant, or does not want any more children.

Sterility and infertility

Many couples want to have their own child but cannot do so for any number of reasons. However, this problem, which used to be irreversible and had a series of emotional, family, and psychological consequences, can now be overcome thanks to scientific and technological progress.

Is sterility the same as infertility?

Traditionally, infertility and sterility have been considered synonymous and represent the difficulty the couple has in achieving pregnancy or successfully continuing a pregnancy to term after having sexual relations for a year without using any kind of contraception. However, in fact infertility means that the woman does succeed in becoming pregnant but does not achieve birth, and sterility applies to a woman who cannot achieve pregnancy at all.

Sterility and infertility can be classified as follows:

• Primary infertility, when the couple achieves a pregnancy, but it does not continue to term, and secondary infertility, when after achieving a normal

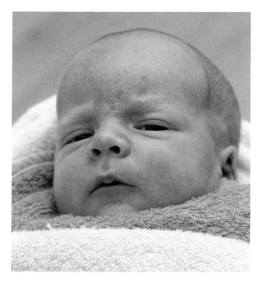

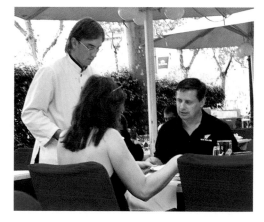

Difficulty in conceiving a child should be understood as the problem of both members of the couple. Traditionally, it used to be the woman who felt the social pressure and obligation to "start a family," and was held responsible for any difficulty in conceiving. If she never succeeded in conceiving children, society considered the woman incomplete. However, the problem of infertility affects men and women equally.

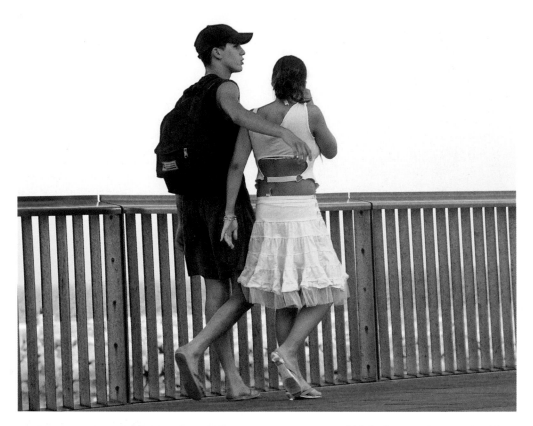

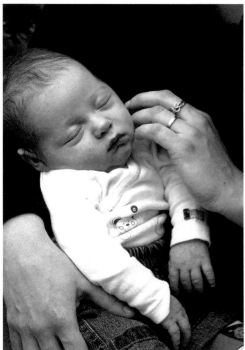

pregnancy and birth, the couple cannot achieve a further pregnancy, or that further pregnancy does not continue to term.

• Primary sterility, when, after having active sex for eighteen months without using any contraception, the couple has not achieved a pregnancy, and secondary sterility, when, after having a first child, the couple does not achieve a second pregnancy within two or three years of having sexual relations without using contraception.

The decision to visit an assisted conception clinic is not an easy one. These clinics are usually consulted by men and women aged between 35 and 40 who have been trying to achieve pregnancy for many years without success. As a rule they have tried the traditional control methods of basal temperature, uterine mucous, etc. with no result.

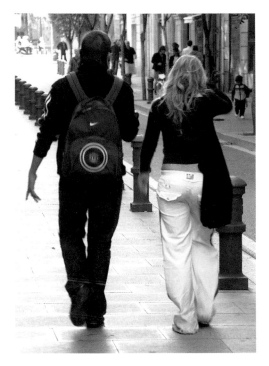

abnormal, there may be testicular irregularities, obstructed tubes, prostate problems, or problems with erection or ejaculation.

Another 40 percent of cases of infertility are due to problems in the woman, such as early menopause, endometriosis (a disease that affects the lining of the uterus), obstructions or lesions in the fallopian tubes, uterine and cervical anomalies, or problems with ovulation. Twenty percent of cases correspond to mixed causes in which both members of the couple are responsible.

Causes of infertility

Physical factors in the woman

• Cervical factor: there can be anatomical or functional irregularities (polyps, cysts, chance or surgical injuries) that interfere with the route taken by the sperm from the vagina to one of the tubes where fertilization of the egg occurs.

• Uterine factor: there can be uterine problems (malformations, benign myomas (also known as

At present, the man is responsible in 40 percent of cases of infertility. The man's sperm production may be inadequate, or his sperm may be

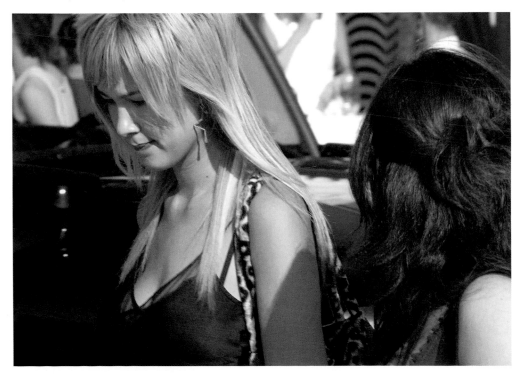

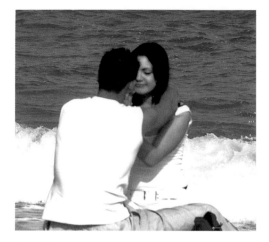

re medication), and coital irregularities (impotence). These factors cause the absence of sperm (azoospermia), or the scarcity or inadequate quality of sperm (oligospermia).

Lifestyle-related factors

In both men and women, stress, diet, or the intensive practice of certain sports can upset the hormonal balance, as can the excessive intake of alcohol and drugs. Environmental toxins and substances such as pesticides influence fertility, as do psychic and emotional factors.

The assessment of a couple consulting a clinic about sterility

It is important to remember that both members of the couple should be studied at the same time. It is pointless to subject a woman to numerous troublesome and sometimes expensive examinations over the years, only to discover that her partner's or sperm count was so irregular that her chances of becoming pregnant were greatly reduced.

The cause of their sterility should be diagnosed quickly, to avoid discouraging and exhausting the couple, thus reducing their desire to start treatment.

In the case of the woman, the various factors involved in fertilization are studied:

• Ovarian factor. The woman's production of oocytes and hormones is assessed, to check whether or not she is ovulating. Indirect indications are considered, such as:

• Measuring the basal temperature. The temperature must be taken anally every morning before getting out of bed, and recorded on a chart to see whether it increases at any time during her cycle.

• Transvaginal ultrasound scan. An ultrasound scan is carried out during the preovulation period, to see whether a reasonably large follicle exists that suggests it is about to burst and release the egg. An examination is also made of the endometrium, the inner lining of the uterus that continually changes its structure, shape, and thickness at various points in the female sexual cycle under the influence of hormones.

• The determination of the hormones during the first days of the cycle enables the doctor to assess the functioning of the ovary, the hypophysis, and the egg reserve.

• Tuboperitoneal factor. For fertilization to take place, the female genital organs that allow the egg

fibroids) or tumors, adhesions to the walls, etc.), or endometrial problems.

• Tuboperitoneal factor: irregularities in the tubes or the space of the ovarian tubes, because of infections (that can obstruct the tubes) or for other reasons, such as endometriosis (the appearance of endometrial (or uterine) tissue outside the uterus [womb], and in the ovaries and ligaments that attach the uterus to the pelvis).

• Ovarian endocrine factor: chronic (as opposed to circumstantial) anovulation. This can be caused by a malfunction of the hypothalamus and the hypophysis, so that the gland does not produce enough of the hormone, gonadotrophin that stimulates the ovaries to generate eggs, or produces too much of it. There can also be ovulation irregularities caused by problems with other hormones, such as an increase in prolactin, or thyroid irregularities.

Physical factors in the man

• Pretesticular factor: irregularities in the hormones that stimulate the testicle. These are infrequent.

• Testicular factor: irregularities in the testicle. These can be genetic, congenital (since birth), or acquired (mumps, exposure to radiation, certain medicines, injuries, varicose veins, etc.).

• Post-testicular factor: This affects the sperm once they have left the testicle, and obstructs the route traveled by the sperm (of congenital origin, such as malformation of the deferent conduits, or caused by injuries, or voluntary ligature, such as vasectomy), seminal infections, the presence of antispermatic antibodies, ejaculatory irregularities (caused, for example, by diabetes or blood-pressu-

to meet the sperm must be permeable. To ascertain this, a hysterosalpingography is carried out. This is a radiographic study in which a contrasting device is inserted through the neck of the uterus to compare the uterine cavities with the fallopian tubes, showing whether or not there is permeability, and the level at which the obstruction, if any, is located.

• Cervical factor. The neck of the uterus is the first point the sperm need to reach. The cervical mucous changes its appearance, fluidity, quantity, and consistency, according to the stage of the cycle, which is dependent on hormonal changes from month to month.

Laparoscopy

Laparoscopy is a study carried out under general anesthesia. A camera is inserted through the wall of the lower abdomen to examine the internal genital organs. This procedure provides information about the anatomy of the ovaries, tubes, and uterus. It enables any adhesions between the organs to be diagnosed, as well as endometriosis, quite a frequent condition in women that can adversely affect the couple's fertility.

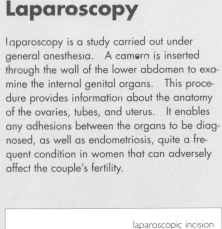

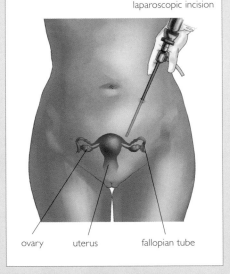

laparoscopic incision

ovary   uterus   fallopian tube

The most usual methods

There are three main types of fertility treatment: ovarian induction, low complexity assisted conception (artificial insemination), and high-complexity assisted conception (assisted conception techniques or invitro fertilization). The method chosen will depend on what caused the infertility.

Ovarian induction (OI)

• This consists of the stimulation of ovulation with hormonal preparations, administered orally or by injections, so as to achieve correct ovulation.

• Ultrasound scans are taken periodically to see the number of follicles the woman is generating.

• After three or four procedures, the cycle is usually ended to avoid multiple pregnancies.

• If fertilization is not achieved naturally, this technique is usually combined with artificial insemination.

• It is indicated in cases of anovulation and to make artificial insemination more effective.

Artificial insemination (AI)

• With this technique, semen is inserted into the neck of the uterus using a fine tube or catheter to facilitate fertilization.

• The semen used can be that of the woman's partner or of an anonymous donor.

• If the semen of the woman's partner is used, it is obtained by masturbation on the day when the insemination is to take place. The couple is recommended not to have active sex or masturbate during the preceding days and before obtaining the semen on the day of the procedure, the man should reach the maximum level of arousal beforehand. This will guarantee a better quality and quantity of semen.

• Sometimes, in men with a low sperm count (oligospermia), or men with transmissible diseases (such as AIDS), the sperm can be washed to eliminate impurities and isolate and concentrate the spermatozoids, to avoid any problem. If this is not possible, a sperm bank can always be used.

• This technique is indicated for couples who have cervical problems, semen or ejaculation irregularities, or anatomical malformations of the male reproductive organs, and whose infertility has unknown causes.

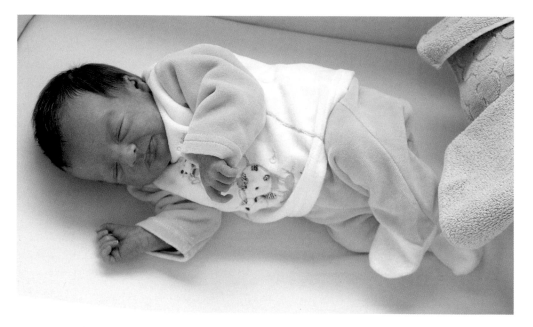

Preimplantation Genetic Diagnosis, or PGD, is a sophisticated technique enabling the embryo to be examined before it is implanted, in order to diagnose chromosome irregularities, principally trisomies (such as the trisomy that causes Down's syndrome). It also enables the sex of the embryo to be ascertained. This is not merely a whim, but a very important matter for couples with hemophilia problems, for whom choosing the sex of the baby may be vital to prevent their child inheriting the disease.

Assisted conception techniques or in-vitro fertilization (IVF)

• This consists of the fertilization of the egg by sperm in an artificial environment, such as a laboratory.

• The ovaries are stimulated first to make them produce eggs that can then be collected.

• During this procedure, the woman is given sedatives, although she can leave the hospital after a couple of hours.

• The rest of the process is conducted in the laboratory, and consists of fertilizing the egg with capacitated sperm.

• Three to five fertilized eggs (zygotes) are implanted in the woman's uterus, 48 to 72 hours after insemination. This does not require anesthesia and is painless.

• Gestation and birth proceed normally.

• If pregnancy does not occur, another attempt is made during the woman's next menstrual cycle.

• This IVF technique includes the intratubal transfer of gametes which requires at least one of the woman's fallopian tubes to be working normally.

• It consists of isolating and extracting eggs directly from the ovary, after ovarian stimulation.

• Three to five eggs are transferred to the fallopian tube, where the semen is also deposited.

• If fertilization occurs, the embryo is then transferred to the uterus.

• Either a general or a local anesthetic is administered, depending on the method used to extract the eggs.

Pregnancy

A woman experiences many changes throughout her life, but pregnancy is the condition when the greatest number of changes occurs in a short time. Many women experience their pregnancies with the sense of never having felt better in their lives, while others find it a difficult time. However, a wanted pregnancy will always bring new emotions with it that enable a woman to confront any difficulties positively.

Pregnancy

A pregnant woman's physical symptoms

• Tiredness is sometimes the commonest symptom and occurs mainly during the first trimester and the last month. During the 4th and 7th months, women usually feel great energy and vitality. It is not usual to feel extreme tiredness throughout a pregnancy and if she experiences it the woman should consult a specialist.

• Nausea and some vomiting often occur in the morning, although some women experience it all day. It normally occurs during the first 14 weeks. Excessive or recurrent vomiting requires medical treatment.

• Acidity (or "heartburn") after meals that can be caused by emotional disturbances, fatty meals, or eating too fast. An acid liquid is regurgitated from the stomach accompanied by a burning pain in the chest.

• A rise in estrogen and progesterone levels. The latter is particularly responsible for causing relaxation of the soft tissues such as muscles and ligaments. This can cause varicose veins and even back pain.

The commonest psychological symptoms

• Emotional sensitivity will increase. From the very first moment when a woman finds out she is pregnant, she has many fears, hopes, and motivations that change, both positively and negatively. It should be borne in mind that the pregnant woman

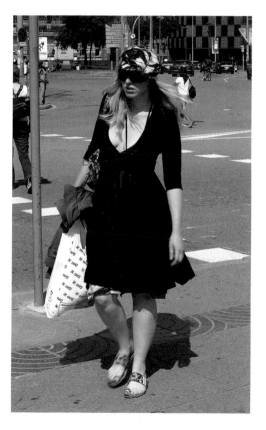

Being pregnant is in no way synonymous with being unwell. Pregnancy is a period in a woman's life for which she needs to be physically and mentally prepared.

Am I pregnant?

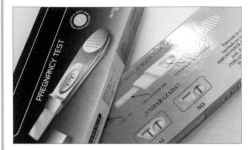

first day after a period is late. It offers high diagnostic precision and, although its results are not definitive, it can be carried out in comfort and privacy at home.

- Firstly, the commercially available urine test, in a few minutes detects the presence of the pregnancy hormone in the urine, from the

- Secondly, the laboratory urine test, which also detects the presence of the pregnancy hormone, and is more precise than the commercially available test, from as early as 7 to 10 days after conception has occurred.

- Lastly, the blood test, which determines the presence of the pregnancy hormone with great accuracy, some 7 to 10 days after conception has occurred.

CAMBIOS EN LA MUJER MES A MES

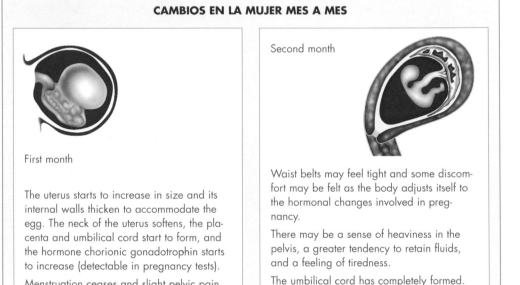

First month

The uterus starts to increase in size and its internal walls thicken to accommodate the egg. The neck of the uterus softens, the placenta and umbilical cord start to form, and the hormone chorionic gonadotrophin starts to increase (detectable in pregnancy tests).

Menstruation ceases and slight pelvic pain may occur, with tiredness, an increase in vaginal secretions, possible nausea and vomiting, and the need to urinate more frequently.

During the first month of pregnancy, the woman focuses on the emotional and physical changes she is experiencing. She may have sudden mood swings and even contradictory feelings about her maternity.

Second month

Waist belts may feel tight and some discomfort may be felt as the body adjusts itself to the hormonal changes involved in pregnancy.

There may be a sense of heaviness in the pelvis, a greater tendency to retain fluids, and a feeling of tiredness.

The umbilical cord has completely formed. The uterus changes from being pear-shaped to a rounder shape, similar to an orange.

The breasts increase in size, and there may be sensations in the nipples, the areola becomes darker and some weight may be lost.

Pimples and other skin disorders may appear because pregnancy causes an increase in fat secretions in the skin.

Third month

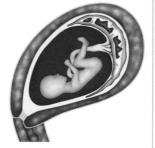

Nausea and discomfort start to disappear, and the pregnant woman's appetite improves, although cravings may persist or appear and certain odors may be found unpleasant.

The uterus is full of amniotic fluid and the placenta is small, but fulfills its function of secreting hormones (estrogen and progesterone) and passing nutrients from the mother to the baby.

The volume of blood of the mother-to-be will increase by between 40 and 50% during pregnancy. As a result, the woman may notice her veins more, especially on her stomach, breasts, and legs.

Marks may appear on the skin because of the hormonal upheaval involved in pregnancy.

Fourth month

The second trimester is the most comfortable and pleasant stage of pregnancy. Most of the most troublesome symptoms have ceased.

The top of the uterus reaches and passes the pubis.

The placenta and the amniotic fluid increase in size and quantity.

As the uterus stretches, some abdominal discomfort may be felt. This is absolutely normal and is known as the round ligament syndrome.

The woman's body begins to prepare to feed the baby. The breasts grow, and the areolas darken and increase in size.

The pregnancy hormones are leveling out, which means less nausea, less frequent urination, and less tiredness.

The woman may suffer from constipation.

Fifth month

Marks may appear on the forehead, cheeks, nose, and chin. These are typical marks produced by the hormones and disappear after giving birth.

It is very usual for the skin to itch and a rash may even appear, as the skin is being increasingly stretched.

Stretch marks may appear. These are easily preventable with moisturizing lotions and oils, which also relieve the dryness and itching.

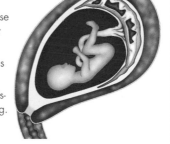

The uterus reaches about the size of a melon, reaching up to the navel. It contains about 2 pints (1 liter) of amniotic fluid.

The line between the navel and the pubic hair darkens (the black line). This pigmentation will lighten after giving birth.

The woman will probably gain more weight now, while the baby continues to grow.

The extra weight may make itself felt with back troubles and pain in the legs.

The ankles and feet may also feel and in fact be swollen. At the end of the day in particular, it is recommended to rest with the feet up.

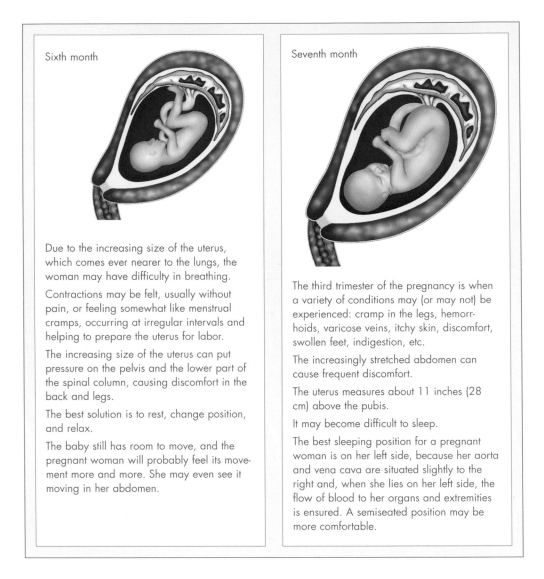

Sixth month

Seventh month

Due to the increasing size of the uterus, which comes ever nearer to the lungs, the woman may have difficulty in breathing.

Contractions may be felt, usually without pain, or feeling somewhat like menstrual cramps, occurring at irregular intervals and helping to prepare the uterus for labor.

The increasing size of the uterus can put pressure on the pelvis and the lower part of the spinal column, causing discomfort in the back and legs.

The best solution is to rest, change position, and relax.

The baby still has room to move, and the pregnant woman will probably feel its movement more and more. She may even see it moving in her abdomen.

The third trimester of the pregnancy is when a variety of conditions may (or may not) be experienced: cramp in the legs, hemorrhoids, varicose veins, itchy skin, discomfort, swollen feet, indigestion, etc.

The increasingly stretched abdomen can cause frequent discomfort.

The uterus measures about 11 inches (28 cm) above the pubis.

It may become difficult to sleep.

The best sleeping position for a pregnant woman is on her left side, because her aorta and vena cava are situated slightly to the right and, when she lies on her left side, the flow of blood to her organs and extremities is ensured. A semiseated position may be more comfortable.

should not magnify the emotions she feels to prevent them harming herself or those around her. Her state of mind is characterized by initial euphoria after hearing the news and the appearance of exaggerated fears throughout the pregnancy.

• Excessive anxiety about the baby's health, before and after it is born. To some extent this is natural provided it does not become an obsession and cause negative thoughts that interfere with her daily life.

• Anxiety characterized by irritability and restlessness.

• Fear of the pain of childbirth, which can cause a minor feeling of anticipated anguish.

Visits to the gynecologist and tests during pregnancy

When a woman wants to become pregnant, she is recommended to visit a gynecologist beforehand. This will increase her supervision and, therefore, ensure that the whole pregnancy will be as satisfactory as possible, minimizing the chances of unforeseen mishaps. The following steps are an indication of medical care during the pregnancy:

The first consultation

The first consultation is recommended when the woman decides she wants to have a baby. Even before becoming pregnant, it is recommen-

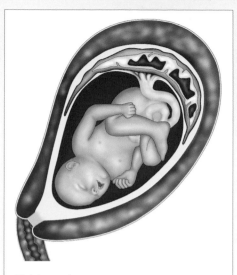

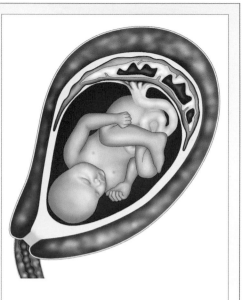

Eighth month

The top of the uterus can be felt about two fingers' width above the navel and presses on the organs more and more, which can cause difficulty in breathing, constipation, and indigestion.

During this period, the woman will gain weight at about 1 lb (500 grams) a week.

Visits to the doctor must become more frequent.

The obstetrician will make an examination to assess the neck of the womb, seek signs of dilatation, and try to ascertain the baby's position.

Ninth month

The uterus reaches the sternum, and the placenta measures some 8 inches (20 cm).

The vaginal fluid becomes increasingly copious, and uterine contractions begin. These may be of two kinds: false and true.

False contractions are irregular and painful, and may be felt in the pelvis and lower back.

True contractions begin at the top of the uterus and extend to the rest of it, growing stronger and more painful all the time, and cannot be alleviated by changing position.

ded to take folic acid, which will reduce the risks of a malformed fetus.

An analysis will also be carried out to specify whether there are any health problems such as diabetes or high blood pressure, in order to establish supervision from the very first moment, as well as authorizing the appropriate medication, so no problems will arise during pregnancy. The analysis will include a blood test for rubella (German measles), toxoplasmosis, syphilis, hepatitis B, and hepatitis C, to ascertain whether or not the future mother is immune.

The second consultation

When the pregnancy test gives a positive result,

the analytical tests of the first trimester will be done. A balanced diet is recommended, and alcohol, drugs, and tobacco are prohibited. The first ultrasound scan is carried out to determine the number of embryos present and where they are situated, as well as their viability.

Weeks 12 to 14

Ultrasound scans are taken to detect any structural anomalies and mental retardation indicators. During the 14th week, a hormonal analysis (triple screening) will be carried out—if the couple wants it—to ascertain the likelihood of Down's syndrome and spina bifida.

THE BABY'S DEVELOPMENT

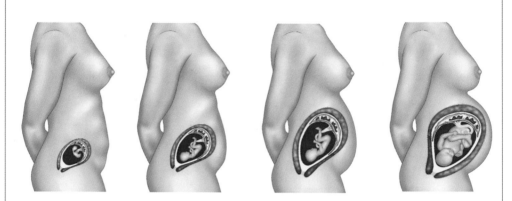

First month

The embryo looks like a disk. The head begins to develop as from the first week and, almost at the end of the first month, the heart begins to beat.   The placenta begins to form around the embryo. It is about 4 mm long and weighs less than 1 gram.

Second month

The eyes form and the arms and legs begin to grow. The internal organs and brain begin to develop. The embryo is about 1 inch (3 cm) long and weighs less than an ounce (3 grams). It floats in a kind of bag filled with amniotic fluid.

Third month

The fetus is now fully formed and moves its arms and legs. It has eyelids and is about 4 (10 cm) long. It weighs about 1 1/2 oz (45 grams).

Fourth month

The skin of the fetus is transparent and fine. Its body is completely covered in fine hair called lanugo. Its intestine begins to fill up with a greenish substance called meconium. It weighs about 6 oz (180 grams) and is a little less than 6 inches (15 cm) long.

Fifth month

The fetus sucks its thumb and begins to develop its defense systems. It already has hair on its head, as well as eyelashes and eyebrows. It weighs a little over 1 lb (500 grams) and is between 7 and 8 inches (18–20 cm) long.

Sixth month

The fetus spends between 18 and 20 hours asleep and, when awake, moves about a great deal. Its face is complete and it can open its eyes. The lungs develop. It is about 10 inches (25 cm) long and weighs nearly 2 1/4 lbs (1 kg).

Seventh month

The fetus responds to outside noise with movements and starts to feel cramped in the uterine cavity.   The first respiratory movements appear, although its lungs cannot function independently until it is born, once the umbilical cord is cut. It is a little under 12 inches (30 cm) long and weighs about 3 lb 5 oz (1.5 kg).

Eighth month

The fetus usually positions itself head downward.   Its skin becomes thicker and begins to turn pinkish.   It is about 13 1/2 inches (35 cm) long and weighs some 5 1/2 lbs (2.5 kg).

Ninth month

The fetus receives antibodies from its mother and its lungs are now ready to function in the outside world. Its skin ceases to be wrinkled and the lanugo falls off almost completely. It weighs about 6 1/2 lbs (3 kg) and is some 20 inches (50 cm) long.

Types of ultrasound scans

Progress has changed and increased the possibility of seeing the fetus and assessing any kind of anomaly during the baby's formation.

But the basic functions of the procedure have not changed and it remains the only way of seeing the fetus in the womb.

Years ago, the first 2-dimensional ultrasound scans offered a new way of monitoring the development of the fetus in the womb, but technology has progressed since then and visibility is improving all the time. Digital 2-dimensional pictures make the transmission of the baby's movements and the visualization of its shape and size look more realistic. And now, with the arrival of 3-dimensional scans, the perception of the fetus is practically like a photograph. The digitally reconstructed images enable the baby's parents to see their child as if he or she were in front of them, with the features and extremities perfectly defined.

Another determining factor is speed. Fetal movements can be observed quite clearly in real time.

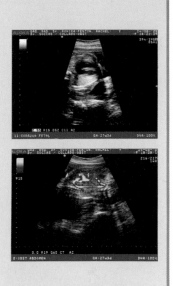

Weeks 15 to 16

This is the right time to perform amniocentesis tests in women who, for genetic reasons, have a history of chromosome irregularities, and in women who are over the age of 35 to 37, as they have a higher risk of congenital deformities than younger women, or those who opt to take the tests voluntarily. This test detects the most frequent genetic problems such as Down's syndrome, Pateau's syndrome and Edward's syndrome. If any genetic family disease is present, these tests will detect it.

Week 20

The scan taken during this week detects possible morphological deformities, and the sex of the baby can usually be seen.

Week 24

An analysis is made during this week to study the sugar curve and detect the possibility of gestational diabetes.

Week 34

A vaginal and rectal culture will be taken at this visit to determine whether any infection is present and to treat it with antibiotics at the moment of birth.

Week 37

An analysis is made to determine whether epidural anesthetic can be administered without risk, assessing it at an anesthesia consultation. From

As from the second visit to the clinic, checkups start to be made every month and usually include an ultrasound scan to determine the growth of the fetus, its condition, the situation of the placenta, and the quantity of amniotic fluid, as well as an analysis to check any kind of problem such as urinal infections, glucose irregularities, etc.

this point on, birth being imminent, visits to the clinic will become weekly, with continuous examinations, so as to ensure that the fetus is as closely monitored as possible, for the greatest possible stability and safety of both mother and baby.

What tests are carried out during pregnancy?

• Placental blood flow test. This is a painless exploration carried out during ecography. The gynecologist obtains fuller information, but for the woman nothing changes. For example, it can check that the blood is reaching the placenta properly and from there is reaching the fetus. As a rule, it is only carried out if it is suspected that insufficient blood is reaching the future baby.

SOME EXTERNAL PHYSICAL CHANGES IN THE PREGNANT WOMAN

Fourth month

Fifth month

Sixth month

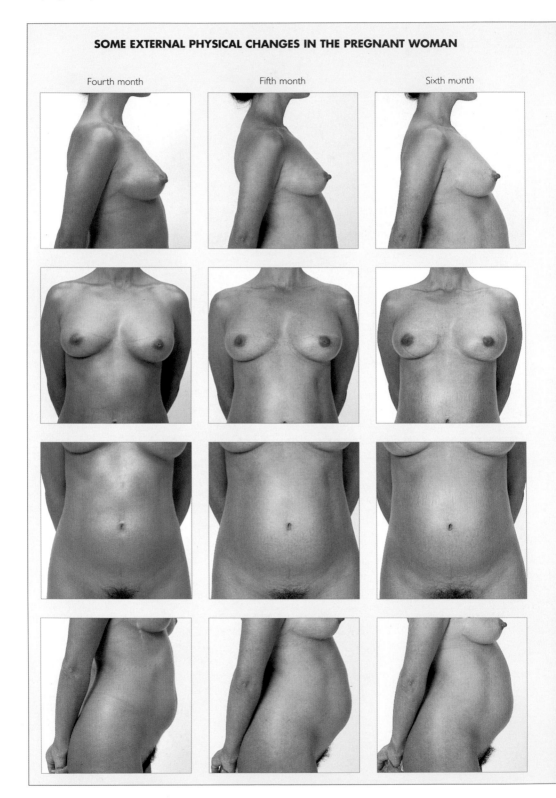

Seventh month   Eighth month   Ninth month

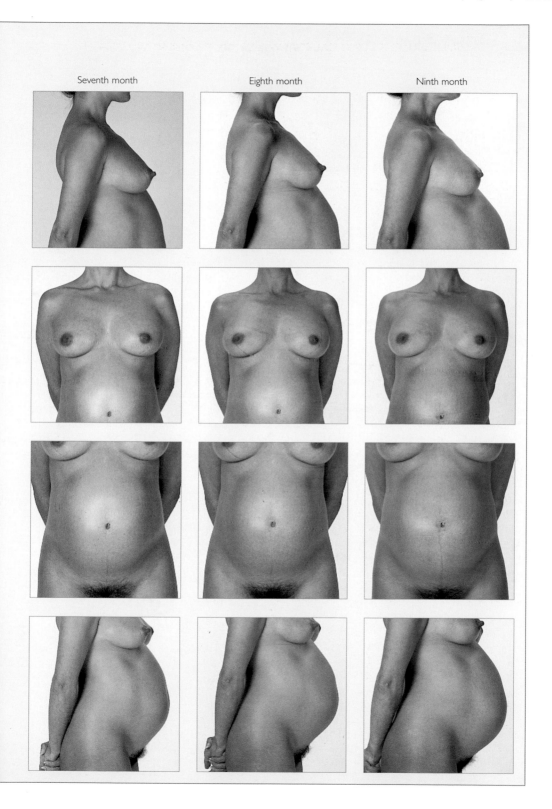

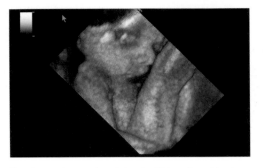

The ultrasound scan taken during the 20th week enables the baby's sex to be seen.

• Triple screening. This is carried out between the 15th and 20th week of the pregnancy and consists of measuring the mother's blood to detect certain biochemical markers (alphafetoprotein and HCG-beta) that are usually found in fetuses affected by Down's syndrome, anencephaly, or spina bifida. The results do not constitute a diagnosis, but merely enable the risk to be calculated. This test does not imply any risk at all.

• Amniocentesis. This test detects anomalies in the chromosomes and, therefore, possible genetic defects. In amniocentesis, a sample of the amniotic fluid is obtained by inserting a needle through the abdomen and into the uterus. The test is done with the help of an ultrasound scan to ascertain the best place to make the insertion. It enables any anomaly in the chromosomes to be detected, such as Down's syndrome, and other genetic defects. It is not a painful procedure, although it can cause some discomfort where the needle has been inserted. A few hours' rest are needed before resuming activity. The risk of spontaneous abortion after this procedure is 1 percent. Therefore, amniocentesis is recommended only if:

- the pregnant woman is over the age of 35, as the risk of having a baby with Down's syndrome increases at that age.

- the couple has had a child or a near relative with neural tube defects (defects of the spine and brain, including spina bifida and anencephaly).

• Chorionic villus sampling (CVS). As with the extraction of amniotic fluid, this procedure enables the chromosomes to be examined before birth, but consists this time of taking samples from the placenta membrane. The advantage of this analysis over amniocentesis is that it can be done from the 8th week, instead of waiting until the second trimester. The placenta is reached with a needle through the abdomen and the uterus, although in some cases samples can be obtained using special forceps through the vagina. This procedure is not used in all pregnancies, as it implies a certain risk to the baby.

• Percutaneous umbilical blood sampling (PUBS). This is used to perform fetal blood extractions or transfusions. One of the blood vessels in the umbilical cord is pierced with a needle, guided by an ultrasound scan. This procedure is used to diagnose diseases in the fetus, such as rubella (German measles), toxoplasmosis, or hemophilia, and can assess the degree of oxygenation of the blood if a serious deficiency is suspected.

Pregnancy and diet

A sensible diet for a woman during this physiological stage is the best weapon against premature birth and even problems related to the newborn child's development, such as low birth weight, reduced resistance to infections, etc.

Foods that must be included in the diet

• Dairy products. Drink about 2 cups (475 ml) of milk and take the rest in the form of low-fat dairy products; 2 yogurts and a little low-fat cheese, for instance. This food group supplies a good proportion of proteins of high biological value, calcium, vitamins B2, A, and D. If the woman is overweight or obese, skim milk products are recommended.

• Meat, fish, eggs, and their derivatives. Meat, less than six times a week—4 to 4 oz (120–130 g) per portion. Fish, at least four times a week—5

The objectives of dietary guidelines

• To cover the nutritional needs of the pregnant woman herself.

• To fulfill the nutritional requirements of the growing fetus.

• To prepare the mother's organism for childbirth.

• To ensure sufficient fat reserves for the production of milk during future lactation.

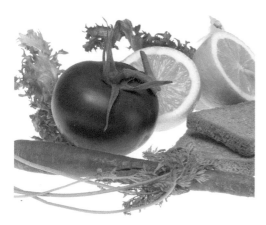

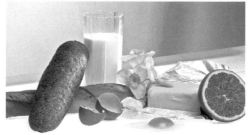

The fact that a woman is pregnant does not mean she must eat more, but she should follow an adequate and well-balanced diet, under the supervision of a gynecologist or dietician.

oz (140 g) per portion, of white and oily fish. Eggs, up to three times a week (1 or 2 eggs per serving). All these foods are basic sources of protein of high biological value and easily absorbed iron, nutrients increased amounts of which are needed, especially in the last months of gestation. Together with dairy products, they provide the essential amino acids (that the body cannot synthesize on its own), necessary for the development of the fetus, the placenta, the increased volume of maternal blood, and for the development of the uterus and breasts. Oily fish provides the omega-3 acids essential for forming the baby's nervous system and retina. Choose lean meat because it contains less saturated fat: skinless chicken and turkey, rabbit, beefsteak, veal, loin of pork, etc.

• Cereals, potatoes, and pulses; bread every day. It is recommended to alternate pasta, rice, potatoes, and pulses at lunch and dinner about two to four times a week. All of them are excellent sources of energy. Cereals and potatoes contain complete carbohydrates and are low in fat (except for wholegrain cereals). The foods in this group are an important source of the B group vitamins that are necessary for the proper absorption of other nutrients in the diet (proteins, fats), to maintain the skin, mucous membranes, and nervous system of the mother and her future baby in good condition. Pulses are rich in complete carbohydrates, vegetable protein, fiber, minerals, and vitamins.

• Green vegetables. As ingredients of starters and main dishes, and to garnish others, and a little salad. Their fiber encourages intestinal movement and provides hydrosoluble vitamins, and salts.

• Fruit. About three portions a day. They provide simple carbohydrates (sweet flavor), vitamins, minerals, and fiber. Eaten raw, they are an important source vitamin C, carotene, and other beneficial substances, and their fiber regulates the intestinal rhythm.

• Sugar and candies. Control the amount of these. Diabetics should not eat them at all.

Diet is very important for a pregnant woman, but she should remember that each woman should be prescribed a specific diet. Thus, a diet that may be good for one may not be so for another. The dietician or gynecologist must tell the pregnant woman which is the right one for her.

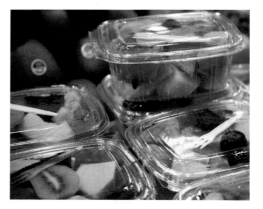

Folic acid

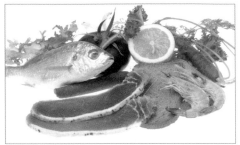

Folic acid is essential for the development of the fetus, especially during the first months of pregnancy. A deficiency of folic acid in the diet increases the risk of genetic problems such as the neural tube defects that affect the spinal column and the skull. Folic acid also helps produce the additional blood the body needs during pregnancy.

To help prevent neural tube defects, 0.5 milligrams of folic acid should be taken every day before and during pregnancy.

It is difficult to obtain all the necessary folic acid from the diet alone, so a supplement should be taken containing the right dose of this vitamin.

Women who have had a child with a spinal column or cranial defect are more likely to have another with the same problem, so they need

higher doses of folic acid. They should begin taking it at least one month before becoming pregnant and during the first three months of the pregnancy.

Women who need 5 milligrams of folic acid should take it on its own, and not as part of a multivitamin preparation.

To obtain sufficient folic acid from vitamin supplements, a woman would also be taking an overdose of other vitamins.

Folic acid is found in various foods:

- Dark green leaf vegetables (such as spinach, curly kale, and beet tops, romaine lettuce, broccoli, and asparagus).
- Wholegrain bread and cereals.
- Fruit and citrus fruit juices (such as strawberries, oranges, and orange juice).
- Dried peas and dried vegetables (such as black beans, white beans, and chickpeas).

▪ The teeth during pregnancy

It is very important for the pregnant woman to receive adequate dental care to prevent complications that could arise as a consequence of the hormonal changes of gestation. This is of fundamental importance for the health of both the woman and the future baby. With a balanced diet and proper dental hygiene, complications and the loss of teeth can be avoided.

During the early months, brushing the teeth often increases the digestive problems that are so frequent during pregnancy, such as nausea or vomiting, which may lead to a neglect of dental hygiene and hence, in association with the hormonal effects of pregnancy itself, may cause gingivitis (inflammation of the gums).

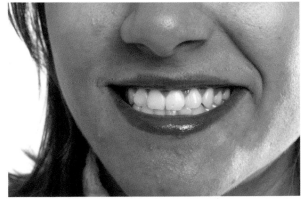

• Added oils and fats. These provide the liposoluble vitamins and essential fatty acids (lineoleic and linolenic acid) necessary to develop the future baby's nervous system, but they should be eaten in moderation.

• Miscellaneous. Occasionally, a moderate amount of cake, pastries, sweetened drinks, tidbits, and snacks. Stimulating and alcoholic drinks are not advisable, even if their alcohol content is low, such as cider or beer.

• Liquids. A pregnant woman should drink between 6 and 8 glasses a day of water, light infusions, soups, sugar-free fruit juices, or fresh vegetable juices, etc. More water is needed than usual: two thirds of the weight gained at the end of the pregnancy consists of water. Moreover, an increased intake of liquids will enable the kidneys to work better and eliminate sodium, thus reducing the risk of fluid retention.

General advice and care during pregnancy

The mother to be should take care of herself during her pregnancy. She should follow all her doctor's advice. Pregnant women should wear loose clothing and comfortable shoes, take some exercise, and rest.

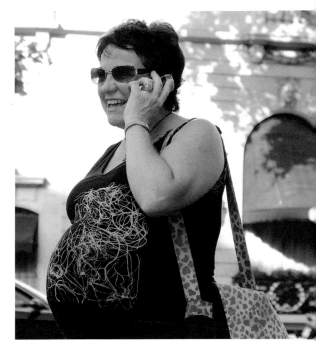

Should a pregnant woman eat for two?

It is true that as from the end of the first trimester of gestation, a greater need for food is felt due to the growth of the fetus, and so the woman usually eats more than before.

Specialists calculate that from the 4th month on, her increased energy needs come to some 350 calories daily more than she would normally eat. It is therefore clear that she should not double her food intake, but that the components of her diet should provide the body with the nutrients essential for the good health of the mother and the healthy growth and development of the future baby.

Some precautions

• Visit the doctor every month so that proper pregnancy checkups can be carried out.

• Prepare for childbirth, finding out about its stages.

• Eat properly and adequately throughout pregnancy and afterward, during breast feeding.

• Never, on any pretext, take medication that has not been prescribed by the doctor.

• Don't take drugs, drink alcohol, or smoke, as these have very serious consequences for both the mother and the child.

• Do physical exercises every day, as recommended by the doctor.

• Rest, relax, and seek forms of activity to control stress and lead as normal a life as possible.

• On experiencing any sign, such as bleeding, pain, colic, fainting, excessive vomiting, headaches, or other problems, visit the doctor immediately and follow her instructions carefully.

• Demand complete respect from the doctor and his assistants.

• Stay calm and carry on working, as it is your right to continue to work.

• Learn how to care for and look after the newborn baby. Both the mother and the father should do this.

The health is reflected in the skin

The best things for the skin are rest, exercise, and a healthy diet. However, during pregnancy some special precautions are needed. As a rule, the skin looks better due to the influence of the pregnancy hormones themselves. Estrogens make the skin more moist, but in some places, such as the thighs, cellulite may appear (sometimes called orange-peel skin). This usually disappears after the birth, always provided the body's fat deposits have not increased excessively.

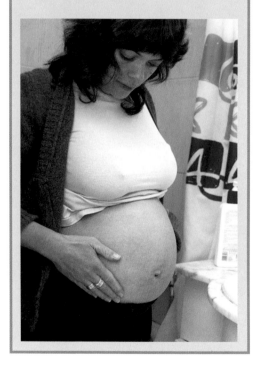

• Organize your life so that the father is equally committed and shares in everything that goes on

Suitable clothing

Looking pretty and being comfortable will certainly make the pregnant woman feel well. Taking care of her appearance during pregnancy will increase her confidence. As pregnant women often perspire more all over the body, clothing made of natural fibers (cotton, wool, linen, silk) is the most advisable, as it allows the skin to breathe better, and is therefore more comfortable. The same applies to undergarments.

Shoes should always be well ventilated and comfortable. High-heeled shoes should be avoided as they can affect posture as well as balance.

Can a pregnant woman travel?

There is nothing against traveling during a normal pregnancy, except by air as from the seventh month, because of the risk that it might set off premature labor or the breaking of the membrane.

Practical travel advice

• Don't drive because it causes unnecessary stress.

• If you travel by car, ask the driver to stop frequently so you visit a restroom and stretch your legs.

• Don't travel by boat during the first trimester, as it can increase nausea and vomiting.

• If you travel to hot places, take great care to avoid contaminated water and food that does not require cooking.

• If you travel to cold places, guard against colds and wrap up warm.

Pregnancy and tobacco

Smoking tobacco during pregnancy is harmful to the fetus, so pregnant women are advised not to smoke. Various studies have shown that tobacco causes a reduction in the weight of the newborn baby of between 7 and 10 oz [200–300 g], either through the direct effect on the absorption of toxic substances such as nicotine or carbon monoxide, or by altering the uterine flow and causing irregularities in the blood gases.

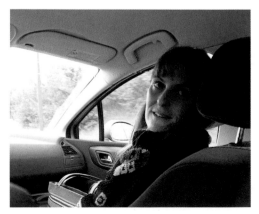

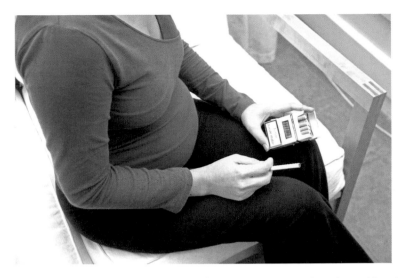

The smoking habit is always harmful, but during pregnancy it is even more so, as it has various damaging consequences for the fetus.

Tobacco can also increase the risks of premature breaking of the membrane, premature birth, bleeding before the birth, and retarded intrauterine growth and, all in all, increases perinatal mortality.

Moreover, effects on the weight of the newborn baby have been described when the mother is a passive smoker.

Tobacco is not related to congenital deformities, except perhaps for a slight increase in hare lips and cleft palates, although there are no important studies in that respect.

Pregnancy and alcohol

Alcoholic drinks should be avoided during pregnancy. Its customary consumption can adversely affect the newborn baby and cause retarded growth or even fetal alcoholic syndrome, characterized by slow growth, cranial and facial anomalies, and nervous system irregularities.

These effects will vary from case to case and it is important to remember that alcohol has different effects in each individual and that alcohol tolerance in females is approximately half that of males.

Multiple pregnancies

In human beings it is normal to conceive only one child at a time. A pregnancy with more than

No alcohol at all should be drunk during pregnancy and lactation, not even drinks with a low percentage of alcohol, such as beer.

one embryo is considered unusual and is classified as a high-risk pregnancy, because it is atypical. This does not mean that there will always be complications, but it is more likely to be associated with certain pregnancy difficulties.

How does a multiple pregnancy occur?

In cases of pregnancy involving two embryos, there are two mechanisms, the first for identical twins (monozygotic), and the second for fraternal twins (bizygotic).

• Identical twins.   After fecundation, it is not known exactly why, the first cell divides into two cells which continue to develop independently, resulting in two embryos of the same sex with identical physical and emotional characteristics, as they share the same genes. They also share the same placenta. Cases of identical twins are less fre-

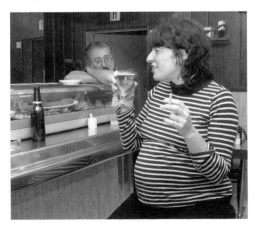

A few statistics

- One in every 80 pregnancies produces twins, one in every 8,000 triplets, and one in every 1 million quadruplets. These figures have changed because of ovulation stimulation treatments and pregnancies resulting from assisted conception techniques, so multiple pregnancies are now becoming increasingly frequent.

- There are factors that predispose a woman to multiple pregnancies, such as heredity, transmitted only through the mother, that is to say that a history of multiple pregnancies in the woman's family only is concerned, not in that of the man.

- It has been demonstrated that when a woman becomes pregnant for the first time after the age of 30, she is more likely to have a multiple pregnancy. The reason for this is not known.

- Also, becoming pregnant in the first month after ceasing to take contraceptive pills increases the likelihood of a multiple pregnancy.

quent (30 percent), and more often lead to complications.

• Fraternal twins. These siblings can be of different sexes and are as like one another as is normal between brothers and sisters. Fraternal twins occur when two eggs are fertilized by two sperms, resulting in two simultaneous pregnancies, but each embryo has its own placenta. These pregnancies are less risky than those in which the twins share a single placenta, and are the most frequent (70 percent).

As a rule a multiple pregnancy is diagnosed by an ultrasound scan or because the size of the uterus is much greater than normal, and sometimes

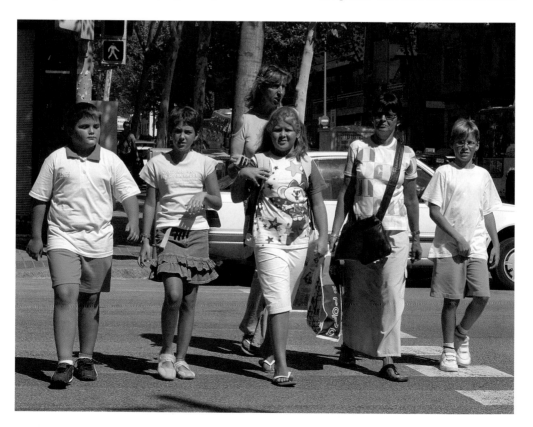

the pregnant woman experiences many more symptoms than usual (especially nausea and/or vomiting). It is normal to suffer more problems with this type of pregnancy, as two placentas produce greater quantities of hormones than one, and this hormonal revolution is responsible for the problems typical of the first trimester of pregnancy.

Ultrasound scans are now performed very shortly after pregnancy begins, so a diagnosis can be made at an early stage.

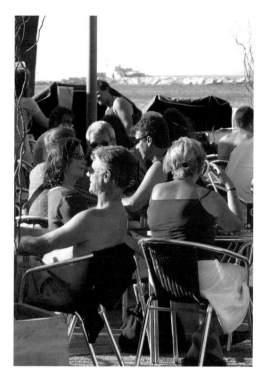

The medical consultation once a month will include ultrasound scans which enables the whole process to be carefully monitored. These scans enable various aspects to be ascertained: shape, sex, development of the fetus, possible deformities, and the detection of certain pathologies, etc.

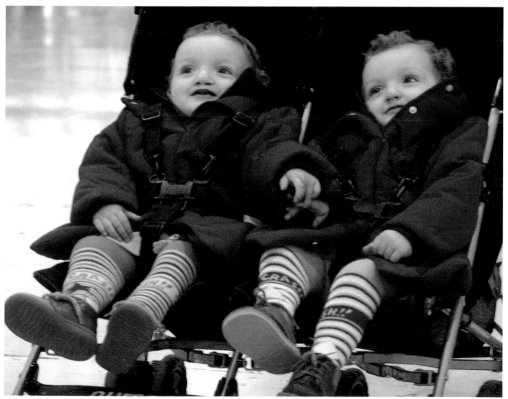

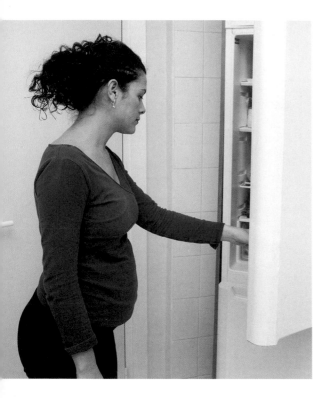

The monthly gynecological checkup in no way means that a woman should not visit her gynecologist as soon as the slightest symptom occurs. In this respect, it is always better to visit the doctor too often than too seldom.

Symptoms of premature birth

A pregnant woman should visit the doctor immediately if any of the following symptoms occurs unless she has completed the 37 weeks of pregnancy:

- Pressure, or feeling of heaviness in the pubis or perineum.
- Pain in the lumbar region that increases in intensity, especially if she has not felt it before, accompanied by contractions.
- Sharp pains or a feeling of emptiness in the depth of the vagina.
- An increase in vaginal secretions.
- A brownish or bloody vaginal flow.
- Breaking of the membrane.
- Vaginal hemorrhage.

Irregularities during pregnancy

It is very important to know about some of the diseases than can appear during pregnancy. These are usually directly associated with gestation. Most of these situations require rest, as well as other kinds of care.

Preterm or premature birth

This consists of a birth that occurs before time, that is to say before completion of the 37 weeks of gestation. It has always been affirmed that the best incubator is the mother's womb, so the longer the baby remains in it the better prognosis it will have. The best therapy for premature birth is to prevent it.

Complications

The most frequent complication is premature birth. Normally, a single-embryo pregnancy lasts 39–40 weeks on average, and in the case of twins, 37 weeks. No reliable statistics exist in cases of more than two babies. Moreover, in premature birth there is a greater risk of preeclampsia and high blood pressure caused by the pregnancy, which occurs more frequently compared with single-fetus pregnancies. This complication also occurs earlier, and it is sometimes more difficult to control it with the customary medications.

The low birthweight of the babies is another of the commonest complications of multiple pregnancies. This complication occurs in about 50% of twin pregnancies. The weight of the babies is lower because they have to share the flow of nutrients they receive from the mother's womb. However, they have the characteristic that, after birth, they gain weight much more quickly than babies born with the weight that corresponds to their gestational age.

Rhesus (Rh) disease

It is very important to know about some of the diseases than can appear during pregnancy. These are usually directly associated with gestation. Most of these situations require rest, as well as other kinds of care.

Rhesus (Rh) disease

Rhesus disease, also known as fetal erythroblastosis, can be a very serious condition for the baby and has been virtually eradicated now. It occurs when the gestating baby inherits from its Rhesus positive father a factor that the Rhesus negative mother does not possess called antigen D. The Rhesus negative mother's immune, or defense, system does not recognize the existence of the D factor, as her blood has no D antigens. She is therefore Rhesus negative.

If, through an incompatible blood transfusion (Rhesus positive), a miscarriage or a voluntary abortion, a Rhesus positive baby is born, or through a procedure or problems during the gestation of a Rhesus positive baby (chorionic villus sampling, amniocentesis, bleeding of fetal origin), the mother's Rhesus negative blood comes into contact with the baby's Rhesus positive blood which contains the D antigen, the mother's defense system will not react when this antigen, which is alien to her, enters her circulation.

As a consequence, the mother's defense system starts to generate antibodies against that antigen, the anti-D antibodies.

This process is called sensibilization and is what usually occurs with vaccinations given to prevent diseases. But, in the case of the Rhesus negative mother, sensibilization causes the formation of antibodies against the factor D in the gestating baby's red blood corpuscles, and consequently the red blood corpuscles of the intrauterine baby are destroyed and the baby becomes anemic.

This situation can develop into serious heart deficiency and the baby will die.

Detached placenta

This happens when there is a hemorrhage in the area between the uterine wall and the placenta, causing the placenta to become detached from it before the baby is born. This hemorrhage coagulates forming a clot of variable size that causes the placenta to become ever more detached.

Clinically, it is manifested by intense pain in the abdomen associated with permanent hardening of

Causes of premature birth

• Maternal diseases.

Diseases of maternal origin are the most frequent causes and can include urinary infections, kidney and heart diseases, diabetes, severe anemias, untreated thyroid problems, and vaginal infections, among others.

• Illnesses due to the pregnancy itself.

Preeclampsia or diabetes associated with the pregnancy (gestational diabetes) can mean that birth has to be induced prematurely to improve the prognosis of both mother and baby, which, if it remains in the uterus, is at greater risk from remaining there than it would be from premature birth.

• Uterine factors.

Actual uterine causes can be myomas (or fibroids) of the uterus, and an incompetent cervix, inadequately attached placenta, deformations of the uterus, and a bicornate uterus can be important factors too.

• Emotional factors.

Maternal anxiety, stress, and tension can predispose a woman to premature birth.

• The mother's age.

The mother's age is important. Thus, a woman aged under 16 or over 35 is more likely to give birth prematurely.

• Fetal factors.

Fetal factors can correspond to multiple pregnancies. Premature breaking of the membrane, congenital malformations, and intrauterine infections are the most frequent.

• Social factors.

Social factors can also increase the risk of premature birth—low socioeconomic level, maternal malnutrition, and excessive physical activity are some of these.

• Toxic maternal habits.

The mother's toxic habits, such as smoking, alcoholism, and taking drugs also increase the risks and are associated with inadequate birth weights (retarded intrauterine growth).

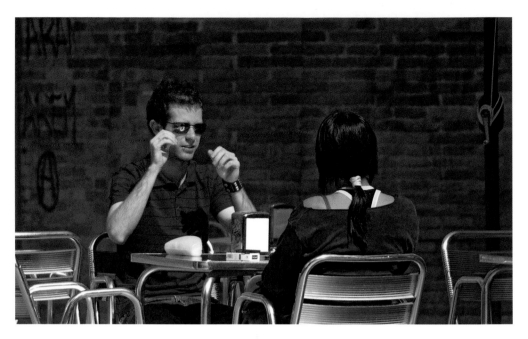

When a couple decides to have a child, both parties are recommended to have a medical checkup beforehand specially designed for that purpose. The checkup will provide a great deal of information about the advisability of a future pregnancy, and/or the care that should be administered if a pregnancy occurs, to guarantee that it proceeds to a successful conclusion.

the uterus. It is sometimes accompanied by a loss of dark blood via the vagina.

It is a serious complication during the last trimester of pregnancy and is associated with preeclampsia in most cases. If the placenta becomes detached before the baby is born, the detached part of it ceases to provide the oxygen the baby needs.

To save the baby from this irreversible situation (the placenta cannot reattach itself, but tends to become completely detached), an emergency caesarian section has to be performed. The mother's health can be endangered too, because the blood clot that forms in the area of the initial hemorrhage can be so big that it uses up the factors that are essential to enable the mother's blood to clot, predisposing her to hemorrhages that are very difficult to treat.

Placenta previa

This term is used to describe a placenta that is located anatomically in front of the baby's head, blocking the outlet at the neck of the uterus. It is a common situation and, at the 20th week of pregnancy, the placenta is in fact located low down in the uterus in 1 in 3 women, but, as the uterus

grows bigger, the placenta moves up to the top. If it is still in this low position by the time labor begins, vaginal birth is impossible, because the placenta is between the baby and the birth canal. Therefore a caesarian section is indicated.

During the last weeks of pregnancy, bleeding may occur because of contractions dilating the cervix. If the hemorrhage is very heavy, both the mother and the baby are at risk unless the problem is treated immediately.

Premature breaking of the membrane

The premature breaking of the membrane is the term used for the evacuation of the amniotic fluid through the vagina, but does not trigger labor in the following 24 hours. It is most common in the last weeks of the pregnancy, but can occur at any time as from the second trimester.

The intact ovular membranes are a barrier against the entry of the germs present in the cervix and vagina. When the membranes break, these germs invade the amniotic fluid and can cause infection in the baby. If it is suspected that the membrane has broken, a doctor or obstetric center should be consulted immediately.

A vaginal examination by qualified staff is essential to confirm that the membrane has in fact broken. It often turns out to be urinary incontinence or vaginal flow.

If the membrane breaks before the 32nd week, the doctor will try to prolong the pregnancy for a few weeks, because the risk of premature birth is greater than that of fetal infection. In that case, he will prescribe rest, medication to accelerate the maturation of the baby's lungs, and antibiotics, laboratory tests being necessary to diagnose signs of infection, in the form of a white blood-cell count, or a culture of vaginal secretion, to identify the germs present.

If infection is suspected, labor will be induced to avoid greater risks to the baby.

Polyhydramnios

This is the name given to an excess of amniotic fluid. It can have normal causes when associated with a big baby or a multiple pregnancy, or be the consequence of a disease in the mother, such as diabetes, or a disease in the baby, such as congenital deformities due to swallowing defects including obstruction of the fetal trachea, esophagus or stomach, or anencephaly, spina bifida, myelomeningocele, or hydrocephalus.

Polyhydramnios can be diagnosed at a routine prenatal checkup and confirmed by an echograph, measuring the volume of the amniotic fluid. An excess of amniotic fluid can also appear without any cause, and the baby may be perfectly normal.

The uterine distension caused by the excess liquid can trigger premature birth or cause the baby to be located in the wrong position for birth, and when the waters break spontaneously a prolapsed umbilical cord can occur.

Oligohydramnios

This means a reduction in the quantity of amniotic fluid. It can be caused by congenital malformations in the fetal urinary tract, usually in the kidneys, or obstruction of the baby's bladder. A severely deficient placenta can also be the cause, combined with a baby of very low weight.

The diagnosis is confirmed by an ultrasound

When planning a pregnancy, a couple should choose a gynecologist in whom they can really trust and, throughout the process, should follow his advice and instructions to the letter.

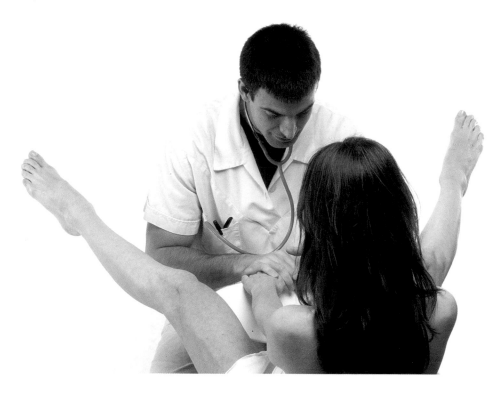

Anemia

The red blood corpuscles contain hemoglobin, the substance that carries oxygen from the lungs to all the body tissues. During pregnancy, the number of red corpuscles increases, but there is an even greater increase in liquid all over the body, resulting in a slight decrease in the concentration of hemoglobin by dilution. If the decrease in hemoglobin is excessive, that is to say, if it falls below 10g dl, anemia will occur.

The symptoms can be tiredness, shortness of breath, and a lack of energy. If anemia is severe, the woman will be unable to take walks or climb the stairs. The baby is not harmed by the mother's anemia. After giving birth, an anemic woman feels exhausted, which can reduce her milk production.

The ideal thing is to prevent anemia during pregnancy. At least two hemoglobin checks should be made during pregnancy and, if the level is lower than 10g dl, treatment should be started.

The commonest causes are nutritional deficiencies. During pregnancy, the baby rapidly uses up the mother's supply of iron.

tion of substances such as thromboxane leading to constriction of the arteries. It develops in women with normal blood pressure or becomes aggravated in a woman whose blood pressure is already high, as from the 20th week of pregnancy.

It is a dangerous disease for both the mother and the baby. In the mother, it can cause a blood pressure crisis, hepatic or renal insulin deficiency, coagulation irregularities, and even convulsions or comas called eclampsia, among other complications.

It can cause slow growth in the baby, or serious complications such as a detached placenta. Blood-pressure checks are one of the pillars of prenatal supervision.

scan and, depending on the problem causing it, prenatal treatment may or may not be given.

Gestational diabetes

This is set off during pregnancy as a consequence of the influence of the hormones in the placenta. The treatment of gestational diabetes is usually a very strict diet, as regards carbohydrates, although sometimes daily insulin injections are necessary.

Any woman who has had gestational diabetes should be rigorously monitored, because she is at greater risk of suffering diabetes in the years following the birth and greater complications with future pregnancies.

Preeclampsia

This is excessively high blood pressure occurring in pregnancy. It is caused by the placenta's produc-

Childbirth

The gestation of a new life is a wonder of nature in itself and can be an immensely happy event for the future parents. However, any new experience can cause anxiety and arouse certain fears, which are natural. Birth itself, especially for a first-time mother, can become a terrifying experience when she is not prepared for it. Knowing all the possibilites it will present, preparing herself with relaxation and breathing exercises, and sharing her fears with other people can help her achieve childbirth as one of the happiest and most positive experiences of her life.

First symptoms of childbirth

In the days preceding the birth, the woman will experience some new sensations or some that have already been experienced will intensify, as the baby wants to descend into its place in the birth canal. The most frequent signs and symptoms that indicate that childbirth is beginning are:

- Pressure on the pubis.
- Pain in the lumbar region.
- Sharp pains or a feeling of emptiness in the depth of the vagina.
- An increase in vaginal secretions.
- A brownish or slightly bloody vaginal flow.
- Expulsion of the mucous plug.
- Breaking of the membrane of waters.

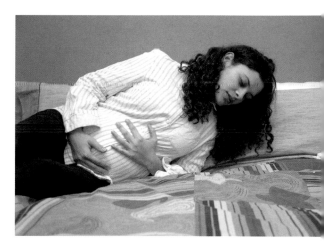

The mucous plug may be expelled before labor begins, or even a few days earlier. The bag of water can also break some days before labor begins. It feels like having urinated.

How to tell that birth is imminent

The most important sign that labor is beginning is the occurrence of rhythmic contractions intense enough to be perceived. They are called rhythmic contractions because each contraction is followed by a period of rest, followed inexorably by another one. There can be no birth without rhythmic contractions, which do not stop, even if the woman rests, relaxes, takes an analgesic, or follows any method she may have learned during her preparation for childbirth.

The duration of labor depends on many factors, and it is difficult to determine the number of hours it requires. The size of the fetus, and whether or not the woman is given an epidural anesthetic, are some of the variables that can shorten or lengthen the process. For first-time mothers, contractions continue for between 12 and 24 hours—the average time is 14 hours—although with subsequent births the time is reduced to 6 hours. Expulsion and suturing are usually much quicker, and the process is complete in 30 minutes.

Why are contractions painful?

During the contraction of the muscle, the blood vessels that irrigate it become short of blood, producing a transitory absence of oxygen in the tissue, or anoxia. Anoxia causes pain. When the muscle relaxes, its blood vessels dilate in order to irrigate themselves, and the pain disappears.

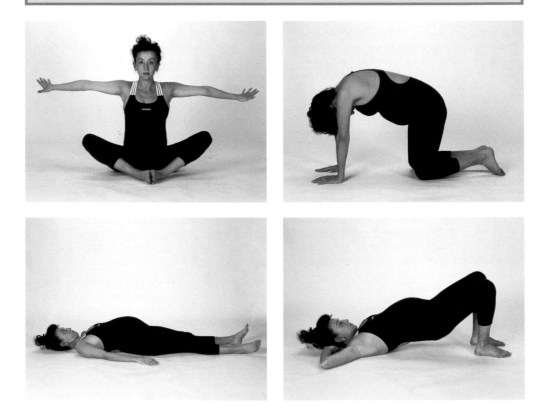

The purpose of birth-preparation classes is to prepare the future mother physically, psychologically, and emotionally for the moment of birth. Programs usually include theoretical and practical lessons and, in some cases, a guide to looking after infants, as well as aspects related to the period following childbirth.

How does childbirth progress?

Broadly speaking, labor can be divided into three stages:

- The first stage, called dilation, in which the neck of the uterus softens and dilates as a consequence of the action of the uterine contractions and the support of the fetal thrust (cephalic or pelvic).

- The second stage, called expulsion, during which the baby is expelled from the uterus through the vagina helped by the push produced by each contraction.

- The third stage, called the afterbirth, when the placenta (or afterbirth) is expelled.

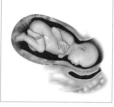 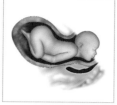 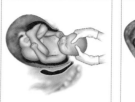 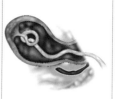

The dilation stage

Anatomically, the neck of the uterus is a cylinder just over 1 inch (3 cm) long, enclosing a channel called the cervical canal with two orifices, an internal one and an external one. Its walls are about half an inch (1 cm) thick. As a result of the contractions and pressure by the fetus, the neck shortens until it is completely eliminated and dilates to reach the circumference necessary to allow the baby to pass through.

At the same time, the baby descends as a result of gravity and the uterine contractions. In order to descend, the baby has to make various movements to accommodate itself to the mother's pelvis. Firstly, it has to decide what pelvic diameter is most suitable for it to enter the birth canal. After making that decision, it has to reduce the diameter of the part of its body it is presenting (head or bottom) as much as possible in order to pass through that bony barrier. When it achieves this, it is said to have "engaged," as it can then no longer return to its previous position.

Next, it has to turn itself round so that a firm part of its body (head or bottom) contacts the pubis and then make a kind of hinge movement which will propel it into the outside world during the expulsion stage.

During this stage, the doctor may intervene in various ways to help, either encouraging the baby's descent by artificially breaking the membrane or increasing the intensity of the contractions, if they are insufficient, with an oxytocin drip or, if the mother is finding the pain intolerable, using an analgesic designed for administration during labor.

The expulsion stage

The expulsion stage is the most longed-for moment of the whole birth process, because it leads to the baby's emergence through the vagina as a result of the mother's push that accompanies each contraction. During this stage, the doctor decides whether an episiotomy is needed. Once the baby's head or bottom can be seen from outside, the doctor makes a series of maneuvers to help the rest of its body pass through the birth canal. When the baby is born, the umbilical cord is clamped and cut, because as from that moment, the baby's circulation system changes and it oxygenates itself with the air entering its own lungs. The baby is then totally autonomous.

Shortly afterward, the afterbirth is delivered, that is to say the placenta and the bag that contained the baby are expelled, as the result of further powerful uterine contractions. This usually happens no more than 30 minutes after the baby was born. It is accompanied by bleeding, called lochia, that lessens a few hours after the birth and continues, much reduced, for a period of 20 to 50 days, commonly called the lying-in period. This bleeding results from the wound left in the uterus by the placenta after it has come away.

If contractions occur

The pregnant woman should call the doctor or go to the hospital if birth contractions occur, that is to say, rhythmic and regular contractions, especially if the predicted date for the baby's birth is still some way off.

If the predicted birth date is close and if, after an hour of trying to make the contractions stop using various techniques (breathing exercises, resting on her left side, or taking an analgesic), the contractions persist, the obstetrician or doctor should be called, as the birth process has begun.

When should the obstetrician or doctor be called?

If the contractions are continuing at the same rate or are becoming more frequent after an hour, the woman should go to the hospital or call the doctor, as delivery is imminent. It should be remembered that 8 to 12 hours can pass from the beginning of labor to the baby's birth, so there is plenty of time for the woman to realize that something is happening to her body. The doctor should also be called if the membrane has broken, if there is any kind of vaginal bleeding, if the woman becomes feverish, is suffering abdominal pain, an acute headache, or vision irregularities.

Birth

Birth comprises the series of events that occur to enable the baby to be born. The process has a beginning, a development, and an end.

• Beginning. Labor can begin spontaneously, when contractions start on their own, helping the baby to descend and the neck of the uterus to dilate, or can be induced, when, for some reason, the pregnancy has to be ended because its continuation could be harmful to the mother or the baby. These are called reasons for inducing labor.

• Development. This can comprise a eutocic delivery, when the doctor simply monitors the events that are occurring naturally, or directed, when the doctor decides to intervene using methods that encourage labor, such as artificially breaking the membrane, an oxytocin drip, or analgesia designed for labor.

• End. This determines how the baby will emerge and can be vaginal or abdominal. A vaginal birth uses the vagina as the birth canal for the emergence of the baby and the placenta. An abdominal birth is one that requires surgery to extract the baby and the placenta, and is called caesarian section. Vaginal birth can itself be either natural, that is to say, produced by the mother's

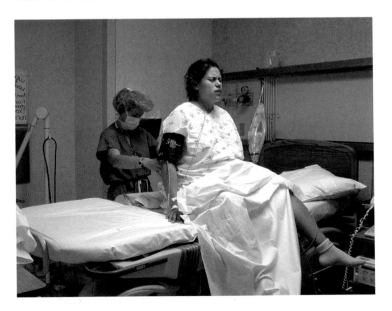

The help the hospital offers is beneficial both to prevent problems and to give the woman in labor confidence. Therefore, when the woman experiences the symptoms indicating that the birth process has begun, she should go to the hospital.

own pushing, or artificial, when various instruments are used to assist the emergence of the baby, such as forceps or a ventouse or vacuum extractor.

What are contractions?

A contraction is a hardening of the abdomen as a consequence of the action of the uterine muscle. Contractions are felt if their intensity is greater than 10mmHg, the usual tone of the uterus. There are different types of contraction.

• Focal contractions. These are caused by the stimulation of only one section of the uterus, usually as a result of movement by the baby.

• Generalized contractions. These start in any sector of the uterus and spread throughout the whole organ. They can be caused by the baby's movements, changes of position (from lying down to sitting up), uterine irritation resulting from a full bladder, or intestinal congestion.

• Braxton Hicks contractions. These begin as from the 5th or 6th month of pregnancy or even earlier, and are characterized because they affect the whole uterus, and are felt from top to bottom (from the top of the uterus to the vagina). They are not painful and the woman merely senses that her abdomen is hardening, with a feeling of abdominal tension when they occur. They come approximately every 30 to 60 seconds. They correspond to an exercise of the uterine muscle preparing itself for labor. Like any muscle, the uterus needs some training in order to confront the work involved in giving birth. When that day comes, it will have to contract for a period of about 9 hours, and if it did not have adequate training it would become exhausted.

• Birth contractions. Birth contractions are different. They are very regular, occurring every two or three minutes, and can last some 90 to 120 seconds each. They do not pass unnoticed, because they are usually painful. They are generally associated with the expulsion of the mucous plug, a gelatinous fluid often including blood, and a new feeling of pressure in the vagina, caused by the baby's head pushing against the perineum and the rectum and producing feelings similar to the desire to defecate. A typical characteristic of labor is that the pain ceases between contractions, enabling the woman to do deep breathing exercises and relax the muscles, helping her to withstand the next contraction.

How can labor pains be alleviated?

The pain of labor varies according to the characteristics of each woman, as the pain threshold is absolutely individual. The most important thing is to know that the more a woman relaxes, the less pain she will feel.

The pain can be controlled by various techniques, including acupuncture, massage, and breathing and relaxation techniques, but there are analgesics that can be used without risk:

• Peridural or epidural anesthesia. This is one of the methods used to alleviate pain during labor and assist its progress. It is also the anesthesia most often used for caesarian deliveries. Using a special needle, the anesthetic solution is injected into the spine, between the 2nd and 5th lumbar vertebrae (about 4 inches [10 cm] from the point where the spinal medulla terminates), and into the peridural space— the space around the channel through which the cerebrospinal fluid that surrounds the nerves giving sensitivity to the legs and the pelvic region passes. The anesthetic liquid compresses the area, suppressing pain caused by compression, so the anesthetic never enters the bloodstream. The dosage is monitored by positioning a plastic catheter in the back through which the anesthetic is progressively administered. The effect starts to be felt 15 to 20 minutes after it is administered.

This type of analgesic enables the woman to push, and to feel the contractions and the baby's descent into the birth canal, but without such intense pain. This type of anesthesia is not used for patients with diseases of the nervous system or severe high blood pressure.

• Meperidine. Sedative injections such as meperidine can be given, although they can cause fainting, nausea, and disorientation. This preparation crosses the placenta and can make the baby sleep after it is born, an effect that lasts about 2 to 6 hours, but does not damage its health.

• Local anesthetic. There are two possibilities with this type of anesthesia: paracervical anesthesia and local perineal infiltration.

• Paracervical anesthesia. This is applied during the dilatation stage of labor and consists of anesthetizing the depth of the vagina and acting on the nerves that sensitize the perineal area.

• Local perineal infiltration. This is the injection of an anesthetic in the area where the episiotomy is performed.

THE NEWBORN BABY'S FIRST MINUTES

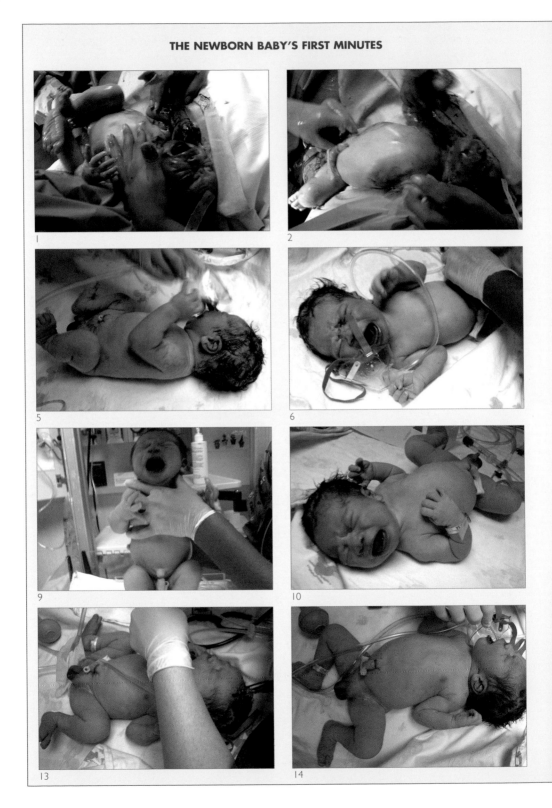

After delivery, the newborn baby requires immediate attention to check that his or her breathing is normal and to cleanse the body of birth fluid and mucous. Very soon after being born, the baby must be given a general examination.

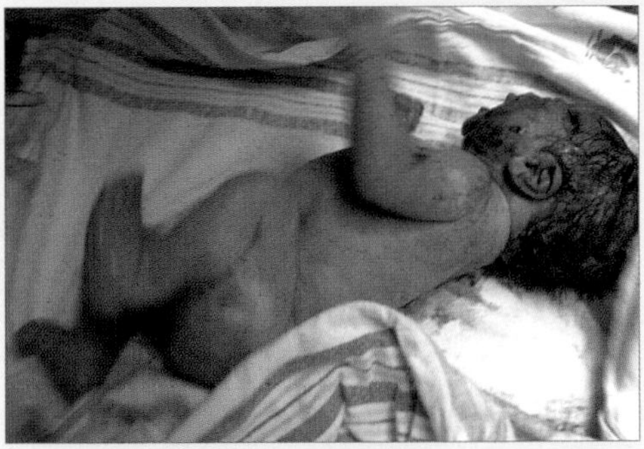

3

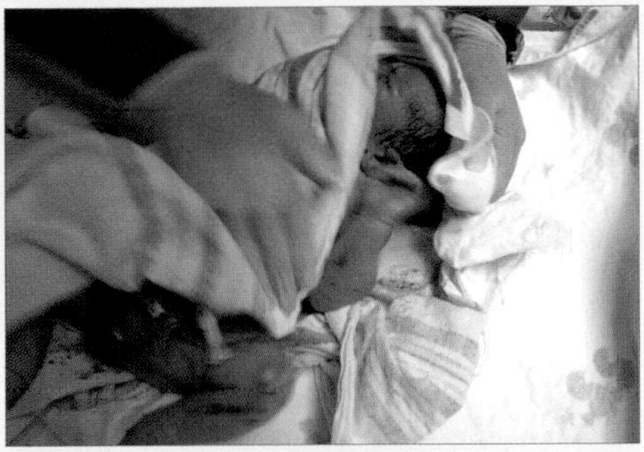

4

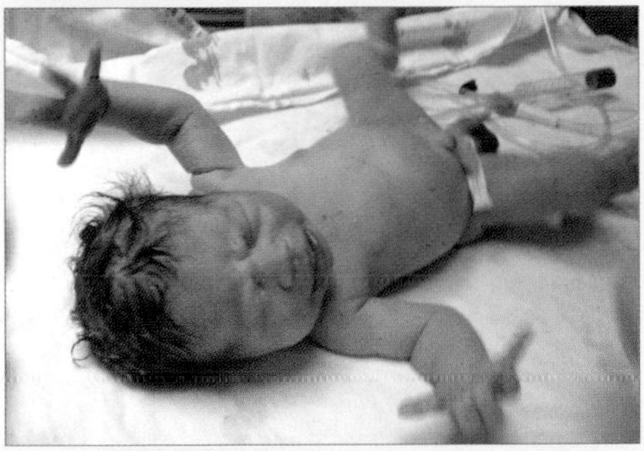

7

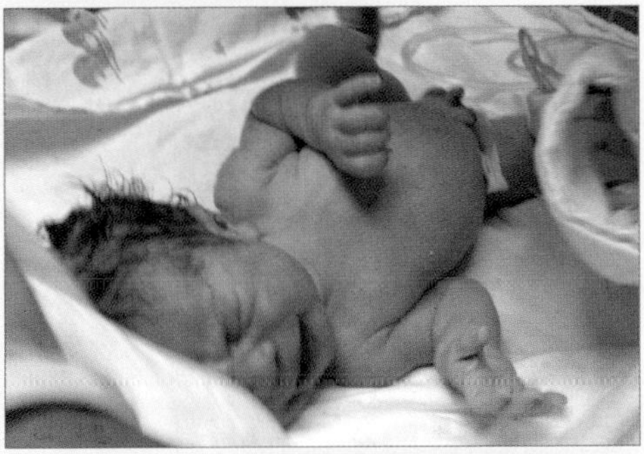

8

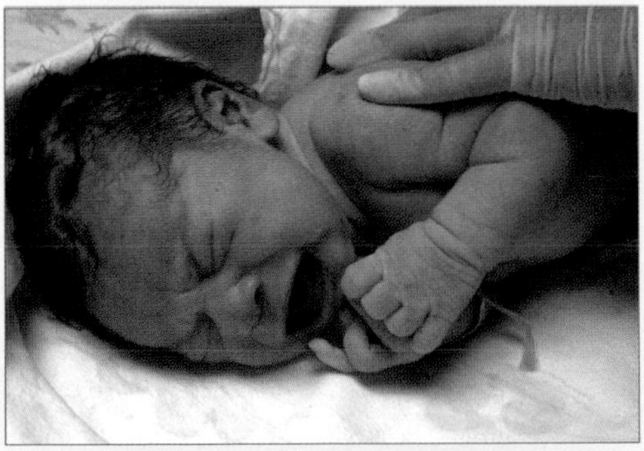

11

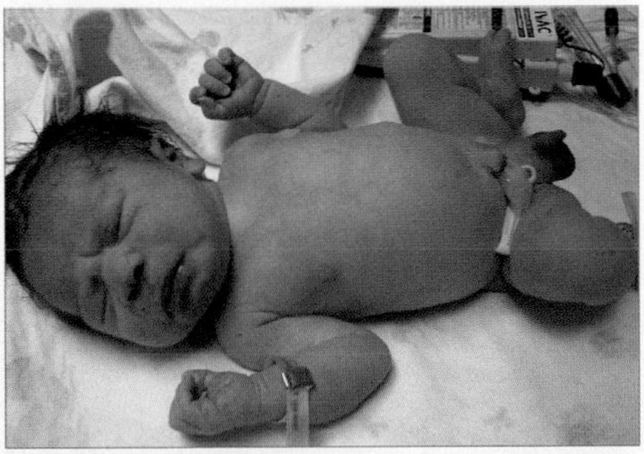

12

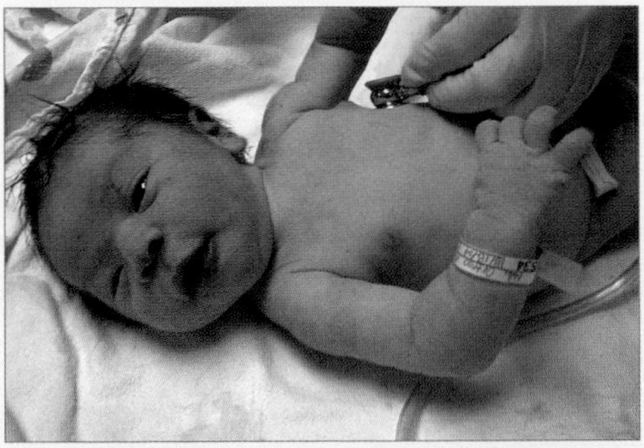

15

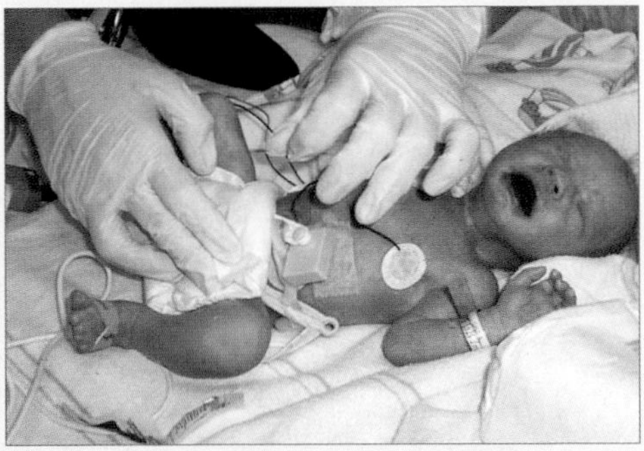

16

And after delivery?

Sometimes symptoms occur after giving birth which mothers can find alarming, but which are totally normal:

• Vaginal bleeding. For the first few hours after giving birth, it is normal for vaginal bleeding to occur, accompanied by blood clots. This bleeding is much more copious than during menstruation. It is called lochia, and is caused by the separation of the placenta from the wall of the uterus. This separation leaves a bleeding wound which initially starts to close as a consequence of the uterine contractions that immediately follow delivery and then of the release of the oxytocin that is triggered by breastfeeding. The liquid lost is red for the first 3 or 4 days, and then becomes brownish. It continues for a total of about 40 days, and during this time only sanitary towels should be used, never vaginal tampons.

• Extreme tiredness. Naturally, for the first few days after delivery the woman feels physically exhausted. Labor is very intense and, after delivery, the newborn baby occupies many hours of the day, making it difficult for her to get more than 3 or 4 hours' continuous sleep.

• Facial hematomas. The effort of pushing for a long time during labor can leave some transitory marks on the face, such as small hematomas in the eyes or on the cheeks. These should not cause alarm, as they will disappear within 24 to 48 hours.

• Pains. After giving birth, the body aches.

• The episiotomy or caesarian incision. The area of the episiotomy or caesarian incision is also painful for the first few hours. It is advisable to take analgesics and use ice as a local painkiller.

• The muscles of the birth canal. In vaginal births, the distension of the birth canal muscles usually causes small lacerations that can be troublesome. Analgesics also help to relieve these problems.

• Afterbirth contractions. These very powerful contractions make the uterus retract, thus preventing hemorrhages. They are painful in women who have had more than one labor, as the uterus is more fibrous and sensitive to pain. They are only painful for the first two or three days and are usually an accompaniment to breastfeeding.

Natural childbirth

Natural childbirth can take place at home or in a hospital or maternity home. It is the personal choice of the mother who decides to give birth in an intimate environment with the help of a midwife— accompanied by a mobile emergency unit very close at hand in case birth complications occur. There are many different forms of natural childbirth, precisely because its principle is that the woman should adopt the position in which she feels most comfortable:

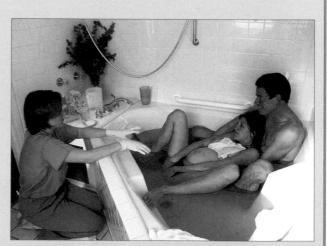

• Many women in labor choose the vertical position (the woman sits, squats, kneels, etc.). For many women, this is the ideal position for delivery, because the force of gravity will help the baby move down the birth canal. This age-old position encourages the woman to participate in labor, as she can watch its progress.

• Another method of natural childbirth is the "birthing pool" which is becoming more widely accepted nowadays.

The baby's suckling causes the release of a hormone called oxytocin which induces contractions. This mechanism also helps the uterus to return to its normal size before pregnancy. An ice pack applied to the suprapubic area helps relieve these problems.

• Perineal area. Pain in the perineal area is frequent, especially in women who have not had an episiotomy. A baby weighing on average 6¹/₂ lbs (3 kg) does not pass through the birth canal unnoticed. Even without an episiotomy, the stretching of the muscles and the vaginal mucous sensitize the area, and some discomfort is felt there for a few days.

Episiotomy

This is a cut in the perineum (the skin between the vagina and the anus) which is sometimes made to enlarge the vaginal opening so the baby can emerge more easily.

Episiotomy causes pain during the healing process and because the area is constantly being rubbed by clothing. Healing takes about 10 days. While the woman is in the hospital, a nurse will check that it is progressing normally and that there are no signs of serious inflammation or infection.

It is important to change the sanitary towels at least every 4 hours, and they should be removed from front to back, to avoid anal germs coming into contact with the vagina. The area should be washed using neutral soap three or four times a day, drying it thoroughly afterward. The local application of ice is beneficial when the area is painful. For sitting, the woman can use special cushions with a hole in the center so as not to press on the episiotomy area.

• Difficulty in urinating. For the first hours after delivery it is sometimes difficult to urinate. The woman may feel an irrepressible urge to do so, but be unable to, or may feel a burning sensation the first few times. This is caused by:

- The bladder returning to its usual size.

- The bladder's capacity returning to normality after delivery, because the baby's head that prevented its normal expansion is no longer there.

- The bladder, hurting from the pressure exercised by the baby's head, may be paralyzed for a few hours. It may be full of urine but the need to urinate may not be felt.

- The bladder may have been sensitized by anesthesia.

- Pain in the perineum impedes the emptying of the bladder because it may cause a spasm in the urethra that prevents it from emptying.

- It is essential for the bladder to be emptied during the first 6 or 8 hours after delivery. If this does not happen, complications can occur, such as a hemorrhage. It can also cause urinary infections.

These urinary upsets disappear of their own accord within 24 hours. It should also be remembered that it is important to drink large amounts of liquid during the first days after delivery. This will help produce milk and also create a larger amount of urine, which is important to prevent infections of the urinary tract.

• Difficulty in defecating. At some time after delivery, the bowels will have to be emptied. Many women feel terrified that doing so will cause pain or burst the episiotomy stitches. There is no need to worry about this, as the vagina and the rectum are two separate organs. There are factors that make emptying the bowels difficult. The abdominal muscles, distended by pregnancy, do not have their usual propulsive strength, and the rectum will certainly have been emptied before or during the birth and, therefore, there is nothing to empty. If hemorrhoids have appeared, they can be alleviated with special creams or suppositories.

When is a caesarian section required?

• Bad position and bad presentation of the baby. When the baby is presenting itself in a pelvic (seated) or transverse position (lying crosswise), and if any serious disease or anatomical anomaly is present in which vaginal birth could be traumatic.

• Multiple pregnancy. In multiple pregnancies with more than two babies, when they are situated in positions that would be dangerous for vaginal birth.

• Genital herpes. If the mother has genital herpes, because of the risk of the baby's being infected as it passes down the birth canal.

• Placenta previa. In the case of placenta previa, because the baby's way out is blocked.

• Maternal illnesses. In the case of certain conditions in the mother which could put the life of mother or baby at risk, meaning that the baby must be born before the uterine conditions are ready for natural birth. Examples of such diseases are preeclampsia and diabetes.

• Previous uterine surgery. If surgery, such as a previous caesarian or a myomectomy, have been

What is a caesarian section?

A caesarian section is a surgical procedure performed to extract the baby and the placenta from the mother's uterus when, for some reason, vaginal birth is not possible. This procedure is increasing in Western countries, not only for medical reasons but also in response to societal demands.

Caesarians can be programmed, or performed in an emergency.

• Programmed caesarians. Here, the reason for this procedure is known before labor begins and it is often possible to arrange a convenient date and time for it.

• Emergency caesarians. Here, the reason for the procedure arises during labor, when urgent measures are required to resolve a problem and avoid risks to the health of the mother or baby.

performed on the mother's uterus before, a caesarian is recommended to prevent the uterine scar breaking.

When is a caesarian section a matter of urgency?

• Placental problems. Before labor begins, the detachment of the placenta and placenta previa with copious bleeding can be reasons for performing an emergency caesarian.

• The size of the baby. During labor, babies can turn out to be too big for the size of the mother's pelvis (cephalopelvic disproportion).

• Fetal distress. The fetal heartbeat can deteriorate so that the baby cannot withstand the shortage of oxygen caused by each contraction and so cannot wait long enough for vaginal birth to occur. This is called acute fetal distress.

• Twisted umbilical cord. The umbilical cord can wind round the baby very tightly and prevent the blood in the cord flowing normally, which also causes the baby distress.

• Prolapsed umbilical cord. The umbilical cord can slip through the neck of the uterus in front of the baby's head and cause compression that prevents the flow of blood through it and does not allow the baby to oxygenate itself normally.

• Stoppage of labor. Other reasons for performing a caesarian during labor are the stoppage of labor, inadequate dilatation, or because the baby is badly positioned, preventing its descent down the birth canal.

After having a caesarian, is a vaginal birth possible?

At present, 60 percent of pregnancies ending in a caesarian section require another caesarian for the next one. The principal risk for patients who have had a previous caesarian is uterine breakage in the area of the caesarian scar, which can be a serious complication for both mother and baby. In all cases, detailed questions must be asked about the reasons for the previous caesarian, and the doctor must assess each case individually and issue very clear warnings about individual risks. He should always listen to the opinion of the couple in order to reach a clear understanding and achieve a successful outcome.

Breastfeeding

Mother's milk is the best food for the majority of babies. It contains the nutrients the baby needs to grow and develop healthily for the first six months of its life. Breastfeeding is also beneficial to the mother's health, as, among other things, it enables her to return to her weight more quickly before becoming pregnant again. Moreover, the special relationship that is established between mother and baby is reflected in emotional benefits for both.

Mother's milk

Breast milk is the natural way of feeding the baby. During breastfeeding, mother and child are in intimate contact with one another.

Mother's milk satisfies all the baby's needs for adequate growth during the first 4 to 6 weeks of life.

It protects the baby from certain diseases, as the mother's antibodies (or defenses) are passed on in her milk.

The secret of successful breastfeeding is for the pregnant woman to be informed from the early months of her pregnancy of all the advantages of maternal breastfeeding and for her to begin it as early as possible, as soon as she has her first contact with her baby. Only if suckling is not correct is there a risk of any problem arising in the breast, such as cracked nipples or mastitis.

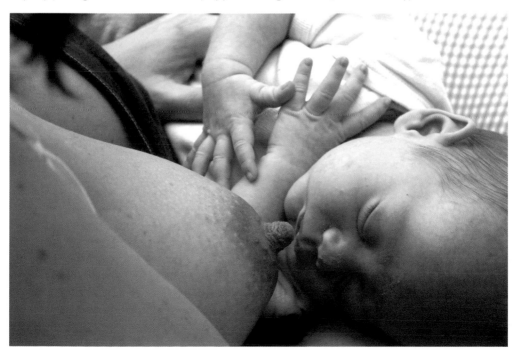

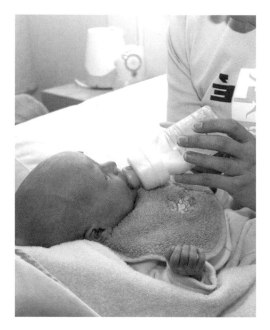

Any woman should be capable of feeding her child exclusively with her own milk. The difference between large or small breasts is caused almost entirely by the fat they contain and not the quantity of milk-producing glands. Moreover, the reasons for not breastfeeding (certain diseases or medicines) are very rare and virtually exceptional. Nowadays, almost all maternal diseases can be treated in a way that does not require the suspension of breastfeeding (the pediatrician should always be consulted).

The baby is born with a natural instinct that leads it to the nipple. Generally, the mother only has to offer it to the baby properly to enable it to suckle effectively without having to make any effort.

■ Duration and frequency of feeds

• The time needed complete a feed varies from child to child and mother to mother, and also depends on the baby's age. It can also vary from feed to feed.

• Moreover, the composition of the milk is not the same at the beginning and end of a feed, or during the first days of the baby's life, or when the baby is 6 months old. The milk is more watery at the beginning of a feed, but the milk at the end of a feed contains most of the proteins and sugars. The milk at the end of a feed is less copious, but contains more calories (the fat and vitamin content is greater).

• Both the number of feeds a baby has a day, and the time each feed takes, vary greatly, so no fixed rules should be established. It is better to offer the breast than to wait for the baby to ask for it. A child may want to suckle only 15 minutes after a feed or, conversely, may wait more than 4 hours before asking for the next one, but during the first 15 or 20 days of life, it is best to try to give the newborn baby at least 8 feeds every 24 hours.

• The mother should not be advised to limit the duration of each feed. Only the baby knows when he is satisfied, so it is important that for him to receive the milk at the end of the feed. Ideally, a feed should last until the child withdraws from the breast of his own accord.

• Some babies receive all the milk they need from just one breast, while others take it from both.

• In the latter case, the baby may not completely empty the second breast, so the next feed should begin with the one that was not completely emptied. The important thing is not for the child to suckle from both breasts, but for each breast to be emptied completely in turn, to prevent an accumulation of milk causing the mother to develop mastitis, and for the mother's body to adjust her milk production to her child's needs. It is therefore recommended to allow the baby to finish with one breast before offering the other

• Even if the baby takes the breast very often or suckles hard on it at every feed, it does not mean that cracked nipples will occur if the baby's position and attachment to the breast are correct.

Other recommendations

- The only hygiene the mother's breast needs is a daily shower or a thorough wash.

- It is not necessary to wash the breasts with soap after each feed. They can be washed with plain water and dried.

- Later, absorbent breast pads can be useful. These should be changed as often as necessary.

- The mother does not need to change her eating or drinking habits. She may feel thirstier, but it is not necessary to drink excessive amounts. Only in the case of allergies may it be necessary to eliminate certain foods from her diet.

- Hard or stressful work can interfere with maternal lactation, so any help the mother can be offered to relieve her of other tasks is very beneficial, either by the father or by other family members.

- The help, support, and understanding of the father and other family members (grandmother, sisters, friends) are essential for breastfeeding to proceed satisfactorily.

- It can sometimes be useful for the mother to learn to express her milk, either to store and enable someone else to feed the baby, or to relieve the problems caused by excessive milk accumulation when the baby's appetite declines, thus avoiding mastitis. Milk can be extracted manually or using a milk extraction pump (consult your pediatrician, midwife, pediatric nurse). Mother's milk can be kept in the refrigerator for 2 days and frozen for 3 to 6 months, depending on the temperature.

- If the mother still smokes, this is the time to give it up. If giving up is impossible, it is preferable to smoke immediately after a feed and not to do so in the child's presence. It will always be better than giving the baby artificial milk. Babies who remain in a smoky atmosphere suffer more frequently from respiratory infections and asthma.

- The same can be said of alcohol, although, if the mother drinks only occasionally and in moderation, she will probably have no difficulty in giving it up completely.

Getting started

It is important for the baby to be offered the breast early, if possible in the first half hour after birth. After the first hour, the newborn baby usually sleeps for a few hours. During that time it is recommended that the baby remains close to the mother, although perhaps showing no interest in suckling, the contact between the skin of both of them is stimulating. Thus, the baby can be offered the breast as soon as he or she looks ready to suckle (mouth movements seeking the nipple, nuzzling, etc.) and not only just when crying begins. Crying is a late sign of hunger.

The principal stimulus that induces milk production is the child's suckling. Therefore, the more frequently the baby is put to the breast, and the more the breast is emptied, the more milk the mother will produce. The amount adjusts itself to how much the baby takes and the frequency with which the breast is emptied each day. The quality also varies according to the child's needs as time goes by.

During the first few days, the milk is somewhat yellow (colostrum) and contains a large amount of protein and antibodies. Later, the mature milk appears. It may look watery, especially when first taken, but its fat content increases toward the end of a feed. However, no mother's milk is of poor quality. It is always adequate for the baby and is all his or her needs.

A healthy newborn baby does not need any liquids other than what is obtained from the mother's milk. It is not necessary or recommendable to offer water or glucose solutions. Before giving the baby supplements or any food other than mother's milk, a pediatrician should be consulted.

The child's position at the breast and his or her grasp of the nipple

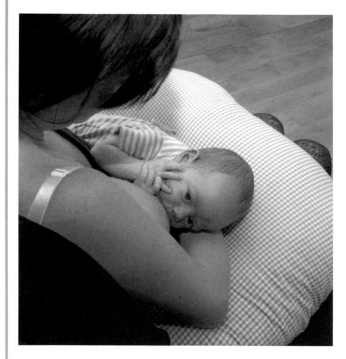

In mothers with flat nipples, the child's suction is sufficient to make the nipple into a teat, as already explained, so the use of nipple shields is not helpful in most cases.

- Most problems with breastfeeding occur because the baby is not being held in the right position, is not grasping the nipple correctly, or a combination of the two. The right method prevents the occurrence of sore or cracked nipples.

- Feeding from the breast is not the same as feeding from a bottle. The mother's milk passes to the child through a combination of active expulsion (the ejection reflex or rising of the milk) and active extraction by the baby (suckling). To suck the breast effectively, the baby must make it into a teat, formed approximately of one-third nipple and two-thirds breast tissue.

- When sucking the nipple, the baby plays a fundamental part, as it is the movement of the tongue, using peristaltic waves (from front to back), that works the breast, which is where the milk accumulates once that movement has occurred. For this to be possible, the newborn baby has to grasp the breast effectively.

- Regardless of what position the mother adopts (sitting or lying down), both mother and child must be comfortable and very close, preferably with the whole of the baby's body in contact with the mother.

- The wrong position can cause problems and back pain. The baby's grasp of the nipple is helped if the mother holds him turned toward her, with his head and body in a straight line, without his neck being excessively turned or extended, and facing the breast with his nose opposite the nipple.

- In the seated position, the mother should keep her back straight and her knees slightly raised, with the child's head resting on her forearm, not in the crook of her elbow. It is also helpful to support the baby's buttocks and not just the back.

- Once the baby is properly positioned, the mother can stimulate him to open his mouth by rubbing his lips with the nipple and then moving him gently toward the breast. The baby will grasp the nipple more easily if it is presented from below, directing it toward the upper third of his mouth, so he can reach the breast by tilting his head slightly backward. Thus, his chin and lower lip will touch the breast first, while his mouth is wide open.

- The intention is that the baby should take as much of the breast into his mouth as possible and have his lower lip attached to the base of the nipple. In the case of large breasts, it can be helpful for the mother to support the breast from below, taking care to do so from its base, close to the chest, so that her fingers do not make it difficult for the baby's mouth to grasp the breast. Similarly, care must be taken to see that the baby's arm does not come between him and his mother.

- If the baby is properly attached, the lower lip will be well below the nipple and most of the areola will be in his mouth. It is almost always possible to see more of the areola above the child's upper lip than below the lower lip. The child's chin touches the breast and the lips are everted (turned outward). In this way the mother can be sure that the breast is well inserted into the baby's mouth and that the suction and milk production movements are effective.

- The baby usually works his jaw with a rhythmic movement that extends to the ears, and the cheeks do not hollow but look rounded. When the baby suckles in this way, the mother feels no pain, even when her nipples are sore or cracked.

- The breast should not be squeezed with the fingers (as when holding a cigarette), as this stretches the nipple and prevents the baby from coming close enough to hold it in his mouth. If the nose is pushed very close to the breast, the head may be too bent. All that is needed is to move the baby slightly toward the other breast to resolve this problem.

Difficulties with breastfeeding

In some cases, breastfeeding can be more difficult, but not impossible, either because the baby has already been bottle-fed, has been given a pacifier, experienced nipple shields, or because of some other specific problem: prematurity, twins, hare lip, Down's syndrome.

In these cases, the mother should consult her pediatrician, midwife or pediatric nurse.

It is possible to feed twins exclusively on mother's milk. One breast can be offered to one twin and the other breast to the other twin, in turn.

When there are more than two babies, it may be more difficult to feed them exclusively on mother's milk, and the mother will probably need more help.

Formula feeding should be reserved only for cases in which it is specifically medically prescribed. One disadvantage is that it is an expensive item in the family budget. Another is that, in spite of the excellent quality of all existing milk formulas, none of them can transmit natural immunities to the baby.

When preparing baby bottles, it is very important to keep to the measurements and proportions indicated by the pediatrician and to read the instructions on the packaging very closely. This will prevent the baby's having digestive problems (diarrhea, constipation, dehydration, and tummy aches).

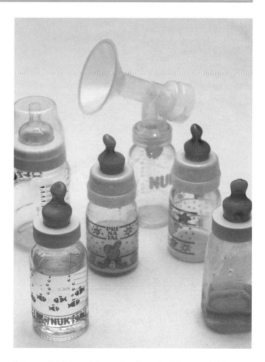

If the pediatrician advises using formula, it is essential for your child's health to follow a series of steps for the correct preparation and administration of the bottle.

How to prepare baby bottles

• Wash your hands thoroughly and sterilize the bottle, cap, and teat for 10 minutes.

• The hole in the teat should be exactly the right size to enable the milk to flow out drop by drop without shaking the bottle.

• Then boil the water you are going to use and let it cool to body temperature.

• Put the amount of water recommended by the pediatrician into the bottle and then add the amount of formula indicated on the container, using level spoonfuls without pressing.

• Shake the bottle thoroughly to eliminate any lumps.

• Before giving the baby the bottle, check the temperature of the milk by dripping a few drops on to the back of your hand. If it is too hot, cool it a little by putting the bottle into cold water without wetting the teat.

• It is advisable to prepare a bottle for each feed. Never use anything that has been left over from the previous feed, and don't leave prepared bottles in the refrigerator, as they could lose some of their nutritive properties or become contaminated. Don't keep any previously boiled water in the refrigerator either.

• During the feed, the bottle should be held at a good angle, so that the teat is full, to prevent the baby swallowing any air there might be in the teat.

• When the feed is over, expel any air swallowed by holding the baby with his or her head on your shoulder, gently patting and rubbing the back.

Some babies regurgitate more than others and some go on doing so throughout their first year. It is important to know the difference between regurgitating food and vomiting. Vomiting causes the baby great distress and is much more copious than regurgitation.

■ Hiccups, burping, and regurgitation

• Hiccups. Most babies have hiccups now and then. This is normally unimportant unless it happens while they are feeding. Change the baby's position and try to get him to burp or relax. Don't try to feed him again until he has stopped hiccupping. If he doesn't stop within 5 to 10 minutes, try giving him sips of water. This is normally the solution. If the baby often has hiccups, try to feed him when he is calm or before he gets too hungry.

• Burping. This is more frequent in bottle-fed babies. The best thing is to delay the feed until the baby calms down. Otherwise, he may swallow more air, feel more uncomfortable, and even vomit. It is best to make him burp frequently, even if he doesn't seem to be uncomfortable, and, when you stop and change position, the baby will feed more slowly and reduce the amount of air he swallows.

• Regurgitation. Babies often regurgitate the food they have received. This may be because they have eaten more than their stomach can contain. They may sometimes regurgitate while they are burping or dribbling. In most cases this is nothing to worry about, but always consult your doctor or pediatric nurse if you are concerned.

Pregnancy in adolescence

Unwanted pregnancies are one of the principal risks associated with having active sex in adolescence. These days, people are starting to have sex at an ever younger age. It is not the person's age that matters, but the degree of maturity with which this new stage of life is approached.

Pregnancy

Pregnancy at any age is a very important biological and psychosocial event, but in adolescence it implies a series of situations that can damage the mother and the child. It can become a health problem that should not be viewed only in terms of the present, but also of the future, because of the complications that may result. The medical risks associated with pregnancy in adolescent mothers, such as high blood pressure, anemia, low birth weight, inadequate nutrition, etc., lead to a high maternal death rate and an estimated infant death rate two to three times greater than that in

Pregnancies in women aged under 19 are called "adolescent pregnancies" and there is a very wide range in this birthrate category across industrialized countries, which is probably the result of the varied cultural norms, religions, and economies.

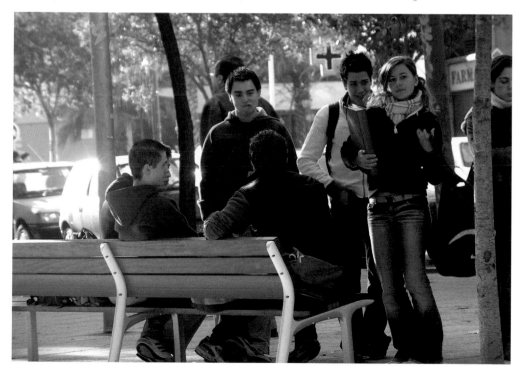

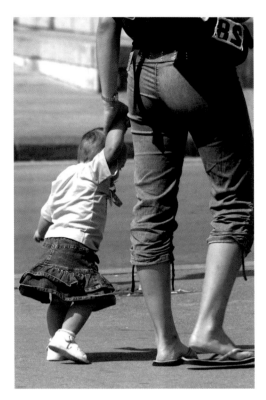

Women who have their first child in adolescence are more likely to have more children in total, and those children are also less likely to receive the full support of their biological parents, complete their education, work in a vocational job, and establish the independence and financial security to provide for themselves. Married adolescent mothers are more likely to divorce than married women who delay their pregnancy until at least the age of 20.

Advice for parents

- Parents should try to leave behind antiquated ideas that prevent them from communicating openly with their children.
- It is important to start talking to them about sexuality from an early age.
- Supervise their activities, while accepting that they are no longer children, but young people who need a degree of independence.
- Parents have the right to know with whom their children are associating.
- It is important to realize that children can read and listen.
- Parents should help them to set standards for the future.
- Children should be given the opportunity of studying and practicing sport.
- Children should be motivated.

pregnancies of women between the ages of 20 and 29.

In adolescents, the increased comparative risk observed does not seem to be due to particular physical conditions, but rather to the sociocultural variables, and the care and medical attention they receive. Adolescent pregnancy is often viewed as an unwanted or unplanned event, the product of a casual relationship between the couple, producing an attitude of rejection, or concealment of the condition for fear of the family's reaction, and leading to delayed or inadequate prenatal supervision.

A common mechanism has developed which could explain various conditions specific to pregnancy that appear more often in adolescent pregnancies, such as: maternal high blood pressure, premature birth, delayed intrauterine growth, and premature placental detachment. A defect in the physiological mechanisms that adapt the circulatory system to pregnancy has been postulated, known as poor circulatory adaptation syndrome, whose various clinical manifestations can occur separately or together in the mother and/or the fetus.

Pregnancy

Leaving aside the obvious cause of a pregnancy's resulting from a sexual relationship, it can be affirmed that the causes of adolescent pregnancy are much more complex.

- Inadequate sexual education. This is the first and most important cause. Many adolescent girls reach this age without information about their sexual functions, relations between the sexes, and how to prevent pregnancy. However, information alone is not enough. True education does not consist only of information, but also of a set of values that make sense of it and allow a person to build a life plan for themselves. Within such a plan, sex, the partner, marriage, and procreation can be freely and responsibly chosen.

Pregnancy in adolescence is associated with a higher risk of illness and death, for both mother and baby. A pregnant adolescent has a higher risk of complications, such as toxemia, high blood pressure, anemia, premature birth, and placenta previa, among others.

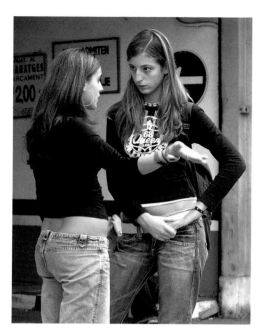

• Family inadequacy. Lack of values is mainly due to family inadequacy. Some homes do not take an open and understanding attitude to sex. Many parents, dominated by myths and fears, reject the responsibility of informing their children about sex, even though they suffered that same problem in their own families. Official educational systems also often fail to offer adequate training on this and other personal development matters.

• Over-emphasis on sex. To this should be added the over-emphasis on sex that exists in modern society. Today's adolescents grow up surrounded by a culture in which television, films, music, videos, advertising, and the places where they meet for amusement, bombard them with messages in which casual sexual relationships are presented as commonplace, accepted, and desirable.

• Lack of information about contraception. Available information about contraceptive methods for those who decide to be sexually active can be sparse and often may be erroneous. In areas of poverty and low social aspiration, this lack is aggravated by the near impossibility of obtaining condoms or other methods of avoiding pregnancy.

• Alcohol and drugs. The growing use of alcohol and drugs at an increasingly early age also has a negative effect. When under the influence of these substances, adolescents are less capable of preventing pregnancy.

There are many ways of preventing adolescent pregnancy that have been tested with varying degrees of success.

Some people preach abstinence in the hope of delaying the start of sexual contact until the person is mature and skilled enough to manage sexual relations without the risk of unwanted pregnancies. Others believe adolescents should be allowed to have sex as soon as they feel the desire to do so, and should therefore have adequate information about their bodies and contraceptive measures. In any case, opting for the values of responsible love and respect for the new life that may be conceived will be the nucleus of prevention, not only of adolescent pregnancy, but also of the many pathologies caused by the transmission of sexual diseases, among which HIV/AIDS and Hepatitis B have taken on new importance nowadays.

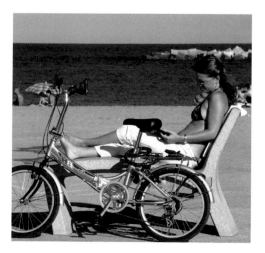

Termination of pregnancy

Abortion is the expulsion of the fetus during the first months of pregnancy and can be spontaneous, natural, or induced. A pregnancy can be terminated by the voluntary decision of the woman, or on medical advice and indication, and occurs before the pregnancy has developed to term.

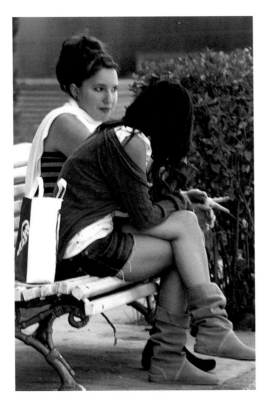

The termination of a pregnancy before the 12th week is less complicated and risky to a woman's health than giving birth, provided it is performed in suitable conditions by specialized staff.

Voluntary termination of pregnancy

Voluntary termination of pregnancy can be performed up to the 22nd week of gestation. Depending on its purpose and the circumstances, terminations of pregnancy have been classified into the following types:

• Elective abortion. This is an abortion performed under the presumed right of the mother to interrupt her pregnancy. A series of motivations are given—the most frequent being economic or social. The fact that the pregnancy is unwanted will be considered a sufficient reason.

• Eugenic abortion. This is performed with the intention of eliminating a fetus when it can be predicted that it will probably or certainly be born with a defect or disease.

• Abortion for medical or therapeutic reasons. This is the voluntary termination of a pregnancy before the fetus is viable, for maternal health reasons.

• Selective abortion. This is what is known as selective fetal reduction and is designed to eliminate some embryos in the case of multiple pregnancies, to enable the others to have a better chance of survival.

Precautions to be taken before and after termination of pregnancy

The decision to terminate a pregnancy is complex, so the fullest possible support and information about its physical and psychological aspects is necessary.

◗ Methods of terminating pregnancy

The methods used to terminate pregnancy vary according to the stage gestation has reached. The earlier it is performed, the less will be the risk of complications.

The most frequently used methods are:

- Aspiration. This is performed before the 10th or 12th week of pregnancy. It does not necessitate hospitalization and is normally carried out under a local anesthetic, the risks being minimal in this case. It can sometimes be performed with a general anesthetic, which will imply hospitalization.

- Dilatation and curettage (scraping). This is a surgical procedure sometimes performed at the same time as aspiration to ensure that the uterus is completely emptied. It is usually carried out under general anesthetic.

- Induction. This is used to interrupt pregnancies of more than 14 weeks' duration. It is com-

plex, and sometimes requires hospitalization. It can be combined with medication that induces the expulsion of the contents of the uterus.

- Chemical method (for example RU 486 – oral/vaginal prosta-glandins). This is a legal method of voluntary termination and is therefore governed by legal indications and limitations. It can be used only for pregnancies that have lasted less than 7 weeks, that is to say, in women in whom less than 49 days have elapsed since the first day of their last menstrual period. It is not available in pharmacies, or even on prescription. Therefore, the patient must attend the clinic with her documentation in order, or with her parents or legal guardian, if she is under age and the state requires it.

After the procedure, the woman should be monitored by specialized staff. Her treatment should include a gynecological checkup (carried out 10 to 30 days after the termination), and the necessary psychological attention. The gynecologi-

cal checkup is the right moment to choose the most suitable method of contraception.

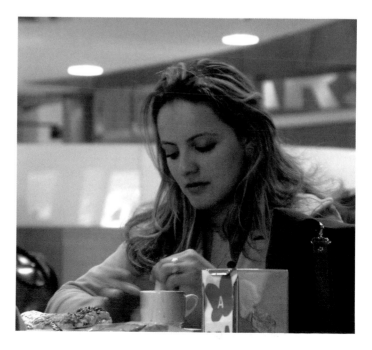

What can a woman do when faced with a possible termination of pregnancy? The most important thing is to seek advice as early as possible from a health center, family planning clinic, or women's rights information bureau. These services will tell you about the legal situation in each set of circumstances, and the medical, psychological, and social consequences of a termination, and advise you about where to apply and what formalities have to be completed.

The commonest complications

- Continuation of the pregnancy (if aspiration is not performed very early on).
- Incomplete abortion.
- Hemorrhage.
- Uterine perforation
- Infections.

- Cervical tearing.
- Postabortion syndrome (bleeding in the uterus).
- If a microcaesarian section has been performed, all the complications of major surgery.

◢ What you should never do

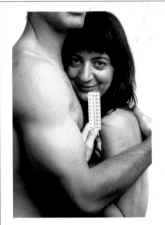

- Allow yourself to be handled by untrained staff or in conditions that do not comply with the essential standards of hygiene.
- Use household methods to induce an abortion.
- Self-medicate.

These practices are ineffective and also endanger your life and your health.

Termination of pregnancy is not a method of contraception. Effective contraceptive methods are the pill, the IUD, and the condom, among others, when used properly. They are very safe for sex with penetration, and prevent unwanted pregnancy.

Spontaneous abortion, or miscarriage

- A pregnancy can terminate itself naturally, before the fetus is viable.
- The percentage of pregnancies that end spontaneously is not known exactly, but it is estimated at between 10 and 30%.
- The most frequent causes of miscarriage are chromosome anomalies in the embryo's development.
- There are other factors that adversely affect the uterine environment, such as viral or bacterial infections (mycoplasma, chlamydia, brucellosis, listeriosis), radiation, chemical factors, or chronic maternal diseases (discompensated diabetes, hyperthyroidism or hypothyroidism, high blood pressure), and uterine deformities (fibroids of the uterus).
- Even physical or psychic trauma and stress can cause miscarriages.
- Although it is not very frequent, the loss of the pregnancy for immunological reasons should be mentioned, as it occurs when the mother's body rejects the pregnancy in the same way as it would an organ implant.

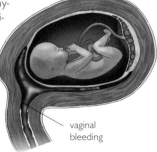

vaginal bleeding

Rheumatism

The word rheumatism is used to describe pain and stiffness in the joints or other muscular and bony structures. It is not a specific disease, but a set of symptoms caused by other problems, such as arthritis or fibrosis.

Rheumatism

The generic use of the words rheuma or rheumatism refers to distinct inflammatory processes of the joints and their components, and of the muscles and bones, which occur accompanied by pain, limitation of normal function, and even deformation of the structure of one or more parts of the musculoskeletal system.

Other symptoms experienced by people suffering from rheumatism are usually inflammation, hypersensitivity, and stiffness of the affected part.

All these symptoms tell us little about the underlying problem, as they are very common in a wide range of diseases involving the joints and their associated structures, the bones and muscles.

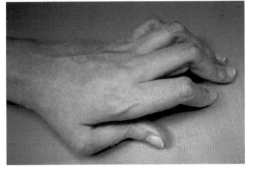

There are two types of rheumatism, depending on the part of the body where it occurs: articular and nonarticular. Articular rheumatism is localized inside the joint itself, affecting the cartilage or the synovial membrane. Nonarticular rheumatism is caused by inflammation of the structures surrounding the joints, such as tendons and muscles.

Rheumatoid arthritis

This is a chronic, deforming disease that causes pain, stiffness, swelling, and loss of function in the joints, and can also be accompanied by inflammation in other organs. Although the cause

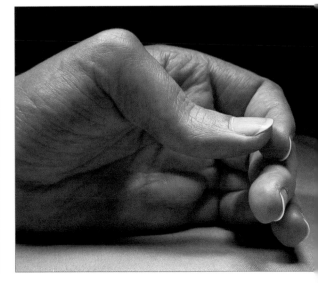

Diagnosis of arthritis

Arthritis is an autoimmune disease, that is to say, the sufferer's own immune system attacks the joints because it does not recognize them as its own, and they therefore become inflamed. There seem to be certain proteins (markers) in the surface of the cells that are transmitted by heredity and predispose a person to this disease.

◢▰ Causes of rheumatism

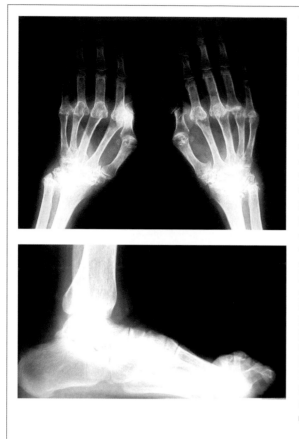

Whenever we move, we use one or more joints and notice almost at once if there are problems in any of them, whether because of the pain or the inability or difficulty of making certain movements. All the joints are linked by fibrous bands, called ligaments, which surround the fibrous capsule of the joint and the synovial capsule, a thin membrane that lubricates the joint. Where the ends of bones come into contact with one another, their surfaces are covered with a fine, strong substance called articular cartilage.

In old age, joint pain is very frequent and there is a link between the way in which a joint has been used at each stage of life and the tendency to develop rheumatism, although how this happens has not yet been demonstrated. Rheumatism can appear in the course of many diseases, known as rheumatic diseases. For example, osteoarthritis, rheumatoid arthritis, juvenile arthritis, and ankolising spondylitis cause articular forms of rheumatism. Nonarticular rheumatism can be caused by bursitis and fibrositis, which is an inflammation of the muscle tissue. Other ailments, such as gout and lupus erythematosis, can also cause rheumatic pain.

of rheumatoid arthritis is still unknown, considerable progress is being made in research into inflammatory immune mechanisms that lead to arthritis and joint damage.

Treatment of rheumatoid arthritis

The aim of treatment is to improve joint mobility and reduce joint pain. Nonsteroid anti-inflammatory drugs are administered for this, and if they do not produce a good response, medication is used that modifies the immune response, such as gold salts, methotrexate, chloroquine, sulphasalazine, azathioprine, and D-penicillamine.

Sometimes, combinations of these and associated steroids are used, especially if other organs of the body are affected. To keep the joints working, it is also recommended to follow a good program of rehabilitation exercises. In the severest cases, and if the disease causes functional incapacity in certain joints, a synovectomy is performed or a total replacement of the joint with a prosthesis (very usual for hip and knee joints).

Arthrosis

Arthrosis, or degenerative joint disease, is the commonest of the joint diseases. It occurs most often in middle-aged or elderly people, affecting the neck, lumbar region, knees, hips, and finger joints. Approximately 70% of people over the age of 70 show radiological evidence of the disease, but only half of them develop symptoms.

The study of arthrosis is one of the areas of what is normally known as rheumatism. Arthrosis defines the progressive deterioration of the articular cartilage and other alterations that occur in the surrounding tissues as a consequence of the original injury. Although all the articular structures can be affected, most anatomical changes are located in the articular cartilage and bones adjacent to the joints.

Arthrosis can also affect joints that have been previously damaged by prolonged overuse, infection, a previous accidental injury, or a previous rheumatic disease.

Patients with arthrosis suffer pain and functional deterioration.

Arthrosis appears when the articular cartilage degenerates. This deterioration has many causes. Some forms of arthrosis are hereditary, including the commonest form, which causes deformed knuckles, for which a specific genetic anomaly has been found. This anomaly causes a change in one of the basic components of the proteins called amino acids, leading to premature cartilage deterioration. Much research concerns this genetic anomaly, as well as new ways of studying the cells, chemistry, and working of the cartilage. All these efforts are rapidly increasing our understanding of the condition.

- Diagnosis: Arthrosis is suspected when pain occurs in the joints that are typically affected by this disease. This suspicion has to be confirmed by a physical examination, X-rays, and the exclusion of other types of joint disease. It should be remembered that, because arthrosis is a very common complaint, it can occur at the same time as another rheumatic disorder.

- Treatment: The treatment of arthrosis includes pharmacological and nonpharmacological measures aimed at relieving pain and improving joint function. Pharmacological treatment must start with simple analgesics (for example, Acetaminophen), to which nonsteroid anti-inflammatory drugs can be added, or the intermittent intraarticular administration of corticosteroids. Nonpharmacological treatment includes teaching the patient exercises to restore joint movement and increase muscular strength and aerobic capacity, reduce weight on the painful joints, and apply heat and cold to lossen pain.

In seriously damaged joints, repair or replacement surgery (joint replacement) may be necessary to eliminate pain and restore function.

Symptoms of arthritis

The most characteristic symptoms are:

- Suffering from arthritis for more than 6 weeks.
- Stiff joints in the morning.
- Presence of nodules (small swellings) on the skin.

If these symptoms are present, blood tests and X-rays are performed, and the results supporting the diagnosis are observed:

- Joint erosion visible in an X-ray.
- Positive rheumatoid factor (in more than 75% of cases).

Menstrual problems

Menstruation is part of the normal menstrual cycle in a healthy woman of fertile age. The menstrual cycle lasts some 28 days, but is also considered normal if it lasts between 21 and 35 days. It starts on the first day of bleeding (known as the period) and ends on the day before the following period.

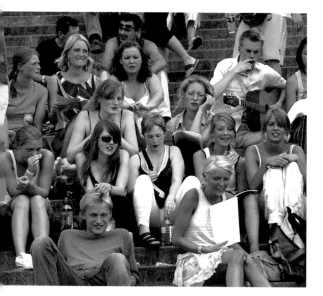

Menstruation

When women become accustomed to having periods, they learn to distinguish the signs of each phase of their menstrual cycle, even if only vaguely.

Symptoms can vary according to the menstrual cycle:

• During the preovulation phase (the days following the period), a woman will feel fulfilled, with renewed energy and strength.

• During the ovulation phase (some two weeks after the period), an acute pain is often felt on one side of the lower abdomen, and an increase in vaginal secretion, or flow.

• The postovulation phase (a few days before the period) produces more physical and psychic changes, to the point that some women may suffer premenstrual tension (PMT). In this syndrome, the commonest symptoms are a feeling of tearfulness and melancholy, difficulty in concentrating, a swelling of the lower abdomen, and an increase in oil in the skin and hair.

• During menstruation, or bleeding, hemorrhage is the principal characteristic, and can last between 3 and 7 days. The amount of blood lost varies from woman to woman, but the average loss would be equivalent to the volume of a teacup. Ninety percent of it is expelled during the first three days of a period. Other symptoms of this phase are: a cramping pain in the lower abdomen, pain in the back and legs, feeling faint, nausea, vomiting, and diarrhea.

Premenstrual syndrome

Not all women suffer PMT, although they may feel discomfort in the days preceding a period. For PMT to be present, there must be specific problems in addition to the feelings of tearfulness and tension characteristic of the premenstrual phase. Its symptoms have both physical and psychological aspects. The physical group includes:

• Tension in the breasts.
• Swelling (head, abdomen, fingers).
• Headache (migraine).
• Appetite changes (craving for candies).
• Acne or urticaria.
• Constipation or diarrhea.
• Palpitations.
• Changes in sexual interest.
• Changes in sleep pattern.
• Muscular stiffness.

Painful periods

One third of women suffer dysmenorrhea, or very painful periods. The pain is like a cramping sensation, but more intense, and can be accompanied by nausea, vomiting or feeling faint. The best treatment for each case must be decided by a doctor.

Some studies indicate that dysmenorrhea may be related to the production of too much prostaglandin. Some women obtain relief by taking a warm, relaxing bath, or having a relaxing massage of the abdomen when the first signs of pain occur.

- Back pain.
- Asthma.
- Rhinitis.

The psychological changes the woman may suffer are:
- Depression.
- Feeling of tearfulness, melancholy.
- Tiredness.
- Tension or restlessness.
- Anxiety.
- Irritability and aggressiveness.
- Difficulty in concentrating.

The symptoms usually appear during the days preceding menstruation and disappear when bleeding starts. They are more frequent in women aged 30 and those who already have children, for reasons unknown.

The most acute cases of premenstrual syndrome may need medical treatment. For other women the following remedies may be useful. If in any doubt, a doctor should be consulted.
- Diet. Eat a healthy diet, rich in fruit and green vegetables. Reduce your salt intake to avoid swelling, and eat a little more sugar than usual, as it may help regulate your glucose level when you feel short of energy.
- Exercise. Exercise regularly.
- Relaxation. Avoid stressful situations as far as possible. Learn relaxation methods. It also helps to read an absorbing book or take a walk.

Menstrual problems:

The most frequent irregularities

- Amenorrhea. The absence of two or more consecutive menstrual cycles.
- Proiomenorrhea. Cycles that last less than 25 days or if menstrual bleeding starts more than 5 days late.
- Opsomenorrhea. Cycles that last more than 35 days or if the period starts more than 5 days early.

Duration irregularities:
- Polymenorrhea. Menstrual bleeding lasting more than 8 days.
- Oligomenorrhea. Menstrual bleeding lasting less than 3 days.

Quantity irregularities:
- Hypermenorrhea. A considerable increase in the customary amount of menstrual bleeding.
- Hypomenorrhea. A marked decrease in the amount of menstrual bleeding.

Irregularities in the rhythm of blood loss:
- Periods that start very intensely. These arise from lesions that bleed of their own accord and usually originate from the uterine cavity.
- Nictomenorrhea. Menstruation that occurs predominantly at night has been considered a symptom of cancer of the uterus.
- Periods that are interrupted for one or more days. The most frequent type consists of menstruation that stops for 24 to 72 hours after 3 to 5 days and then starts again, usually sparsely, for one or two days more. Its cause is usually endocrine related.

Abnormal uterine bleeding (metrorrhagia).

Very heavy periods

Some women have very heavy periods. Excessive bleeding need not mean anything is wrong. It sometimes happens when a woman has omitted to take a contraceptive pill, or after a birth, or in women close to menopause. If a heavy period occurs suddenly for no obvious reason, a doctor should be consulted. Moreover, if a woman feels particularly tired during a menstrual period, she may be anemic.

Irregular menstruation

Few women have a menstrual cycle of exactly 28 days. In fact, many have longer or shorter cycles, and anything between 21 and 35 days is considered normal. When the cycle lasts longer than 6 weeks, it is considered abnormal, although this is nothing to worry about during the first years of menstruation, because it takes some time for the cycles to become regular.

These unusually long cycles are sometimes diagnosed as oligomenorrhea (an excessively low number of periods in a year), or amenorrhea (absence of periods). Oligomenorrhea can be caused by hormonal imbalance, but it may simply be that particular woman's normal cycle. To rule out the possibility that a disease is the cause, the woman should consult a gynecologist who will carry out the pertinent examinations and analyses.

The usual reason for amenorrhea, if the periods have always been regular, is pregnancy, but it can also be related to dietary changes, excessive physical activity or very acute stress.

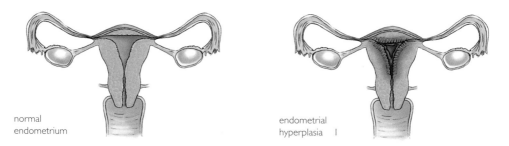

normal
endometrium

endometrial
hyperplasia   I

There are various causes of irregular menstrual periods, such as endometrial hyperplasia, endometrial polyps, fibroids of the uterus, and abnormal functioning of the thyroid and pituitary glands. The endometrium is the tissue that lines the inside of the uterus. When it becomes abnormally thick, the condition is called endometrial hyperplasia, and can cause profuse and prolonged menstrual bleeding.

Periodical uterine bleeding:
• Anovulatory menstruation. This affects women who lose blood with a frequency, duration, and rhythm identical to normal menstruation but who have demonstrated the absence of ovulation and, therefore, of a menstrual cycle.
• Periodical intercalary hemorrhage. This is characterized by losses of blood that occur around the time of ovulation (intermenstrual bleeding). Its cause is unknown.

Arrhythmic uterine bleeding
There are five types:
• Metrorrhagia that continues after menstruation. Prolonged bleeding that starts on the date when the period was expected. It can last from a week to two or three months.
• Premenstrual bleeding. A small amount of bleeding that precedes the period.
• Bleeding following a period of amenorrhea:

- Pregnancy complications.
- Complications following childbirth.
- Injury, malignant tumors, infections.
• Bleeding that is atypical, irregular, and nonrhythmic, and occurs at random. This occurs after menopause.

Breast pathologies

The breasts produce milk for feeding infants, but, in the human species, they also constitute secondary sexual organs that play an important part in sexuality and eroticism. The importance of the breasts from the gynecological point of view lies in the frequency of the appearance of pathologies and how accessible they are to early detection and diagnosis.

The breast

The breast is made up of two basic kinds of tissue: glandular tissue and supporting (stromal) tissue). The glandular part of the breast includes the lobules and the ducts. In lactating women (who breastfeed their babies), the cells of the lobules produce milk that is carried to the nipple through the milk ducts. The supporting tissue of the breast includes adipose tissue (fat) and fibrous connective tissue that determine the size and shape of the breast and support it. Any of these areas of the breast can undergo changes that cause symptoms.

The two principal types of change in the breast are benign conditions (noncancerous) and cancerous tumors. The commonest benign tumors are

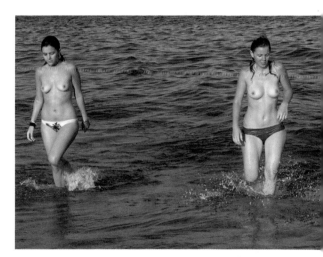

Although breast cancer is one of the pathologies that causes the most deaths in women, that fact should never make you believe that any anomaly you may detect in your breasts is a sign of a malignant tumor. What is important—very important—is that as soon as you notice any anomaly, however small it may be, you should consult a gynecologist at once to ascertain its nature.

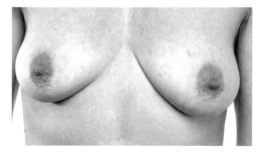

Women view their breasts as especially delicate organs. Their medical care should always be a priority and, therefore, periodical checkups should not be postponed. Prevention is always better than cure.

The most frequent breast diseases

• Fibrocystic breast disease. This is a change in the mammary tissue that gives the breast a dense, irregular consistency, usually more marked in the outer quadrants of the breast. This varies with the menstrual cycle. It is associated with pain (mastalgia) and is sometimes accompanied by nodules or cysts that do not require major treatment. Its cause is not exactly understood, but it seems to be associated with ovarian hormones, because the nodules usually disappear with the menopause. It is estimated that more than 60% of women aged between 30 and 50 have the condition. It does not increase the risk of developing breast cancer.

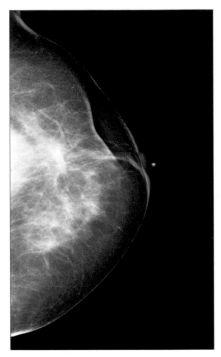

• Microcalcifications of the breast. This is the deposit of calcium secondary to normal processes such as lactation, resulting in inflam-mation, small lesions, and cellular destruction that are detectable in a mammogram. In a small percentage of women, microcalcifications have particular characteristics that may indicate a malignant disease, meaning that more specific studies need to be carried out.

• Infection of the breast (mastitis). This involves the infection and inflammation of the mammary gland, sometimes associated with lactation. The gland becomes swollen, producing pain, increased volume, reddening, and a rise in skin temperature.

• Fibroadenomas. These tumors, that occur frequently in young women, are benign, with a smooth, flat surface, moveable, without adhesions, and not deep. They are produced by a proliferation of tissue round the mammary lobule and feel rubbery to the touch. If a woman is in any doubt about the diagnosis, she can undergo a biopsy.

• Breast cancer. This is an uncontrolled growth of the mammary tissue cells which, when they combine, form a tumor. This disease and the numerous ways in which it manifests itself develop very differently from woman to woman. In some, it may remain within the breast for years and in others it can spread to the lymph glands, even before there is a nodule that can be felt.

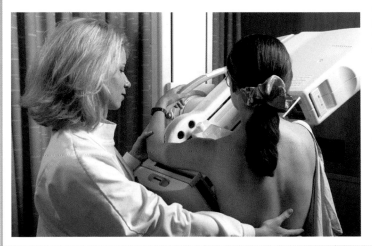

fibrocystic changes, benign breast tumors, and inflammation of the breast. Benign breast conditions are very common. If the breast tissue is examined under a microscope, these changes can be detected in 9 out of 10 women.

Unlike cancerous breast tumors, benign breast conditions are never life threatening. Only in exceptional cases do these conditions cause troublesome symptoms. Moreover, some benign conditions are associated with a greater risk of contracting breast cancer.

The main risk factors in the development of breast cancer

• Sex. Being a woman is the greatest risk factor, as the probability of developing breast cancer is 100 times greater than in men.

• Age. This disease is very rare before the age of 30 and increases progressively with age, 80 percent of cases being diagnosed in women aged over 50.

• Personal history of breast cancer. If cancer has developed in one breast, the risk of its developing in the other is 3 to 4 times greater.

• Genetic predisposition. The incidence of breast cancer varies from country to country. The United States, Canada, and northern Europe have the highest frequency, while Asia has the lowest.

• Motherhood. Women who have not had children or whose first pregnancy occurred after they were 35 years old are at greater risk.

• Estrogens. The longer the period of exposure to estrogens, the greater will be the risk. Thus, women who had their first menstrual period (menarche) before reaching the age of 12, or their last one (menopause) after reaching the age of 55, are more exposed to them.

• Family history. Women whose mothers, aunts,

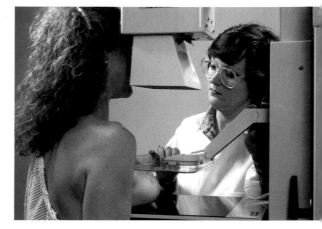

To confirm the diagnosis, all women over the age of 40 are recommended to have a mammogram taken regularly on the advice of the doctor who examines her breasts. In women with a family history of breast cancer, this check should be initiated 10 years earlier than the age at which breast cancer was diagnosed in the family member. Mammography has been shown to reduce death from breast cancer by between 25 and 30%, because it enables tumors to be detected two years before they can be felt.

or sisters have had breast cancer are at greater risk of developing it. This risk increases if the disease was diagnosed before their relatives reached the menopause. For a woman with a close relative with this disease, the risk doubles. If more than 2 relatives have had it, the risk is multiplied by 5.

• Uninterrupted combined hormone replacement therapy (HRT) for more than 5 years. A woman who has taken estrogens and progesterone for prolonged periods is at increased risk and should undergo periodical medical examination.

• Race. Caucasian women more often develop this disease, compared with those of black and Hispanic race.

• Tobacco. Smoking significantly increases the risk of developing this disease in women with a family history of breast or ovarian cancer.

• Alcohol. Consuming more than 2 alcoholic drinks a day increases the risk of developing breast cancer by 20 percent, compared with women who don't drink.

If many nodules are found (cystic fibrosis of the breast), count them and note their size, so their number and size can be checked every time, and possible changes observed.

Remember that 41 percent of cancerous nodules are found in the upper lateral quadrant of the

Symptoms of breast cancer

• A tumor that can be felt in the breast or armpit.

• Blood in the nipple.

• Retraction in the nipple or areola areas.

• Changes in the skin of the breast, orange-peel skin, changes in color, formation of tumors.

Self-examination of the breasts

- The breasts should be examined 3 to 5 days after menstruation has ended, when they are less sensitive.
- If the woman has passed menopause, she is recommended to examine her breasts on the same day of each month.
- If she is breastfeeding, she should likewise examine her breasts on the same day of each month, after a feed.

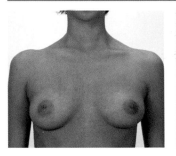

1- You should examine yourself every month, 2–3 days after menstrual bleeding has ended. If you do not have periods, you should examine your breasts on a fixed day every month.

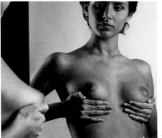

2- Stand in front of a mirror with your body erect. It is essential to be in a good ligh, as no detail must go unnoticed during the exploration.

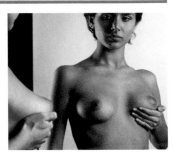

3- Standing in front of the mirror, let your left arm hang loose. Meanwhile, with your right hand, slowly feel the right breast, looking for any anomalies.

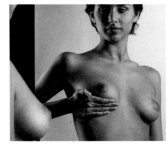

4. Reverse the position of the arm and hand and repeat the operation on the left side.

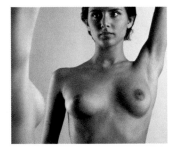

5.Rest your forearm on your head. In this position, look at the outline of your left breast. Repeat the operation with the other arm. Then, raise both arms at the same time and examine your nipples, which should move upward and be at the same height.

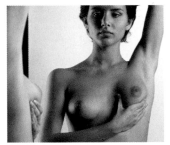

6. Raise your right arm and place your hand on your head, while you feel the right breast and the whole right armpit with your left hand, looking for lumps, protuberances, or inflammations. Repeat the exploration on the other side.

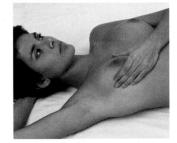

7. Lie on your back with your right hand behind your head. With your left hand, feel the whole lower part of your right breast. Move the hand over the upper part and the center of the breast. Grasp the nipple and areola at the same time, and press lightly. This is to detect anomalies, see if it causes any pain or observe whether any liquid emerges from the nipple.

8. Repeat the operation on the other side.

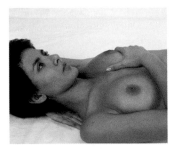

breast (toward the shoulder), 34 percent in the upper middle quadrant (toward the neck), 14 percent in the lower middle quadrant (toward the navel), and 6 percent in the lower lateral quadrant (toward the elbow).

The earlier that breast cancer is discovered, the easier it is to treat. For that reason, many experts recommend all women over the age of 20 to examine their own breasts each month to check the presence of new lumps or other changes. However, self-examination has limitations and is not a substitute for regular medical examinations. It is recommended to talk to a doctor about the pros and cons of self-examination. If the woman examines her own breasts, she should do so 3 to 5 days after the end of the menstrual period when they are less sensitive and have fewer protuberances.

▪ Treatment of breast cancer

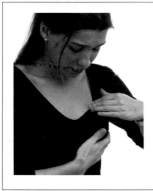

- Treatment depends on the stage at which the cancer is diagnosed.
- When possible, the tumor and surrounding area of normal tissue will be surgically removed and, if necessary, the lymphatic ganglia in the armpits will be emptied.
- It is sometimes necessary to perform a mastectomy (removal of the breast), with immediate or deferred plastic reconstruction.
- Surgery is usually followed by radiotherapy to destroy any cancerous cells that may remain in the breast.
- The treatment may be combined with chemotherapy and/or hormone therapy.

▪ Breast pain

This defines any pain or discomfort in the breasts, such as premenstrual sensitivity.

Breast pain can have many causes. For example, hormonal fluctuations related to menstruation or pregnancy are often responsible for sensitive breasts. Some degree of inflammation and sensitivity just before a period is normal. It all depends on how bearable or unbearable the person finds it. Although many women who suffer pain in one or both breasts rightly fear it, breast pain is a very unusual symptom of breast cancer.

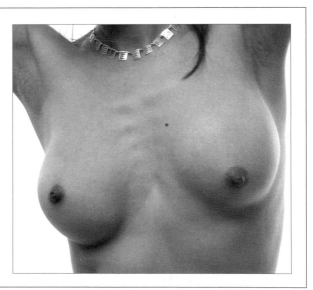

Ovarian cancer

The ovaries are the principal female reproductive organs. They are located in the pelvis, one either side of the uterus. Each ovary is about the size and shape of an almond. They produce the eggs and the female hormones (the chemical substances that control the way each cell and organ works).

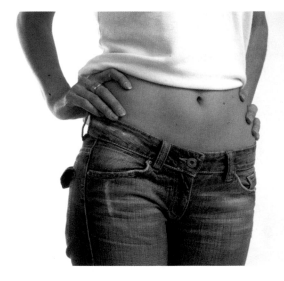

Cancer of the ovaries

Tumors that originate in the ovaries are usually benign, but some are true malignant processes. They can be cystic or solid, and originate from cells that are undergoing a malignant transformation and start growing in a disordered and uncontrolled manner, invading and destroying the tissues around them.

Causes of ovarian cancer

It is not at present known why ovarian cancer occurs. However, it is known that several hormonal and reproductive factors can favor its appearance, such as infertility or a small number of pregnancies. Genetics are a determining factor in only 10 to 15 percent of cases. Those cases are asso-

ciated with breast and ovarian cancer in the same family, or even in the same person.

It is also suspected that certain environmental factors, such as diet, some viral infections, or even using talcum powder may be of importance in the appearance of this disease.

Types of ovarian tumor

As a rule, ovarian tumors are named according to the type of cells from which the tumor originated, and whether it is benign or cancerous. There are three main types of ovarian tumor:

• Germ cell tumors. These originate from the cells that produce the eggs.

• Stromal cell tumors. These originate in the

Which women are at greatest risk?

• Women with a family history of cancer of the ovary, colon, and breast.

• Women who carry the BRCA1 and BRCA2 gene.

• Women who have never been pregnant or taken the contraceptive pill.

• Women who have had estrogen replacement therapy for a long time (more than 10 years).

• Women who are infertile or have taken medication to treat infertility.

◼ Important aspects

- Although most cases of ovarian cancer occur in women aged 50 or over, it can also appear in younger women.
- Its commonest form, epithelial tumors, is usually diagnosed in women aged 40 or over.
- The risk of contracting any form of this disease starts to increase after the age of 40.
- It accounts for 4% of all cancers affecting women.
- It is difficult to diagnose.
- The possibility of finding evidence of a pre-malignant lesion in an ovary is very small.
- There is little information about how it grows and metastasizes (or spreads).
- In 75% of patients diagnosed as suffering from this condition, the tumor extends outside the ovary.

There are three basic types of malignant tumor. The commonest are the ones that form on the surface of the ovary and are called epithelial cancers. Cancers can also form in the egg-producing cells and the tissues surrounding the ovary, but these are much less frequent.

cells of the connective tissue that supports the ovary and produces the female hormones estrogen and progesterone.
- Epithelial tumors. These originate in the cells that cover the outer surface of the ovary.

Prevention of ovarian cancer

Ovarian cancer is less frequent in women who have had several children and those who have taken oral ovulation inhibitors (the contraceptive pill) for several years. However, no study has

Although ovarian cancer is the fourth most frequent in gynecological oncology (after cancer of the breast, endometrium, and cervix), it is still the leading cause of death. This is because it is very difficult to diagnose early and 65% of it is diagnosed when it is already at an advanced stage.

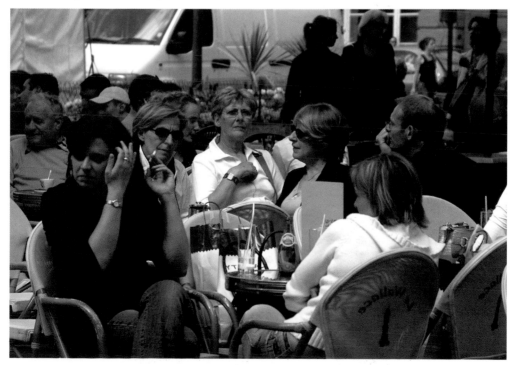

Treatment of ovarian cancer

The treatment of this cancer depends on the patient's age and how long she has been ill. It is more successful when treated early.

Treatment can include:

- A surgical operation to remove the cancer from the ovaries and surrounding tissue
- A hysterectomy is sometimes necessary (removal of the uterus) combined with the removal of both ovaries and the fallopian tubes.
- Chemotherapy. This is the administration of medication to destroy the cancerous cells.
- Radiotherapy.

shown that this reduced probability of ovarian cancer in women, who have taken contraceptives, is offset by other secondary effects such as an increase in the occurrence of cardiovascular diseases and, possibly, other tumors. The use of the contraceptive pill as a preventive measure in the general population is therefore not justified.

A special case is high-risk women who are affected by a hereditary breast and/or ovarian cancer syndrome (BRCA), in whom the protective role played by ovulation inhibitors is being studied. In certain cases, it may be necessary to remove both the patient's ovaries at the age of 35 if she has already had all the children she wants.

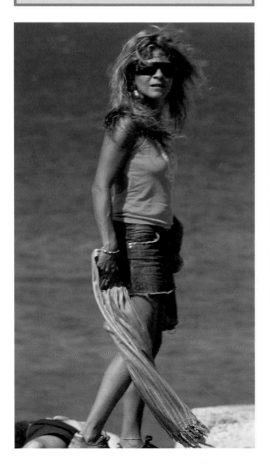

Symptoms of ovarian cancer

There is no detection test for this cancer. It is difficult to detect at an early stage because its symptoms are often imprecise and can be confused with those of other diseases. If any of the symptoms listed below continues for longer than two or three weeks, the woman should consult a doctor to determine the cause:

- Pelvic or abdominal pain or discomfort.
- Inflammation or a feeling of fullness in the pelvis or abdomen.
- Persistent nausea or indigestion.
- Diarrhea or constipation for which no other explanation can be found.
- Pain during the sexual act.
- Anomalous (nonmenstrual) bleeding from the vagina.
- Persistent back pain and tiredness.

Cancer of the uterus

The uterus or womb is an organ located in the woman's pelvis in front of the rectum and behind the urinary bladder. It is a cavity lined by the endometrium. Until the menopause, the endometrium renews itself each month with menstruation. Cancer of the uterus can develop as a result of changes in the cells of the endometrium. It usually occurs in the last years preceding the menopause or thereafter, and is infrequent in women under the age of 40.

Cervicouterine cancer

One of the cancers that causes most deaths in women is cervicouterine cancer (the appearance of abnormal cells in the neck of the uterus). It is considered a public health problem and occupies first place as the cause of death among women between the ages of 25 and 60.

The uterus consists of two parts: the body of the uterus, located at the top, which is where babies develop, and the neck of the uterus, located at the bottom, which connects the body of the uterus to the vagina.

Cancer of the cervix (or neck of the womb) does not appear suddenly. In the early stages, some cells start to change from normal cells into precancerous cells and then into cancerous ones. This change can take several years, although it sometimes develops more quickly. In some women, precancerous changes can disappear without any treatment. However, they usually require treatment to prevent them turning into a true cancer.

Causes and risk factors

A risk factor is anything that increases the likelihood that a person will contract a disease. Some risk factors, such as smoking, can be controlled. Others, such as a person's age or race, cannot.

Cancer of the uterus is the principal cause of death in women aged between 25 and 60, and can be prevented if it is detected in time by a simple procedure called the Papanicolau (cervical smear, or Pap) test.

There are several risk factors that increase the likelihood of suffering cervical cancer.

• Human papilloma virus (HPV). The principal risk factor is infection by this virus. The disease can be transmitted from person to person during sexual relations. Having unprotected sexual relations, especially at an early age, increases the likelihood of becoming infected by this virus. Moreover, women who have many sexual partners (or who have had sexual relations with men who have themselves had many sexual partners) are at greater risk of contracting HPV. Infection by the AIDS virus can also be a risk factor for this type of cancer. Carrying the HIV virus reduces the capacity of the immune system to combat both the human papilloma virus and cancers in their initial stages.

• Smoking is another risk factor for cervical cancer. Tobacco smoke can produce chemical substances that can damage the DNA of the cervical cells and make them more likely to become cancerous.

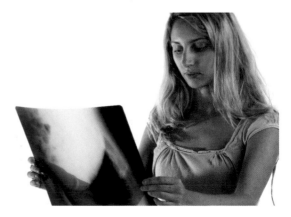

Women who smoke have twice the risk of contracting cervical cancer than those who do not.

• Cancer of the uterus is the principal cause of death in women aged between 25 and 60, and can be prevented if it is detected in time by a simple procedure called the Papanicolau (cervical smear, or Pap) test.Unlike many other types of cancer, which rarely affect young women, cervical cancer can affect women in their 30s and even adolescents.. Although the risk of cervical cancer does not increase much after the age of 40, it does not decline either. Many mature women are unaware that they have the highest risk of contracting cervical cancer and that it is important to go on taking the smear test.

• Race. Several ethnic groups have a higher mortality rate from cancer of the uterus.

Cervical precancers and cancers in their initial stages often present no indications or symptoms. It is therefore important for women to take a smear test regularly. Symptoms usually appear when the cancer has already progressed. If any of the following symptoms appears, a doctor should be consulted immediately:

• Any unusual vaginal flow.

• Spots of blood or light bleeding that is not that of a normal menstrual period.

• Vaginal bleeding or pain during active sex.

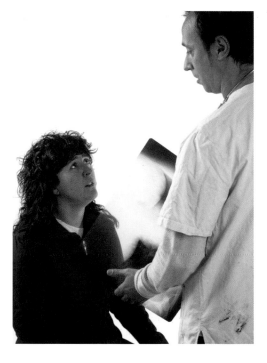

■ Precaution

Most cases of cervical cancer can be prevented. There are two ways of avoiding this disease:

The first is to prevent it, and the best way of doing so is to avoid risk factors, such as:

• Not starting to have sex early.

• Women of all ages can protect themselves from becoming infected by HPV if they use condoms during casual sexual intercourse, if they limit the number of sexual partners they have, and if they avoid having sex with men who have had many sexual partners themselves. HPV does not always cause warts or other symptoms, so it is difficult to know whether a person is infected. Condoms do not protect people against HPV, but they do help prevent infection by HIV, that is to say they give protection against HIV, that develops into AIDS, and other diseases.

• Women who smoke should try to give it up.

• The second way of preventing cervical cancer is to take a cervical smear test regularly. This test can detect HPV infections and cellular alterations. The treatment of these problems can stop the development of cervical cancer before it becomes invasive.

Of course, the appearance of these symptoms does not mean that a woman has cancer, as they can also be the result of a different situation. However, a doctor should be consulted to check what is really happening. If the results of the smear test are suspicious, the doctor will want the woman to take other tests, such as:

• Colposcopy. The observation of the neck of

There are two principal types of cervical cancer: between 85 and 90% of cases are carcinomas of the squamous cells, and between 10 and 15% are adenocarcinomas. If the cancer has the characteristics of both types, it is known as a mixed carcinoma. There are also other rare types of cervical cancer. Cervicouterine cancer is preventable and curable if it is detected early on.

Cancer of the uterus can develop from changes in the cells of the endometrium. It usually appears in the years just before menopause or just following it.

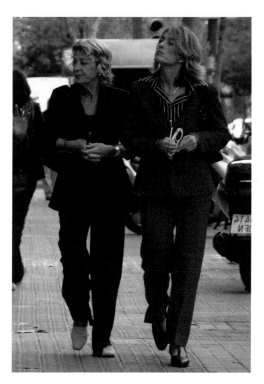

the uterus through an instrument called a colposcope, rather like a pair of binoculars. This test is not painful, has no side effects, and can be carried out even if the woman is pregnant. Various treatment methods can be used if abnormal areas are found during this examination. Some involve the extraction of some tissue with a hot wire or a nitrogen-chilled metal probe. Others consist of using laser surgery to destroy the abnormal cells. These treatments almost always destroy the precancerous cells and prevent them becoming true cancers.

• Biopsy. A biopsy is the extraction of a sample of tissue to see if it contains cancerous cells. It is the only way of ascertaining whether a precancerous condition or a true cancer is present.

▪ Treatment

The three principal types of treatment to combat cervical cancer will depend mainly on the result of the biopsy. They are surgery, radiation, and chemotherapy.

• Surgery. This will depend on the size of the lesion. In some cases, a cone shaped piece of tissue is removed from the cervix (conization), or the uterus only is removed (simple hysterectomy), or the uterus, ovaries, and fallopian tubes are all removed (hysterectomy with bilateral salpingo-oophorectomy). If the cancer has spread outside the uterus, it may be necessary to remove adjacent tissue as well.

• Radiotherapy is a treatment that uses high-potency rays (such as X-rays) to destroy or reduce cancerous cells. This radiation can originate from outside the body (external radiation) or from radioactive materials that are placed directly on to the tumor (internal radiation or implant). Treatment in the pelvic area can make the vagina narrower, due to the formation of scar tissue. This can lead to pain during active sex.

• Chemotherapy. This refers to the use of medication to destroy the cancerous cells. The medication is almost always administered orally or by injection. Once the medication has entered the bloodstream, it spreads throughout the body. Sometimes, several different kinds of medication are administered simultaneously. Chemotherapy can cause side-effects, which will depend on the type of medication, the amounts administered, and the duration of the treatment.

Cardiovascular diseases

Cardiovascular diseases, which include heart disease, high blood pressure, and strokes, account for a third of female mortality throughout the world. Cardiovascular diseases are responsible for 50 percent of the deaths of women aged over 50 in developed countries.

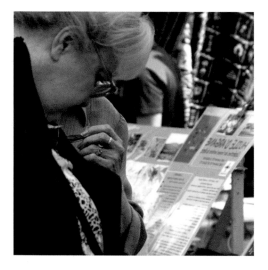

Cardiovascular diseases

Among the main causes of death in women are cardiovascular diseases, tumors, and diseases of the respiratory system, a situation similar to that of men, accidents and injuries being less significant. As a rule, these causal groups are generally identified as chronic nontransmissible adult diseases.

Chronic nontransmissible adult diseases, headed by cardiovascular diseases, represent the principal causes of death in women. For women, this is a major health factor, as they can be prevented, because they depend partly on the individual's lifestyle and risk factors. These risk factors are shared by all women although their relative importance may be different for each disease. The specific mechanism of each factor is not totally clear, but it is not necessary to understand it in order to make the decision to avoid the damage they cause.

The most important risk factors for cardiovascular diseases in women are: addiction to tobacco, high blood pressure (including isolated systolic hypertension), high cholesterol (LDL), diabetes mellitus, obesity, a sedentary lifestyle, an inadequate diet, being over 55 years of age, and/or the menopause (particularly early or surgically induced menopause), psychosocial factors, and a history of premature coronary disease in close relatives.

Other risk factors are also significant—osteoporosis, stress, genetic factors, age, sex, and race—and share in giving rise to these diseases, but their contribution to the damage is difficult to evaluate and is less well known, or simply cannot be altered.

Heart attacks and strokes take more lives, among women, than all female cancers combined. Of the more than 16 million people who die every year from heart and cerebral problems, more than half are women.

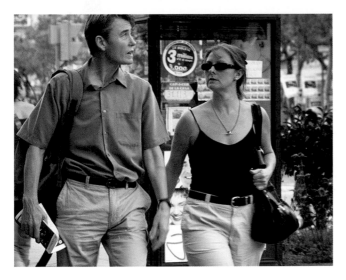

According to mortality statistics, the leading cause of death in women aged over 50 is cardiovascular disease, the second is malignant neoplasias (cancer or tumors), and the third is diabetes or respiratory ailments.

Before menopausal age, the greatest frequency of cardiovascular diseases is observed in men, but after it, their frequency is similar in both sexes—sufficient reason for women to take care of their cardiovascular health.

Although many cardiovascular risk factors are similar for both women and men, differences have been observed, particularly in diabetes and high cholesterol. Whereas the cardiovascular disease and stroke indices are comparable in both sexes, the problem begins later in women, probably because of the protective action of estrogens. There is a significant and specific low risk of coronary disease for women in comparison with men according to age. The risk of dying of a cardiovascular disease in women is similar to that in men 10 years younger, but this risk equalizes between the ages of 65 and 70.

Most women fear cancer, particularly breast cancer, but do not take the same precautions to protect themselves against heart diseases, although they are much easier to prevent. Heart and brain diseases have recently become true epide-

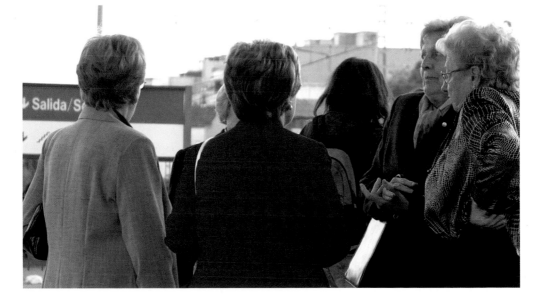

◢▪ Risks that can be controlled

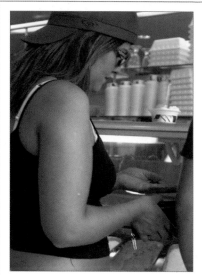

• High blood pressure. Blood pressure increases with age, and high blood pressure is much more frequent in people who are overweight.

• Smoking. A woman who smokes is twice as likely to have a heart attack than one who does not, and is also more likely to die if she has a one. Young women who smoke and take the contraceptive pill are also at significantly greater risk

• High LDL cholesterol. An increase in cholesterol and trigliceride levels. Cholesterol increases with age, obesity, and lack of exercise, and as a result of eating an inadequate diet.

• Diabetes mellitus. A high level of sugar in the blood is a predetermining factor in cardiovascular diseases.

• Obesity. Being overweight makes the heart work harder and causes a greater tendency to high blood pressure and diabetes.

• A sedentary life. Lack of physical exercise generates problems of obesity, reduces the level of good cholesterol and raises the level of bad cholesterol (LDL).

mics and account for more deaths than diseases that used to be considered as a primary factor of sickness and death generally.

◢▪ Risks that cannot be controlled

• Age. The most obviously unavoidable risk factor is that everyone is aging. The number of deaths caused by cardiovascular diseases in women increases by about 5 times after the age of 65.

• Menopause. The occurrence of menopause, whether naturally or surgically (owing to a hysterectomy or the removal of the ovaries), quadruples the risk of suffering heart disease.

• Family history. Unfortunately, an individual cannot control her own genes. A family history of heart disease in young, close relatives is influential in its development.

Medical efforts have been directed at preventing health problems. Much has been learned in the sphere of oncology (cancers) with the development of early detection methods for frequent cancers in women. In the last decade, cardiology has succeeded in developing early detection methods and calculating the probabilities of developing a pattern of cardiac performance over time.

Heart disease manifests itself in people aged over 40, but it begins to develop at an early age, depending on dietary habits, lack of cardiovascular exercise (walking, aerobics, dancing, swimming, etc.), and the consumption of toxic substances, such as tobacco and alcohol.

To achieve cardiovascular health in old age, the good, healthy habits that have been shown to be beneficial need to be adopted from an early age.

Sexually transmitted diseases (STDs)

These include various types of disease that are usually transmitted during sexual relations. The principal means of transmission are the mucous membranes of the mouth, the genital organs, and the anus during sexual relations.

Sexually transmitted diseases

Sexually transmitted diseases are mainly caused by viruses, bacteria, and fungi. Some sexually transmitted diseases cause virtually no appreciable symptoms at first, meaning that the infected person can continue spreading the disease for a long time without even being aware of it. Moreover, sexually transmitted diseases can affect a woman repeatedly, because they do not generate any immunological protection, and there are no vaccines against them. If left untreated, many STDs can

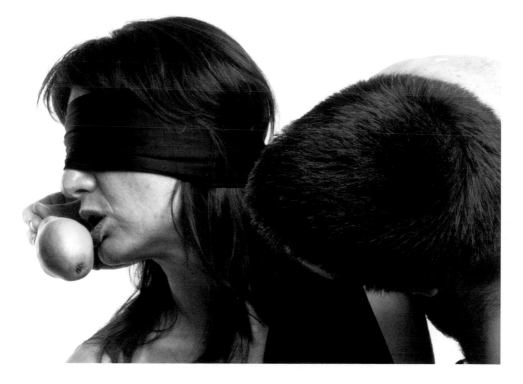

■ Which are the most frequent STDs?

The most frequent STDs are:

- **Gonorrhea** or **blenorrhagia** (caused by the gonococcus bacterium).
- **Syphilis** (caused by Treponema pallidum).
- **Condyloma acuminata** or **genital warts** (caused by the human papilloma virus, HPV).
- **Genital herpes.**
- **Infection by HIV (AIDS)**.
- **Various infections of the vagina and urethra** caused by other microorganisms (Chlamydia trachomatis, Trichomonas, Gardenerella vaginitis, etc.).
- There is another group of diseases that can also be transmitted through sexual relations, including **Hepatitis B** and **genital pediculosis** (pubic lice or "crabs").

have serious and permanent consequences such as blindness and sterility. Many of the symptoms are hard to detect and, with time, can spread to different parts of the body. It is important to consult a doctor in the case of any strange symptom in the lower abdomen or genital area. The symptoms they cause are very similar to one another, and they may not even cause any symptoms, so a person can transmit a disease without realizing it. Some of the symptoms are:

- Flows and secretions in unusual quantities and consistencies.

- Inflamed ganglia in the groin, and difficulty in urinating.
- Itching.
- Small wounds and ulcers in the genitals.
- The appearance of warts (herpes).
- Pain in the lower abdomen and difficulties in having sexual relations.

If you suspect you may have contracted a sexually transmitted disease, you are recommended to follow the guidelines below:

- Visit a doctor if you have any unusual symptom in the lower abdomen or genital area.
- Don't have sex until you are diagnosed and the particular STD treated satisfactorily.
- Advise your sexual partner to visit the doctor to see if he or she has become infected. If treatment is needed, the couple will have to be treated simultaneously.
- Don't hide the disease from the doctor or wait for it to clear up on its own.

Early treatment is of crucial importance as, the sooner it is begun, the less risk there will be of permanent problems. All STDs (except AIDS) can be cured, and diagnosis and treatment are not usually either painful or expensive. To obtain help, visit your doctor, or a specialist in gynecology, obstetrics, dermatology, or urology. You can also seek help at family planning centers and clinics specializing in STDs.

If an STD is diagnosed, it is important to inform the person or people with whom you have had sex recently and tell them what disease you have and the possibility that they may have caught it, even if they have no symptoms. They should be urged to visit the doctor and follow the given instructions and prescriptions.

Preventive measures

The preventive measures that should generally be adopted are:

- Using a condom during sex when there is a suspicion or risk of infection.
- Women who change sexual partners frequently should systematically use a condom and visit the doctor periodically, even if they have no symptoms.

- In the case of the slightest suspicion, the doctor should be consulted. If quickly diagnosed and properly treated, these diseases clear up completely. If not, they can cause sterility, paralysis, dementia, and other serious health problems.
- Pregnant women should take special care to prevent this type of disease and follow the foregoing recommendations, as these diseases can affect the fetus and cause the newborn baby serious damage and deformities.

Prevention is the best way of avoiding STDs. The condom, for both men and women, is the most effective method of preventing these diseases, because it acts as a barrier.

Candidiasis

Candidiasis is caused by the fungus *Candida albicans*, a very long microorganism normally found in small quantities in the vagina, mouth, digestive tract, and skin, without causing any disease or symptoms. The symptoms appear when the number of fungi increases and becomes disproportionate to the other microorganisms normally present in the vagina. These fungi usually appear after treatment with antibiotics prescribed for another condition, as antibiotics upset the normal balance of the vaginal flora.

They can also appear in association with other conditions such as diabetes, pregnancy, taking the contraceptive pill, or problems that affect the immune system (AIDS or the human immune deficiency virus, HIV).

The commonest symptom of this infection is itching in the labia or vagina (pruritis). Occasionally, there is a whitish vaginal discharge. Physical examination will reveal an inflamed vagina and dry, white patches on its walls. Vaginal candidiasis is not considered an STD, but 12 to 15 percent of men

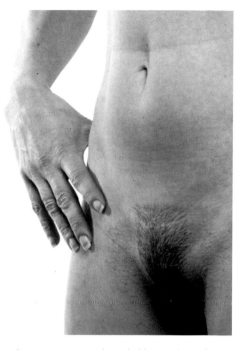

acquire symptoms such as itching and pruritis in the penis after sex with an infected partner.

The development of vaginal candidiasis should be watched carefully, as infections that are repeated or do not clear up could be a first sign that the person is infected with HIV. In men and women with HIV who have developed AIDS, infection by candida can be disseminated, including oral candidiasis (in the mouth), esophageal candidiasis (in the esophagus), and cutaneous candidiasis (in the skin).

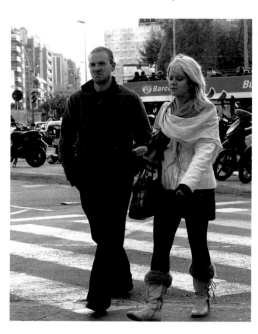

As well as being a contraceptive, the condom for both men and women prevents the transmission of this type of disease as it forms a barrier between the couple's genitals.

Cystitis

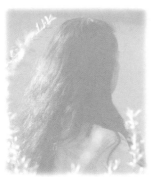

Many women suffer pain and discomfort when urinating, which can be due to a typical female infection, cystitis, and can be treated very effectively with antibiotics, although prevention is always better.

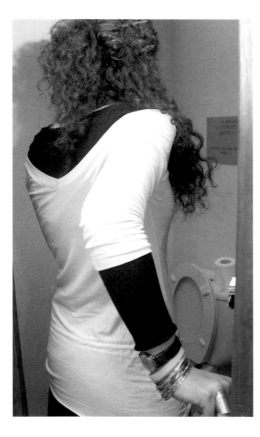

This infection affects most women at some time in their lives, but is not serious if treated in time, although it is very uncomfortable. Two in every hundred people suffer from cystitis, and most of them are women. This inflammation of the bladder and urinary tract can be most uncomfortable.

Cystitis is an infection of the urinary tract produced by the penetration of bacteria into the urethra or bladder and causing inflammation and irritation. As a rule, the urethra and bladder contain no bacteria and, if bacteria enter, they are eliminated in the urine. However, if for some reason bacteria do succeed in entering and are not expelled in the urine, they grow and multiply easily, causing infection.

Escherichia coli bacteria are the common cause of most cases of cystitis (over 90 percent). They usually lodge in the gastrointestinal tract and, although they are harmless to the intestines, when they enter the urinary tract they cause cystitis, with the aggravating factor that, if not treated in time, they can spread to the kidneys.

Cystitis is most frequent in women because of their anatomy. In women, the communication tube

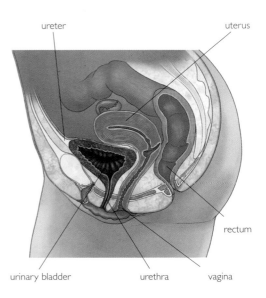

ureter

uterus

rectum

urinary bladder   urethra   vagina

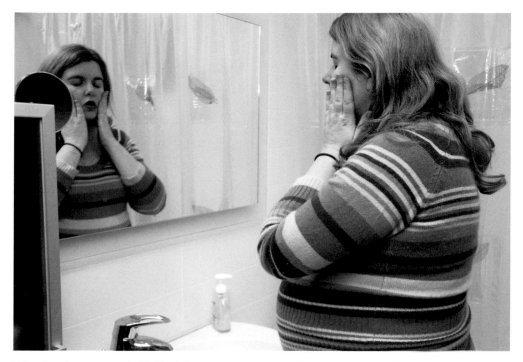

When there is pressure on the bladder during pregnancy or active sex, bacteria can enter the bladder through the urethra, or from using a diaphragm, increasing the risk of cystitis.

between the bladder and the outside world is shorter and straighter than in men and the space between the urethra and the anus is smaller. In men, cystitis usually affects the old, because of the enlargement of the prostate gland. The obstruction of the urine flow thus caused prevents the bladder from emptying completely, so it is more likely to become infected.

Some risk factors increase the likelihood of suffering this infection of the urinary tract:

• Constipation.

• Taking certain antibiotics (analgesic nephropathy).

• Not drinking enough liquids during the day.

• Abnormalities in the urinary system that obstruct the normal operation of the bladder or urethra: irritation caused by crystalline urine deposits (calculus or stones), urine flowing back toward the kidney (reflux neuropathy), etc.

• The insertion of instruments into the urinary tract, such as catheterization or cytoscopy.

• Diseases such as diabetes, multiple sclerosis, or other neuromuscular conditions that affect the bladder, etc.

• In women, pressure on the bladder during pregnancy or the sexual act, when bacteria can enter the bladder through the urethra, or using a diaphragm, can increase the risk of cystitis.

• In old men, the risk of contracting cystitis rises to 33 percent. This is because of incomplete empt-

■ Symptoms

The principal symptoms experienced with cystitis are:

• A burning sensation when urinating.

• Frequent urination.

• Wanting to urinate, even when the bladder is empty.

• Pain in the pubic area.

If the condition does not clear up at once, it can cause the following complications:

• Shivering and fever.

• Blood in the urine.

• Pain in the lumbar region, indicating a kidney infection.

Treatment and recommendations

Once the cause of the cystitis has been ascertained, and if no anomalies are found, it can be treated with antibiotics (for a month or more) to eliminate the infection. Minor cases of acute cystitis can disappear spontaneously if the patient drinks plenty of liquid, which stimulates frequent urination, helping eliminate bacteria from the bladder. However, as there is always a risk that the infection will spread to the kidneys, sufferers are recommended to have it treated with antibiotics for as long as the doctor prescribes.

The doctor will take a urine sample to determine the cause of the infection, and may prescribe antibiotics before obtaining the results of the analysis if the symptoms are very acute.

Not all cases of cystitis are the same or equally serious. The commonest are:

• **Occasional.** When the condition is temporary and its effects disappear within a couple of days, especially if the patient has drunk plenty of water. Keeping a wet bathing suit on for a long time or poor hygiene at certain times are the usual causes.

• **Recurrent.** When at least two episodes of infection have occurred within six months, or three within a year. Tests must be conducted to rule out any physical anomaly.

• **Interstitial (IC).** When the causes of the chronic inflammation of the bladder wall are unknown. Unlike ordinary cystitis, it is believed that IC is not caused by bacteria, because it does not respond to traditional treatment with antibiotics. It is one of the most serious types, as it is difficult to treat.

• **Honeymoon cystitis.** When the symptoms of cystitis and painful urination occur after sex, hence its name. The symptoms usually last one or two days and can reoccur when sexual relations are resumed. It is really a form of chronic urethritis, as it is the urethra rather than the bladder that becomes inflamed. The sufferer should consult a specialist, as the infection may be due to a sexually transmitted disease caused by the bacterium *Chlamydia trachomatis*.

ying of the bladder associated with a narrowing of the urethra, not drinking enough liquids, intestinal incontinence, or inadequate mobility.

Sufferers are advised to see a doctor if the symptoms do not disappear within two or three days, or earlier if fever, shivering, or back pain occur, and also if there is blood in their urine. Pregnant women and people with diabetes, high blood pressure, or kidney problems should consult a doctor at once to avoid the infection causing complications. Cystitis is frequent in women with multiple sclerosis or other neuromuscular diseases that affect the bladder.

How to prevent cystitis

• Drink plenty of liquids, 8 or 9 glasses of water daily.

• Women who often suffer from cystitis should drink a glass of water before having sex and urinate afterward. This helps evacuate any bacteria lodged in the urethra.

• Don't sit around for long in a wet bathing suit.

• Avoid using vaginal deodorants, douches or other irritants, and if you use a diaphragm to prevent pregnancy and experience any of the symptoms mentioned, it might be advisable to change to another contraceptive method.

• After defecating, wipe yourself from front to back so as not to contaminate the entrance to the urethra with fecal remains, and wash yourself with water and soap after defecating whenever possible.

Pelvic pain

Chronic pelvic pain is pain in the pelvic area, that is to say the lower abdomen, that lasts more than 6 months. It is probably the most frequent reason for a woman to consult a doctor. Its characteristics can vary as regards both location and intensity, and it is a symptom of various conditions.

The pelvis, which contains the uterus, fallopian tubes, ovaries, vagina, urinary bladder, and rectum, is the lower part of the trunk located beneath the abdomen and between the hips. Women often feel pain in this area and it is sometimes difficult to ascertain the cause. Frequently, but not always, pelvic pain is associated with reproductive problems. Other causes of pelvic pain concern the intestines or urinary tract. Psychological factors can also worsen the pain or even provoke a painful sensation without the presence of any underlying organic problem.

The causes of this pain can be gynecological, digestive, urinary, bone-related, muscular, joint-related, vascular, and nervous.

Diagnosis

Pain that persists for more than 6 months must be investigated from both the physical and psychological points of view. Thus, the investigation of the problem cannot be considered complete until a number of questions have been answered and all the possible variants reviewed:

• An extensive and precise series of questions must be asked and answered.

• A thorough clinical examination is essential, with a detailed laboratory analysis.

• It may be very difficult to carry out a pelvic ultrasound scan, and a vaginal probe may work better.

• Finally, as a last resort, there is the possibility of carrying out a laparoscopy, a simple surgical procedure generally conducted under a general anesthetic that enables the pelvis to be examined directly.

• Other investigations, such as magnetic resonance imaging (MRI), can be useful.

• Sometimes a laparoscopy is recommendable for the direct examination of the pelvic viscera.

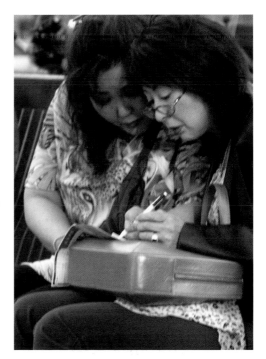

Pelvic pain is a problem that can be, and sometimes must be, handled in a multidisciplinary way, with the participation of other specialists (urologists, gastroenterologists, and traumatologists).

TYPE OF PAIN	POSSIBLE CAUSE
Localized pain	Inflammation
Pain like stomach ache	Spasm in a soft organ, such as the intestine, urethra or appendix.
Pain that starts suddenly	Temporary deficiency in the blood supply, due to an obstruction of the blood circulation.
Pain that develops slowly	Inflammation of the appendix or an
Pain that envelops the whole abdomen	An accumulation of blood, pus or intestinal contents
Pain aggravated by movement or during an examination	Irritation of the lining of the abdominal cavity.

The following are examples of the various types of pelvic pain most commonly described by women, and their possible causes or origin. It is always necessary to consult a doctor to establish a diagnosis.

PELVIC ADHESIONS

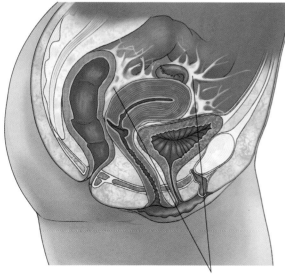

adhesions

Infection, surgery, or injury can cause adherences to form inside the body and in the pelvic region.

Treatment

Once the pain has been correctly assessed, if a specific cause has been ascertained, treatment of that cause is the most important thing for therapeutic success. As a rule, the first treatment will be pharmacological in cases of pain of inflammatory origin. Salicylates should be used first. If they fail, the next therapeutic option is the use of nonsteroid anti-inflammatory drugs. Thirdly, tricyclic antidepressants can be used as an additional therapy. The last option is to use opiates if good results have not been obtained with all the aforementioned types of medication.

In some cases, specific surgery is needed—in situations where an apparent or possible cause of the pain, for instance for releasing adhesions, or securing the uterus, and even hysterectomy. In others, surgery will be performed on the routes taken by the pain, such as the ablation of the uterosacral nerves, presacral neurectomy, cor-

AREAS WHERE GROWTHS ARE COMMON IN THE ENDOMETRIUM (IN RED)

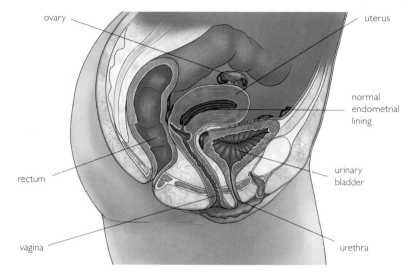

ovary

uterus

normal
endometrial
lining

rectum

urinary
bladder

vagina

urethra

Endometriosis

Endometriosis is a possible cause of pelvic pain. It is a noncancerous disease affecting women of reproductive age and occurs when the endometrium is situated outside the uterus, that is to say, not in its original place. This incorrectly developed tissue can locate itself anywhere in the abdomen, including the strangest places such as the navel or the lungs. The plates that form are called implants when they are small, nodules when they are bigger, and endometriomas when cysts form in the ovaries.

dotomy, or rhizotomy, all of them surgical procedures whose end purpose is to cut the nerves that transmit painful sensations.

Although painful symptoms are often attributed to specific organic causes, it is not easy to classify the causes of chronic pelvic pain simply. Basically, these causes can be divided into two groups, cyclical and noncyclical, that can help discern whether or not the pain is linked to the menstrual cycle.

Predominantly noncyclical causes
- Inflammatory pelvic disease.
- Pelvic adhesions.
- Badly positioned uterus.
- Neoplasias of the genital organs.
- Musculoskeletal disorders.
- Gastrointestinal disorders.
- Urinary pathologies.
- Psychological factors.

- Without demonstrable organic anomalies.
- Ectopic pregnancy.

Predominantly cyclical causes
- Painful ovulation.
- Primary dysmenorrhea.
- Secondary dysmenorrhea.
  - Endometriosis
  - Adenomyosis
  - Endometritis
  - Cervical stenosis
  - Leiomyomas (fibroids)
  - IUD
- Premenstrual syndrome

Fibromyalgia

Fibromyalgia is a chronic disorder in which generalized pain and profound exhaustion occur, as well as other symptoms. Fundamentally, it affects the soft tissues of the body: tendons, ligaments, and muscles. It is most frequent in adult women, but can also affect men, children, and the elderly.

Fibromyalgia

Fibromyalgia is a chronic, nonarticular rheumatic process, characterized by pain, great sensitivity, and stiffness, principally in the muscles, tendons, and ligaments. It is the most frequent cause of generalized pain in the musculoskeletal system that lasts for prolonged periods—months or even years. In the past, it was considered a psychogenic rheumatic disease, possibly because its causes and clinical pattern were not precisely known, but in the last few years it has been discovered that it is a clearly differentiated disease with its own characteristics.

It principally affects women between the ages of 20 and 40, although its cause is still unknown. It has been ascertained that, in situations of tension, stress, inadequate rest, work-related accidents, and

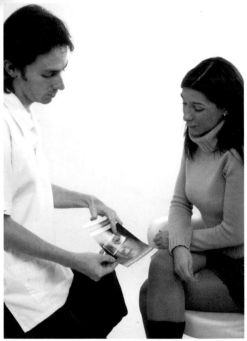

Although women with fibromyalgia suffer pain similar to that caused by a joint disease, fibromyalgia does not cause inflammation, so is not a form of arthritis (which is characterized by swollen joints). Rather, fibromyalgia is a form of rheumatism of the soft tissues.

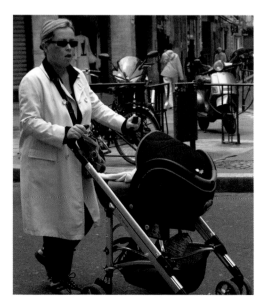

The fibromyalgia syndrome cannot be diagnosed with laboratory tests. The results of X-rays, blood analyses, and muscular biopsies are normal. Diagnosis is therefore based on a clinical examination of a person's symptoms carried out by a doctor.

▪▪ Symptoms and signs

General muscular pain is the most outstanding symptom of fibromyalgia. As a rule, it is felt all over the body, although it may start in one area, such as the neck and shoulders, and spread to other areas after a while. The pain caused by fibromyalgia has been described in various ways, such as: burning, stinging, stiffness, and sensitivity. It often varies according to the time of day, level of physical activity, sleep patterns, the climate, and nervous fatigue. Most female fibromyalgia sufferers affirm that they are always in some degree of pain, mainly in the muscles, and for them the pain can be fairly severe.

exposure to cold or damp climates, the pattern is set off or intensified, chronically stimulating the pain receptors of the nerves and leading to the development of the pattern of fibromyalgia.

It can also occur after viral diseases which set it off.

All these factors cause a kind of dysfunction in the regulation of pain, as they adversely affect the neural transmission system.

Fatigue and deterioration in sleep patterns

About 90 percent of women with fibromyalgia experience moderate or severe fatigue, reduced resistance to effort, or the exhaustion typical of flu or lack of sleep. Sometimes, the feeling of fatigue is more problematical than the pain. Most women with fibromyalgia sleep badly. Although they can fall asleep without much difficulty, they sleep very lightly and wake up frequently during the night. They often rise in the morning feeling tired, even after sleeping throughout the night. The resulting tiredness can range from apathy and reduced resistance to complete exhaustion. The level of fatigue experienced can vary from day to day.

• Symptoms of the nervous system: People with fibromyalgia have frequent mood changes. Many individuals feel sad or depressed, although those suffering from clinical depression account for only 25 percent of the total. Patients with fibromyalgia can also feel anxious. Some researchers believe there may be a connection between fibromyalgia and some kinds of chronic anxiety and depression. However, any woman suffering from a chronic disease, not only from fibromyalgia, may feel depressed at times, when fighting against the pain and tiredness she is feeling. She may also have difficulty in concentrating or carrying out simple mental tasks.

• Other problems: Headaches, and muscular pain in particular (tension), and migraines are common symptoms of fibromyalgia. Abdominal pain and switching between constipation and diarrhea

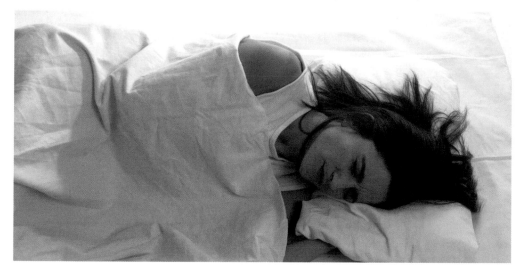

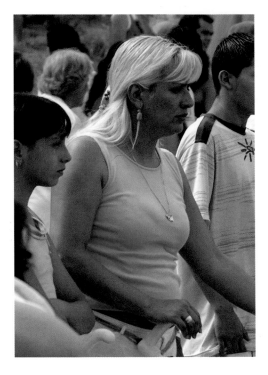

◢■ Treatment

Some female fibromyalgia sufferers have slight symptoms and need little treatment, once they understand their disorder and what makes it worse. Others, however, need a complete care program and training in techniques to alleviate the pain.

The options for treating fibromyalgia include:

- Medication to reduce pain and improve sleep.
- Antidepressive medication.
- Exercise programs to stretch the muscles and improve cardiovascular capacity.
- Relaxation techniques to alleviate muscular tension and anxiety.
- Educational programs to help them understand and control fibromyalgia.

(called irritable bowel syndrome) are also common symptoms. Bladder spasms and irritability can frequently cause an urgent need to urinate.

Exercise and physical therapy

Two ways of treating fibromyalgia are stretching and exercising the tense and painful muscles and increasing cardiovascular capacity (aerobics). Low impact aerobic exercises, or exercises with no impact, such as walking, cycling, dancing, aquatic aerobics, or swimming are usually the best ways of starting a program of this kind.

The attitude to adopt

As a rule, female fibromyalgia sufferers have undergone numerous tests and consulted many specialists in search of a solution. They are often told that, as they look well and the test results are normal, they are not suffering from any real disorder. Friends and relatives, as well as doctors, may also doubt the reality of their complaints, which can make them feel even more isolated and misunderstood.

Both the patient and her family must accept that fibromyalgia causes chronic pain and fatigue. An active part must be played in the control of fibromyalgia, exercising regularly and learning about pain, the use of relaxation techniques, and the control of nervous fatigue.

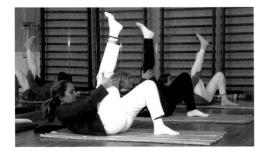

Many women can benefit from learning certain techniques to alleviate and control the pain. These techniques include learning muscular relaxation exercises, meditation, and bioretro-dietary techniques.

Hemorrhoids

Hemorrhoids, or piles, are one of the most frequent health complaints, and most people will suffer from them at some time in their life. Although the complaint is considered commonplace, it can be very troublesome and painful.

Hemorrhoids

Basically, hemorrhoids consist of dilatations of the veins in the rectal cavity that extend to the anus, that is to say the hemorrhoidal veins. These veins, like those in the legs, can dilate for various reasons, so losing the capacity to return the blood circulating inside them.

Thus, they form varicose strings and nodules that can be internal or external. Hemorrhoids that form inside are called *internal* and those that emerge from the anus are called *external*.

Hemorrhoids are dilatations of the veins of the blood-transporting tissue of the mucous membranes of the rectum or anus. If the affected tissues are those of the upper plexus, which are called *internal*, they are situated above the anal duct and are covered in mucous.

Those of the lower plexus are situated below the junction between the rectum and the anus and are covered in external skin.

Diagnosis

For hemorrhoids to be diagnosed, the characteristic symptoms of blood and secretions when defecating must be present. An external anal, or rectoscopic, examination will be carried out to confirm the presence of dilatations in the rectum. An analysis must be made to check the possible presence of anemia. As rectal bleeding is the commonest symptom of internal hemorrhoids and also occurs with various tumors of the colon and the rectum, a rectosigmoidoscopy is recommended, so as to rule out other diseases.

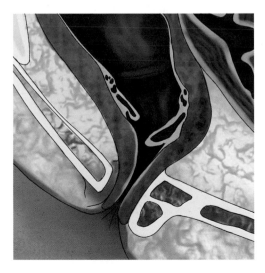

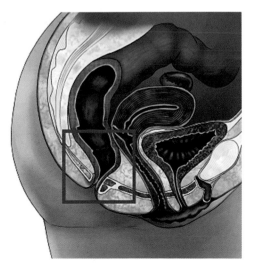

Causes

Some causes that predispose a person to hemorrhoids are:

- There is frequently a family history which would suggest a hereditary basis or predisposition.
- Constipation which, by forcing the feces to pass, compresses the hemorrhoidal veins.
- Diarrhea which can cause irritation.
- Pregnancy, especially in the final weeks.
- Certain anomalies of the microcirculatory system with demonstrable communication between veins and arteries can also be a cause.

Treatment

General measures

- Maintain good anal hygiene and avoid scratching or rubbing the hemorrhoids, to help prevent infections.

- Correct constipation by adding fiber to the diet: fruit, green vegetables, whole-wheat bread, and abundant liquids.
- Avoid diarrhea.
- Avoid highly spiced meals and alcohol.
- Avoid straining when defecating to reduce bleeding and prolapse as much as possible. Reduce defecation time. Use soft toilet paper or clean the anal area with warm water.
- Apply ice and hot compresses during the acute phase of the problem: the cold will reduce the swelling.
- Bathe the area with warm water twice or three times a day. This cold-hot sequence is a way of temporarily alleviating the pain of external hemorrhoids.
- Asymptomatic hemorrhoids do not require treatment.
- Suppositories and rectal oils are not very effective in the treatment of internal hemorrhoids. They have a merely transitory anesthetic effect.
- If the prolapsed hemorrhoids can be reduced, they should be gently pushed back into the rectum. The patient should lie down and reduce their prominence whenever necessary. After reduction, the external inflammation will disappear.
- Hemorrhoids that appear after giving birth or during the early days of motherhood should

Pregnancy

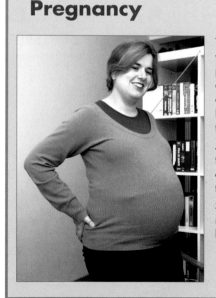

This is the commonest cause of hemorrhoids in young women. The greater frequency of hemorrhoids during pregnancy is believed to be due to the increased pressure exerted on the iliac veins by the growing uterus, causing a rise in venous pressure inside the middle and lower hemorrhoidal veins whose job is to drain the blood from the internal iliac veins.

After pregnancy, hemorrhoids tend to disappear, although they can worsen progressively with subsequent pregnancies or with age. As a rule, hemorrhoids precede constipation, which usually follows them, and not vice-versa.

Sedentary occupations, physical effort during work or sport, standing up for long periods, and certain dietary habits are other causes of hemorrhoids.

Symptoms

The principal symptoms are the appearance of sparse rectal bleeding and difficulty in defecating, with mucous rectal secretion.

The most typical characteristic is being able to feel the hemorrhoids in the anus, and the patient can even reduce them manually.

Hemorrhoids can have the complication of becoming strangulated and dark in color, due to the underlying thrombosis, and they can worsen, fine wrinkles appearing in the mucous membrane, which loses its luster and looks dead. Anemia can be an occasional side effect of abundant hemorrhoids or of the persistent loss of small amounts of blood from them.

not be treated surgically. Sufficient time should be allowed to see whether or not they persist.

Sclerotherapy

• This treatment uses injections of chemical irritants (sometimes freezing can be used) into the tissues surrounding the internal hemorrhoidal varicose veins. The scarring resulting from the inflammatory reaction produces fibrosis of the hemorrhoidal varicose veins.

• The condition recurs in 50 percent of patients. This treatment is indicated if the hemorrhoids are just starting, not complicated, and internal. The complications of treatment with injections are infection and acute prostatitis.

Surgical treatment

• Surgery involves cutting out all the mucous membrane surrounding the hemorrhoids, produ-

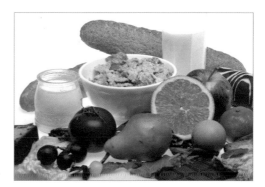

cing an excellent result in the long term. Recurrence is very rare after proper surgery. External hemorrhoids that cannot be reduced, are thrombosed, inflamed, or gangrenous, must be surgically treated.

• Surgery offers a quicker solution to the symptoms, and convalescence is brief.

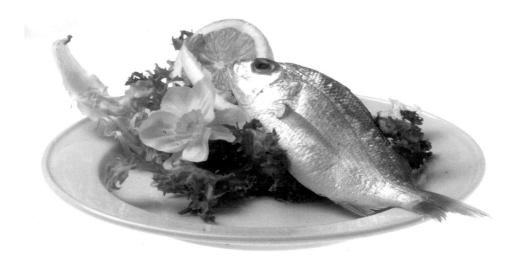

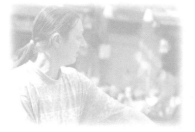

Urinary
incontinence

Urinary incontinence, which consists of an involuntary loss of urine, although typically considered a geriatric complaint, also occurs in younger adults, particularly women. It is calculated that a fifth of the population aged over 65 suffers urinary incontinence.

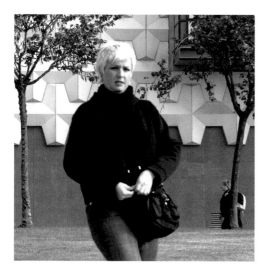

Urinary incontinence

The function of the lower urinary tract, bladder, and urethra is to store the urine formed in the kidneys and to eliminate it periodically. The elimination phase begins with a relaxation of the muscle enfolding the urethra, while the detrusor muscle of the bladder contracts. Thus, the intravesical pressure is greater than the urethral pressure, and the bladder is emptied.

For continence to be maintained, intraurethral pressure must be greater than intravesical pressure. When this pressure ratio is lost, urinary incontinence occurs, and can be due to a reduction in intraurethral pressure (the most usual cause), or to

an increase in intravesical pressure. Occasionally, it is caused by a combination of the two.

In women, the urethra is shorter. For continence in women, the urethral musculature farther from the bladder is of more importance, which contributes to the musculature of the perineum. In men, the musculature close to the bladder is of more importance, the perineal musculature playing a minor role.

Attitude to incontinence

The involuntary loss of urine should not be a reason for shame or concealment. A doctor should be consulted, as for any other condition. Most cases nowadays can be effectively treated. Although each type of incontinence has its own treatment, some general rules should be followed in all cases.

■ Types of incontinence

The commonest types of urinary incontinence that affect women include two large groups: urethral and extraurethral. The type that manifests itself via the urethra, the most frequent type, is called *effort or stress incontinence*. The second type is *urgency incontinence*, and there can be a third category when both types are combined, *mixed incontinence*. The commonest cause of extraurethral incontinence is a genitourinal fistula.

Treatment of incontinence

- The treatment of incontinence is different for each sex. The first thing to do is to see a doctor. In many cases, incontinence has a solution. This is even more important in adult women with minor stress incontinence who maintain sexual relations. In bladder instability, good results are obtained with anticholinergic drugs and electrostimulation.

- In stress or effort incontinence, the commonest type in women, exercises are recommended to strengthen the pelvic musculature, and should be performed several times a day. These consist of sustained contractions of the pelvic floor muscles. Vaginal cones are also used. These are introduced into the vagina for periods of 15 minutes, three times a day,

the weight of the cones being gradually increased. Sometimes, these measures have to be combined with low-intensity electrical stimulation and specific drugs. In some cases, surgery is necessary, the majority of operations producing good results.

- Drugs are usually administered for overflow incontinence. In incontinent old people who do not respond to treatment, the alternative is incontinence pads that should be changed frequently to avoid ulceration and other skin problems and odor.

- Limiting or eliminating certain drinks such as coffee, tea and alcoholic drinks that provoke urination (diuretics).

- Retraining the urination habits. There are ways of doing this.

- In recent years, urodynamic techniques have been developed enabling a very precise diagnosis to be made and the best possible treatment to be

prescribed. There are numerous therapeutic possibilities, including kinesitherapy, electrostimulation, and electromyographic (EMG) biofeedback methods that increase control of an unconscious muscular function, making it conscious and voluntary.

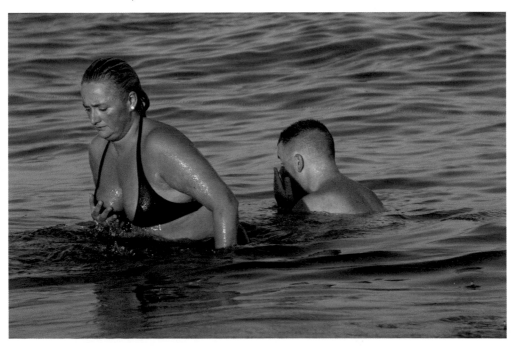

Kegel exercises

Exercises to train women in contracting the muscles of the pelvic floor are called Kegel exercises. They are used mainly to treat people suffering effort incontinence. However, they can also help alleviate the symptoms of urgency incontinence. The principle of Kegel exercises is to strengthen the pelvic floor muscles and hence to improve the functioning of the urethral sphincter.

• To locate the right muscles, try to stop the flow of your urine without using the stomach, leg or buttock muscles. When you succeed in reducing or stopping the flow of urine, you will have found the right muscles.

• Tighten the muscles. Keep them tightened while you count to 10. Then relax them while counting to 10 again.

• Perform this contraction 20 times, 3 or 4 times a day.

• You will probably have to start slowly, tightening and relaxing your muscles for 4 seconds and performing each contraction 3 or 4 times, 10 times a day. Then, keep increasing the number of times.

The success of these exercises will depend on the correct use of the technique and strict adherence to a regular exercise program. Another strategy is to use vaginal cones to strengthen the pelvic floor muscles. The vaginal cone is a device of a certain weight that is inserted into the vagina. The woman must then contract her pelvic floor muscles, trying to keep the device in its place and hold the contraction for about 15 minutes. This exercise must be performed twice a day. Within 4 to 6 weeks of starting this treatment, 70% of women experience some improvement in their symptoms.

▪ Enuresis

Although the word enuresis is used to refer to the involuntary loss of urine in general, it is used nowadays to define nocturnal incontinence during sleep. It occurs especially in children. The following factors influence its occurrence: heredity, anxiety, psychological changes, cerebral immaturity, deep sleep, and functional and organic pathology. There are many theories about the origin of this urinary incontinence, but none is conclusive.

To treat this disorder, the child's social and biological background should be analyzed, as well as the attitude and disposition of the parents. Almost all cases of enuresis clear up with time, and the people affected do not undergo any personality change. Their intellectual capacity is the same as that of other children.

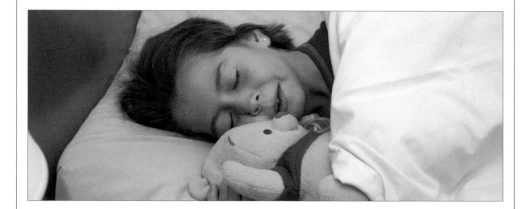

Migraines and headaches

Migraine is a chronic complaint, of unknown cause, that manifests itself in the form of repeated headache attacks with certain characteristics of duration (between 4 and 72 hours), type of pain (throbbing), association with nausea, photophobia (inability to tolerate light), and phonophobia (inability to tolerate noise), sometimes aggravated by physical activity.

A very frequent problem

Headache is one of the commonest forms of pain in the human race. It affects 93 percent of men and 99 percent of women at least once in life, and is the reason for 15 percent of general practitioner consultations and the most frequent

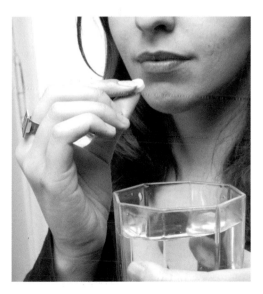

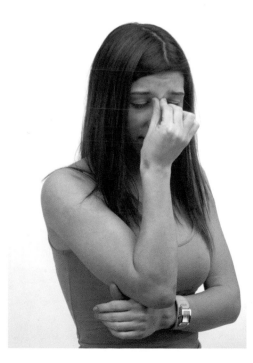

Although both sexes are affected by migraine, it is more frequent in young women, and can occur even in children. This disorder usually starts between the ages of 10 and 35, with a male/female ratio of 1 to 5. Migraine usually starts in adolescence or infancy. A little girl with a propensity to migraine will feel carsick and, in some cases, may even sleepwalk.

Migraine tends to become chronic, although in some cases the condition disappears or becomes sporadic, while in others attacks become very frequent and, at some seasons, can occur every day. There is no way of knowing for certain how the condition will develop. Attacks often vary greatly from one individual to another.

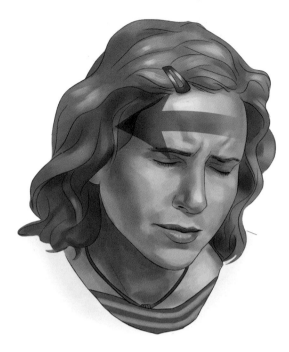

It is best to retire to a dimly lit room and try to sleep. This will often be enough to stop the attack, but in some cases medication will be needed, and the sooner it is administered, the more effective it will be. Therefore in cases of migraine with an aura, medication should be taken as soon as the first symptoms appear. Medication is less effective when the attack is well under way and the arterial and neurochemical processes are working. If nausea and vomiting occur, antiemetics should also be taken to eliminate them.

very changeable pain and, precisely because of that variability in its presentation, localization, intensity, and the factors that cause it, a number of categories have been established for this apparently simple symptom.

The most frequently used classification distinguishes four main groups: migraine, tension headache, cluster headaches, and others associated with various inflammatory, toxic, medication-related, tumor-related, and vascular processes.

The most frequent chronic, persistent, or repetitive types are migraines and tension headaches, which account for about 90 percent of all chronic headaches.

reason for consulting neurologists.

Although it is an everyday problem, it is sometimes difficult to diagnose and treat, and the cause of most headaches can be detected exclusively by taking a complete clinical history, that is to say by analyzing symptoms such as when they occur, how often, what factors trigger them, etc.

Variable symptoms

A headache is not a disease, but a symptom characterized by pain or an unpleasant sensation inside the skull. This pain can be bearable, slight enough not to cause more than a little discomfort, or so severe that it temporarily incapacitates the sufferer. It can last only a moment or continue for hours or days. It can appear very occasionally or be repeated almost every day. It is therefore a

Basic preventive treatment is used to stop attacks when they are very frequent or intense. There are many alternatives, and in most cases, good results have been achieved. As a rule, the treatment chosen by the doctor is administered for a period of three to six months, but although pharmacological treatment is important, there is no doubt that lifestyle is fundamental. Sport, relaxation, a healthy diet, and emotional balance are the cornerstones of migraine control.

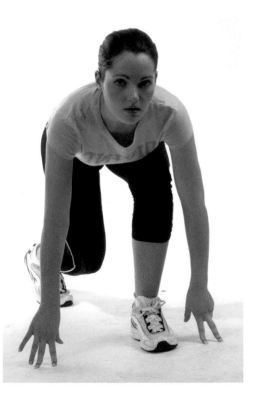

Migraine

Described in ancient times and mentioned in Sumerian records dating from as long ago as 4,000 BC, migraine can be defined as a hereditary disorder characterized by recurrent episodes of headache. Although at first it is localized in one side of the skull, it then spreads and is often accompanied by digestive symptoms such as nausea and vomiting, and a feeling of exhaustion and general discomfort.

Migraine usually produces an intense, throbbing pain (in the forehead, temples, jaw, ears, and around the eyes). In 25 percent of cases, a typical pattern is that 10 to 30 minutes before an attack an aura will be sensed (visual disturbances such as sparks or black spots in the field of vision, patterns of zigzag lines, flashes of light, tingling in the face, etc.).

The headache intensifies after making sudden head movements, coughing, sneezing, and physical effort. The attack lasts between 4 and 72 hours.

Factors that trigger migraine

• The relationship between female hormones and migraine is not clear, but there are indications that there is a connection: many women have a migraine attack with menstruation and ovulation, while attacks disappear with pregnancy. Some women suffer their first attack after the menopause. On the other hand, others, who suffered migraine attacks before the menopause, stop having them. The effects of oral contraceptives on migraines and other headaches are not clear either, although many women find that attacks grow worse, more frequent and more intense, when they take them.

• Stress and anxiety, whether as a result of work, family, or other problems, also cause headaches in many people.

• Intense physical exercise can trigger migraines.

• Lack of sleep, or too much sleep, can be a factor: sleeping for 7–8 hours and going to bed and getting up at the same time each day help prevent attacks. Some people suffer migraines on public holidays, when they usually stay in bed for longer (weekend migraine).

• Drinking alcohol, especially red or sparkling wines, is harmful to some female migraine sufferers.

• Some foods, such as chocolate, eggs, yogurt,

■ Treatment of migraines

> Although all migraines share the characteristic of producing pain, they differ considerably from one woman to another in intensity, frequency, and the factors that trigger them, so their treatment must be personalized.
>
> However, some recommendations apply to all cases:
>
> • Leading a healthy life. As well as sleep and regular rest, moderate physical exercise is advisable. Sufferers should avoid stress and prolonged fasting.
>
> • Once the factors that trigger attacks have been identified, those factors should be avoided as far as possible.
>
> • The aforementioned dietary factors that trigger attacks do not affect all women equally, or do not always affect them, so severe dietary restrictions are not necessary.
>
> • A sufferer should not self-medicate during acute attacks, or take excessive amounts of painkillers in the hope that they will help.
>
> • The treatment the doctor has prescribed should be followed strictly.

nuts, beans, smoked fish, acidic fruit and, especially, sauces containing monosodium glutamate (Chinese and other sauces), tyramine (present in aged, fermented and deteriorated foods, so avoid leftovers, strong cheeses etc.), nitrites, and nitrates (in preserved meats, hot dogs, etc.), can set off an attack, as can prolonged fasting and the consequent drop in glucemia.

• Prolonged exposure to the sun.

• Excessive tobacco smoking.

• Noise, busy environments, lights, beams, and sparkling illuminations can also trigger an attack.

Osteoporosis

Osteoporosis is a disease suffered by older people, especially women. It is calculated that 30 percent of postmenopausal women suffer from it, and its frequency increases with age after the age of 70. Menopause is one of the principal causes of osteoporosis, as a result of reduced estrogen levels.

Osteoporosis

Osteoporosis is a disease of the skeletal system characterized by a reduction in bone mass and the structural deterioration of the bony tissue, making the bones more fragile and likely to break.

Any bone in the skeleton can be injured, except for those in the skull, although the most frequent fractures are those of the hip and wrist, and the vertebrae.

There is much a woman can do throughout her life to prevent osteoporosis, delay its progress, and protect herself from fractures:

• Include adequate amounts of calcium and vitamin D in her diet.

• Calcium. During the years of growth, the body needs calcium to build strong bones and create a reserve. Creating bone mass when young is a good investment for the future. Consuming enough calcium during growth can help delay the occurrence of osteoporosis in later life.

• Whatever her age or state of health, a woman needs calcium to keep her bones healthy. Calcium continues to be essential after growth is completed, because the body loses calcium every day. Although this calcium cannot prevent gradual bone loss after menopause, it continues to play an important part in maintaining bone quality.

▪ Factors

• **Menopause.** The reduced secretion of estrogens that occurs at this stage determines increased bone change. This accelerates the loss of bone mass.

• **Age.** As from the age of 35 to 40, physiological bone loss occurs (about 0.5–1% annually.)

• **Androgens.** The deficiency of this hormone in men.

• **Sex.** When development is complete, women have lower bone mass than men.

• **Corticoids.** High levels of corticoids, whether endogenous (Cushing's syndrome) or exogenous (medication), very frequently imply osteoporosis.

• **Thyroid hormone.** This increases loss of bone mass, so hyperthyroid sufferers are at risk.

• **Diet.** A diet low in calcium and vitamin D, especially during growth.

• **Physical exercise.** Insufficient physical exercise during development makes it difficult to acquire bone mass.

• **Social habits.** Tobacco, alcohol, and coffee favor the development of this disease.

Osteoporosis is an important health problem, contributing to an estimated 1.5 million bone fractures a year. One in every two women and one in every five men aged over 65 will suffer a bone fracture due to osteoporosis. Many of these are painful fractures of the hip, spinal column, wrist, arm, and leg, which frequently occur following a fall. However, even simple household tasks can cause a spinal fracture if the bones have been weakened by the disease.

• Even when a woman has started menopause, or if she already has osteoporosis, increasing her consumption of calcium and vitamin D can reduce the risk of fractures.

• Depending on her age and other factors, the amount of calcium a woman needs will vary. The National Academy of Sciences issues the recommendations on daily calcium consumption shown in the box opposite.

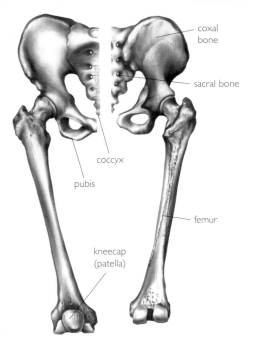

coxal bone

sacral bone

coccyx

pubis

femur

kneecap (patella)

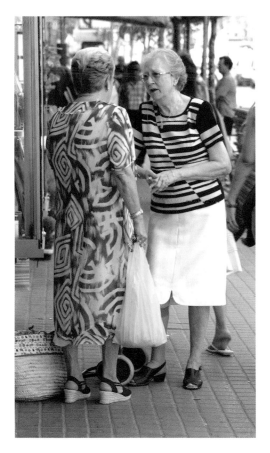

The diagnosis of osteoporosis

Osteoporosis can be diagnosed by a combination of the patient's complete medical history and a physical examination, which will include X-rays, bone-density measurements, and specialized laboratory tests. If the doctor finds low bone mass, he may order additional tests to rule out the possibility of other diseases that can cause bone loss, including osteomalacia (a deficiency of vitamin D) or hyperthyroidism (over-activity of the parathyroid gland).

Treatment

Because lost bone cannot be replaced, the treatment of osteoporosis is aimed at preventing additional loss. While diet and exercise therapy

The most serious fracture due to osteoporosis is the hip fracture (top of femur). After such a fracture, most patients with a fractured hip, who previously lived independently, will require the help of their family or a health professional at home. Any woman with a fractured hip will require help with walking for several months, and about half of them will need walking frames or sticks in order to move about the house or outside for the rest of their lives.

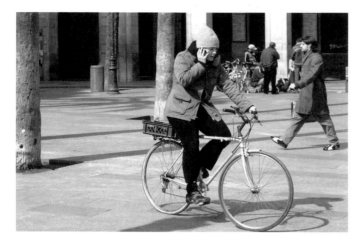

The muscles and bones need exercise to stay strong. At any age, exercise can help reduce loss of bone mass and provide many other health benefits. Doctors state that a moderate exercise plan (3–4 times a week) is effective in the day to day prevention of osteoporosis. Exercise such as running, walking, climbing stairs, dancing, cycling, and lifting weights are the best.

are frequently the main components of an osteoporosis treatment plan, there are other treatments.

• **Hormone replacement therapy (HRT)**. This is often recommended for women at high risk of osteoporosis to prevent bone loss and reduce the risk of fractures. A bone-density measurement when the menopause begins can help decide whether HRT is the most appropriate treatment in each case. HRT is not without risks, as taking it increases the risk of breast cancer.

• **New drugs such as selective estrogen receptor modulators.** These drugs increase bone mass and reduce the risk of spine fractures and breast cancer.

• **Calcitonine.** This is another medication used to reduce bone loss. Administered in the form of a nasal spray, it increases bone mass, reduces spinal fractures, and helps alleviate pain. Many drugs enable osteoporosis patients not only to increase bone mass but also significantly to reduce the risk of fractures, but they must always be prescribed by a doctor. It should be remembered that prevention is preferable to waiting until treatment is necessary.

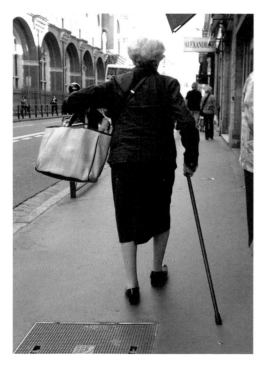

■ Recommended daily calcium consumption

- Girls aged 9 to 18: 1,300 mg per day.
- Women aged 19 to 50: 1,000 mg per day.
- Pregnant or breastfeeding women up to the age of 18: 1,300 mg per day.
- Pregnant or breastfeeding women aged 19 to 50: 1,000 mg per day.
- Women aged over 50: 1,200 mg per day.

Ovarian cysts

An ovarian cyst is a kind of bag containing liquid that develops inside an ovary. They are very frequent in all sexually active women of childbearing age, especially in adolescents whose reproductive systems have not reached full maturity. Their diagnosis is important for ruling out other patterns, such as an ectopic pregnancy, or malignant pathologies such as tumors.

The follicle

Normally, a follicle with an egg inside it starts to develop during each menstrual cycle. This follicle will be expelled to one of the fallopian tubes on the 14th day of the cycle to be fertilized by a sperm. If left unfertilized, the follicle later shrinks and disappears. In some cases, this does not happen. The follicle grows bigger than usual without shrinking, forming a cyst. As these are usually follicles with nothing but a large amount of liquid inside them, many of them are called *functional cysts*, and can produce a greater quantity of female hormones, affecting the whole body.

The necessity for a woman to have a periodical gynecological examination cannot be overemphasized. It should be remembered that many problems can be resolved if they are detected in time.

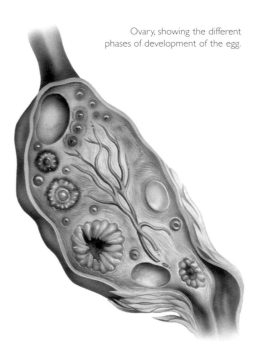

Ovary, showing the different phases of development of the egg.

Nontumorous ovarian cysts

Fifteen percent of ovarian cysts are nontumorous. They occur in the first three decades of life, 80% of them during the reproductive years. Ninety-five to 98% of them are benign. Because of their embryonic origin, their content is strange, being composed of sebaceous material mixed with hair, cartilage, bone, and teeth ("dermoid cysts"). A pelvic ultrasound examination and X-rays are very helpful in detecting the presence of teeth or calcifications. Ovarian cysts are surgically removed.

■ **Nontumorous ovarian cysts**

• **Germinal inclusion cysts.** These cysts are frequent, nonfunctional, small in size, and of little importance. If they are large, surgical removal is recommended.

• **Follicular cysts.** These develop as a result of the over-stimulation of the ovary by the pituitary gland. They usually disappear of their own accord in a few weeks or months. When they persist, they can secrete estrogens (female sex hormones), which can produce irregular bleeding. Treatment: observation, oral contraceptives, and removal of the cyst if it persists for more than 8 weeks.

• **Corpus luteum cysts.** These result from hormonal changes following excessive hemorrhage during ovulation (between two periods). The wall of the cyst can break, producing symptoms very similar to those of an ectopic pregnancy. Treatment: surgical removal if they break.

• **Theca lutein cysts.** These coincide with a disease of the uterus called a hydatiform mole. They are bilateral cysts some 6 inches (15 cm) in diameter. They do not require treatment, and are usually reabsorbed when their primary cause is treated (removal of the mole).

Tumors derived from the coelomic epithelium

• **Serous cystadenomas.** Seventy percent of serous tumors are benign. They are cysts with thin walls and a smooth surface, filled with liquid.

• **Mucinous cystadenomas.** These constitute 15 to 25 percent of all ovarian tumors. 85% of them are benign. They are the biggest ovarian cysts (some weigh 1½–4½ oz/45–130 g) and are sometimes bilateral. They are round or ovoid lumps, with a smooth, grayish-blue surface. Inside, they are divided into sections and contain a thick, viscous liquid.

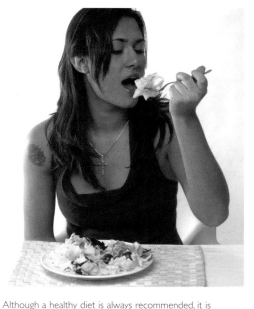

Although a healthy diet is always recommended, it is unrelated to the formation of ovarian cysts.

Diagnosis

• Full physical examination.

• Ultrasound scan of the pelvis.

• Computerized axial tomography ("CAT scan") of the abdomen and pelvis.

• Laparoscopy. Direct examination of the abdomen using fiber optics through a small incision in the abdominal wall, performed under a local anesthetic (epidural). It can be indicated if a serious lesion is suspected.

• Exploratory laparotomy. A surgical procedure on the abdomen to diagnose and, if necessary, treat, ovarian cysts or tumors.

• **Endometriomas.** These can occur singly or in groups, with surface adhesions. They contain a thick, chocolate-colored liquid. If large, they will be treated surgically.

• **Solid tumors.** The most frequent are ovarian fibromas, sometimes associated with an accumulation of liquid in the pleura (the membrane surrounding the lungs) and the peritoneum (the membrane surrounding the intestines), in what is called *Meigs syndrome*.

Treatment

- The treatment for benign ovarian tumors is salpingo-oophorectomy (the surgical removal of the affected ovaries and fallopian tubes).
- In young women, and those who want to remain fertile, the gynecologist will carefully remove the cyst or tumor and then reconstruct the ovary, whenever possible.
- In pre- or postmenopausal patients, the whole womb will be removed, together with both ovaries and the fallopian tubes.

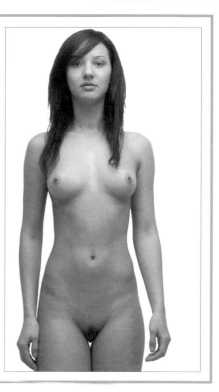

■ Benign breast tumors

The words *tumor, lump and nodule* are generally considered to mean the same thing. Most of these lumps are not cancerous or malignant. Many women have lumps in their breasts and many of these, even when detected by the women themselves, are normal areas of breast tissue that can become more visible or apparent just before a period. The most frequent are:

- **Fibroadenomas.** These are not really a disease, but merely a larger growth in some parts of the breast. They are particularly frequent in women aged under 30, and are considered to be the most frequent breast tumor before the menopause. They are related to hormonal changes in the woman, and are not clearly linked to the use of oral contraceptives. They very rarely turn malignant. They are almost never painful and usually grow slowly. They are very round, can be moved about easily within the breast and can be diagnosed by a combination of clinical examination, mammography, ultrasound scan, and puncture and aspiration of cells using a fine needle.

- **Cysts.** Cysts are smooth, movable lumps. In some cases, their special size makes them visible with the naked eye. They can be painful. They are more frequent in women between the ages of 40 and 50 (that is to say, close to the menopause), fewer cases occurring in women in their 20s, 30s, or 60s.

- **Fibrocystic mastopathy.** This is the most frequent breast complaint in premenopausal women. Its origin is hormonal and its usual symptoms are: pain in the breasts, which may or may not be linked to menstruation, secretions emerging from the nipples, discovering vaguely defined and more or less dense or irregular areas in the breasts, and generally feeling the presence of small lumps. This is also a benign condition and is diagnosed by clinical examination, mammography, and needle puncture.

Thyroid problems

The thyroid gland has an enormous influence over most metabolic processes through the hormones it produces. This is why any anomaly in this gland must be carefully monitored.

Thyroid diseases

Thyroid problems are becoming increasingly prevalent in the female population. Most thyroid diseases are autoimmune in women, which probably means that estrogens play a part in the pathogenesis of thyroid autoimmunity. However, when the thyroid is not working properly, gynecological disorders are likely to arise, which could explain some types of sterility.

There is really no specific diet or physical activity to counteract this type of pathology, except in the case of hypothyroidism, which causes overweight and its accompanying "bad" LDL cholesterol. Patients with this problem should follow a suitable

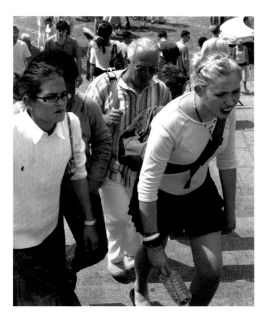

diet and get physical exercise which helps correct these problems. However, certain foods can cause thyroid disorders, such as seaweed, because of its iodine content. This will naturally depend on the person's eating habits and excesses.

The human endocrine system is very complex and its functions are involved in all physical and mental processes. The thyroid gland is a crucial part of that system, and its effect on the body—especially the female body—is the subject of this section.

The thyroid gland

The thyroid gland is a butterfly-shaped gland situated in the front of the neck under the larynx. It produces the thyroid hormones T3 and T4, which tell the body how fast to work and how to use energy. These chemical substances play a vital part in fetal development and, throughout life, govern the metabolic processes of most body tissues.

The thyroid can produce too much of the hormones, in a disorder called *hyperthyroidism*. The body then uses energy faster than it should. Its causes are thyroid autoimmunity, inflammatory diseases, some medications, iodine, lithium, etc.

The thyroid, in turn, is controlled by another gland, the pituitary (or hypophysis), which works rather like a thermostat, telling the thyroid when to start working and when to stop.

▪ The functions of the thyroid glands

- They stimulate basal metabolism and heat production.
- They act on fats, carbohydrates, and proteins.
- They have a marked effect on the heart and peripheral vascular system.
- They encourage the synthesis and action of the growth hormone.

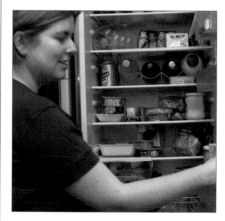

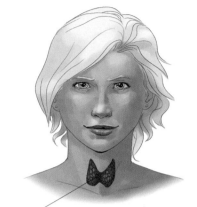

thyroid glands

- They are necessary for the proper functioning of the gonadal steroids.
- They act on the bones.
- They encourage blood formation.
- In the fetus, they develop the nerves and bones.

Possible treatments

- Radioactive iodine, designed to reduce the size of the thyroid gland when it has increased or is producing too much hormone, is used in cases of hyperthyroidism, goiter, and some types of tumor.
- Surgical intervention, in cases of cancer, and also to extract nodules and goiter.
- Thyroid hormone capsules to treat patients with hypothyroidism, goiter, or nodules, or who have had a thyroid operation.
- Antithyroid medication for patients with Grave's (or Basedow's) disease (caused by immune system problems), one of the commonest forms of hyperthyroidism.
- Beta blockers to treat the symptoms of hyperthyroidism, while some of the previously mentioned medications take effect.

In all cases, these treatments must be assessed and strictly prescribed by a specialist, and should never be self-administered.

The most frequent symptoms are a high average heart rate, nerviness, sweating, weight loss, reduction in the quantity and frequency of menstruation, falling hair, etc.

With the opposite condition, hypothyroidism, not enough thyroid hormones are produced, so energy is used more slowly than normal. The most frequent causes are iodine deficiency, medication with an antithyroid action, pituitary (hypophysis) disorders, pregnancy, and the early days of motherhood, etc. The most frequent symptoms are feeling cold, apathetic, depressed, low heart rate,

Symptoms of hypothyroidism

- Fatigue
- Tiredness
- Exhaustion
- Lethargy
- Depression
- Sudden weight gain
- Dry skin
- Itching
- Thickening hair
- Falling hair
- Susceptibility to cold, especially in the legs
- Constipation
- Muscular pain
- Copious menstruation
- More frequent periods

Symptoms of hyperthyroidism

- Nerviness
- Irritability
- Increased perspiration
- Thinner skin
- Fragile hair in poor condition
- Muscular debility, especially in the arms and legs
- Trembling hands
- Rapid heart rate
- Frequent bowel movements
- Weight loss in spite of continuing good appetite
- Reduction in menstrual flow
- Irregular and less frequent periods

In the detection of thyroid problems, as in other diseases, it is important to spot the first symptoms in the early stages. Thyroid problems are diagnosed by measuring the quantity of thyroid hormones in the blood and observing the structure and functioning of the gland.

weight gain, increased menstrual flow, loss of milk from the nipples, infertility, etc.

Thyroiditis is the inflammation of the thyroid, often as a consequence of hypothyroidism. Its commonest form (Hashimoto thyroiditis) increases in women as they age.

Goiter is the enlargement of the neck produced by the increased size of the thyroid gland. The commonest cause is a lack of iodine.

Nodules develop which are benign in 90 percent of cases. Thyroid cancer accounts for only 5 to 7 percent of these nodules.

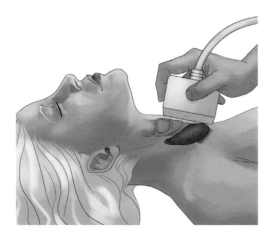

Chronic urethritis

Some women have symptoms of cystitis and painful urination whenever they have sex. The symptoms usually last one or two days and then disappear, only to recur when they next have sex. The problem, known as *"honeymoon cystitis,"* is a form of chronic urethritis, as it is the urethra that becomes inflamed, not the bladder.

Chronic urethritis

Normally, chronic urethritis is caused by a bacterial infection, or a structural problem (the narrowing of the urethra). It can also be associated with a wide variety of systemic diseases, including emotional problems. Urethritis can occur in both men and women.

The principal symptoms of urethritis (painful urination and increased frequency of urination) are very common and account for 5 to 10 percent of all visits to the doctor. Between 50 and 70 percent of the people who experience these symptoms have a bacterial infection in the urethra or bladder (cystitis), either for the first time or recurrently. Ten percent of them are women with vaginitis and the remainder are men or women with urethral

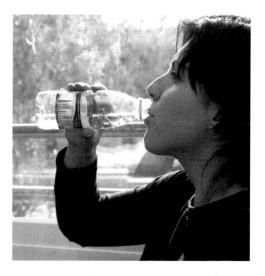

Drinking a large amount of water is helpful. Women with urinary tract infections associated with sexual relations (the symptoms appear within 24 hours of the sexual act) should urinate after sex. Good hygiene is also important, for both the affected person and their partner. Good hygiene is adequate hygiene that is neither excessive nor deficient, and washing should be done with soaps suitable for the genital area that are not too harsh.

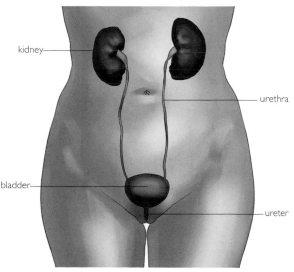

kidney

urethra

bladder

ureter

Diagnosis

- Analysis of the urine, which can reveal the existence of an infection.
- Antibiogram urine culture, to confirm the infection, its cause, and the most suitable antibiotic.
- Urethral exudation or vaginal culture, to rule out any sexually transmitted disease.
- Cystoscopy, to examine the urethra directly. This is not always necessary, although, if the urethritis does not clear up, or its cause cannot be determined, a cytoscopy may have to be performed.

syndrome (they experience symptoms, but there is no evidence of infection).

The group of agents that may cause this condition include all the organisms that produce the wide variety of sexually transmitted diseases (STDs).

As soon as symptoms appear, it is important to take note of them and treat them adequately, to avoid the structural damage that can be caused to the tissues by persistent inflammation or scratching.

The symptoms of chronic urethritis are long-lasting:

- An increase in urinary urgency and frequency.
- A feeling of discomfort when urinating, with burning or tingling in the urethra and the lower abdomen.
- Urethral discharge, which can contain blood or pus.

Treatment of urethritis

- If there is evidence of infection, antibiotics are prescribed and, after all the medication has been taken, a series of cultures are examined to confirm its effectiveness.
- Women who have suffered repeated episodes of urethritis or cystitis can be prescribed a dose of postcoital antibiotics (taken shortly before or after having sex). People with urethral syndrome (symptoms, but no evidence of infection) are prescribed Phenazopyridine to reduce discomfort when urinating if the cause of the problem cannot be ascertained, as there can be many other causes, including vaginitis.

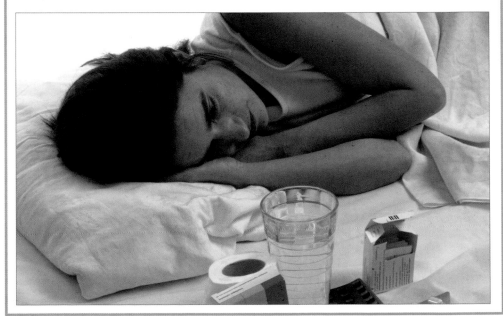

Pyelonephritis

Pyelonephritis, or upper urinary infection, is an infection of the kidneys and the urinary tract—the tubes through which urine passes from the kidneys to the bladder.

When establishing a case of pyelonephritis, the existence of any complications must be taken into account.

• Acute pyelonephritis: The sudden development of a kidney inflammation. Acute pyelonephritis occurs as a result of a common urinary infection (cystitis, or infection of the lower urinary tract) and, although it is much more serious than cystitis, it is not problematical and can usually be cured with antibiotic treatment. It can be much more severe in old people or those with an autoimmune deficiency (for example, people with cancer or AIDS).

• Chronic pyelonephritis. This is a more complex infection of the urinary tract. Some of the most complex problems associated with it are sepsis, or infection, disseminated throughout the body, and renal insufficiency, or the kidney's inability to manufacture urine.

The most frequent symptoms are:

• General discomfort
• Fever
  – over 102.2°F (39°C)
  – persisting for more than two days
• Shivering
• Pain in the back or side
• Abdominal pain (occurs occasionally)
• Nausea and vomiting
• Pain when urinating
• Need to urinate very often, at night, etc.
• Muddy looking or abnormally colored urine
• Blood in the urine
• Very strong smelling urine

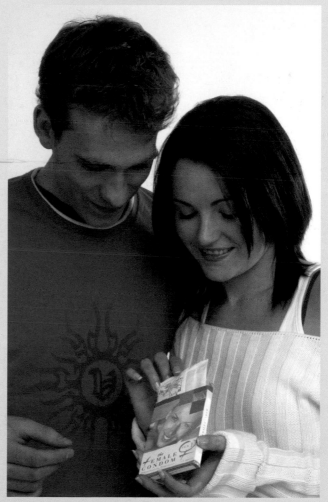

Practicing safe sex can reduce the risk of catching sexually transmitted diseases related to urethritis.

Vaginitis: vaginal infections

Vaginitis is an inflammation of the mucous membrane of the vagina, producing pain, itching, or burning when urinating. Vaginitis is characterized by a secretion, an unpleasant smell, irritation, and/or stinging. The cause of vaginitis cannot always be diagnosed simply from its symptoms or a physical examination. For a correct diagnosis, laboratory tests are usually carried out, such as a microscopic assessment of the vaginal flow. There is a wide variety of drugs to treat vaginitis.

Causes

Vaginitis is often caused by infections that produce discomfort and difficulty. Some infections are associated with other more serious diseases. The commonest vaginal infections are those caused by vaginosis bacteriana, and trichomoniasis, and vaginal infections by yeasts or vaginal candidiasis. Some vaginal infections are transmitted by sexual contact, but others, such as vaginitis candidasica, are not always sexually transmitted.

Vaginosis bacteriana

Vaginosis bacteriana is the commonest cause of symptomatic vaginitis in women of childbearing age. It used to be called nonspecific vaginitis or Gardnerella vaginitis, vaginosis bacteriana being transmitted by sexual activity and reflecting a chan-

Vaginosis bacteriana is the commonest cause of symptomatic vaginitis in women of childbearing age.

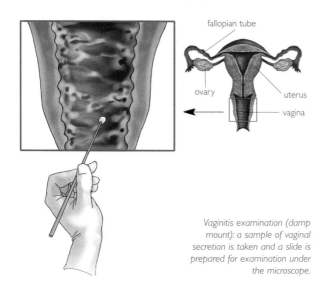

fallopian tube

ovary

uterus

vagina

Vaginitis examination (damp mount): a sample of vaginal secretion is taken and a slide is prepared for examination under the microscope.

Symptoms

The principal symptom of this type of vaginitis is an abnormal, unpleasant smelling vaginal flow. This fishy odor is especially noticeable after active sex and during menstruation. However, nearly half of women with clinical signs of vaginitis bacteriana experience no symptoms. The doctor may observe these signs during a physical examination and confirm the diagnosis by testing the vaginal flow.

ge in the vaginal ecosystem. This imbalance includes changes in the pH balance and appears when different types of bacteria exceed the quantity to which the vagina is accustomed. Thus, instead of a customary predominance of the Lactobacillus bacterium, the number of microorganisms such as Gardnerella vaginalis, Bacteroides, Mobiluncus, and Mycoplasma hominis in the vaginas of vaginitis sufferers increases. Researchers are studying the part each of these bacteria plays in vaginitis, although the part played by sexual relations in the development of vaginitis bacteriana is not yet fully understood. Changing sexual partners and vaginal irrigation, or douching, seem to be risk factors for the acquisition of vaginosis bacteriana.

Diagnosis

The examination of the sample of vaginal flow by microscope enables the presence of the microorganisms associated with the inflammation to be detected. A diagnosis can be made based on the absence of lactobacilli, the presence of many key cells, which are cells of the vaginal epithelium covered in the microorganisms that cause the infection, the fishy smell, reduced acidity, or changes in the pH balance of the vaginal flow.

Treatment

All women with vaginitis should be informed of their diagnosis, its relationship with sexual transmission, and the therapeutic options available to them. Treatment is based on antibiotics such as metronidazol or clyndamicin (also called cleocin) and, generally, sexual partners do not receive treatment.

Complications

Researchers have shown the association between vaginitis bacteriana and the inflammatory pelvic disease that causes infertility and ectopic pregnancies. Vaginitis bacteriana can also produce complications in pregnancy, premature birth, and babies with a low birth weight. All pregnant women are therefore advised to be examined for vaginitis if they have previously given birth prematurely, whether they have symptoms or not.

If a pregnant woman has vaginitis, she should receive oral treatment with metronidazol or clyndamicin. A pregnant woman who has not previously given birth prematurely should receive treatment if she has symptoms or if the laboratory confirms that she has this type of vaginitis.

The disease is also associated with an increased risk of gonorrhea and HIV infection (the human immunodeficiency virus) that causes AIDS (acquired autoimmune deficiency syndrome).

Vaginal candidiasis: vaginal infection by yeasts

Vaginal infection by yeasts, vulvovaginitis candidasica, or vaginal or vulovaginal candidiasis, is a common cause of vaginal irritation. Doctors estimate that 75 percent of all women experience at least one episode of infection symptomatic of yeasts during their lives. Yeasts are normally present in the vagina in small quantities, and symptoms appear when those quantities increase.

Various factors are associated with the increase in this symptomatic infection in women, such as pregnancy, uncontrolled diabetes mellitus, and taking oral contraceptives or antibiotics. Other factors that can increase the incidence of yeast infection are vaginal douches, perfumed feminine hygiene sprays, and topical antimicrobial agents, as well as wearing tight and poorly ventilated underwear.

It is not really known whether or not yeasts can be transmitted sexually. As almost all women have the microorganism in their vaginas, researchers have found it difficult to study this aspect of the natural history of the disease.

Symptoms

The most frequent symptoms of yeast infection in women are tingling, burning, and irritation in the vagina. Difficult and/or painful urination and coitus are common. The vaginal secretion is not always present and can be minimal. It is typically described as thick, grayish-white "curd," although its consistency can range from watery to thick.

As a rule, the sexual partners of women with a yeast infection do not experience any symptoms of infection. However, some report a rash and a transitory burning sensation in the penis after coitus if condoms have not been used. These symptoms are usually self-limiting.

Diagnosis

As few specific signs and symptoms are normally present, this disease is not usually diagnosed by a physical examination of the patient and her history. As a rule the doctor diagnoses a yeast infection by examining the vaginal secretion under the microscope, looking for yeasts.

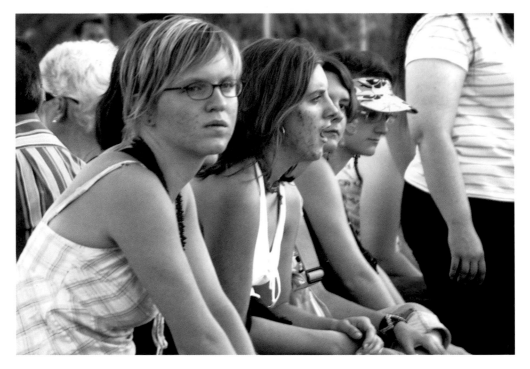

Many women with symptoms of vaginitis do not consult a doctor for treatment, and many with no symptoms reject treatment. Needless to say, that is precisely what they should not do.

Treatment

Several antifungal medications are available for treating vulvovaginal candidiasis. Women can use creams, pills, or vaginal ovules (suppositories) of clotrimazole and other azole derivatives for topical intravaginal treatment, usually after a doctor has examined them.

Other available products contain antihistamines or topical anesthetics which merely mask the symptoms and do not treat the underlying problem. Women with chronic, or recurrent, candidiasis can undergo treatment for long periods, and oral medicines for treating this infection have recently become available. It may be helpful to identify the factors that predispose certain individuals to chronic yeast infections.

Women infected with HIV may suffer more severe candida vulvovaginitis that does not respond to treatment.

Other causes of vaginitis

Although most vaginal infections in women are due to vaginitis bacteriana, trichomoniasis, or yeasts, there are other causes, such as allergies, irritants, and sexually transmitted diseases. Noninfectious allergic symptoms can be caused by spermicides, feminine hygiene products, detergents, and laundry softeners. The cervical inflammation caused by these products is usually a factor associated with abnormal vaginal secretion, but can normally be easily distinguished from true vaginal infection by the appropriate diagnostic tests.

Varicose veins

Heaviness and cramp in the legs, and swollen ankles, are symptoms indicating the presence of venous insufficiency. If they are accompanied by dilatations of the surface veins, varicose veins are present.

The accumulation of blood in the veins and the consequent appearance of varicose veins mainly affects women. This is not merely a matter of esthetics, because women are twice as likely to suffer from varicose veins as men, mainly due to the effects of pregnancy.

There are two vein systems in the legs, the surface veins and the deep veins, that are linked by communicating veins. The surface veins have thinner walls and are surrounded by soft tissues. The deep system contains 90 percent of the venous blood of the legs. These veins have thicker walls that are less capable of distention.

Varicose veins are veins that undergo permanent dilatation and lengthening, becoming snakelike. They are the visible manifestation of chronic venous insufficiency (CVI).

Chronic venous insufficiency (CVI)

This is a pathology in which the return of blood is reduced, especially when the person is standing, and the blood flows in the opposite direction, from the deep system to the surface system. It is the most frequent vascular disorder, affecting 25 percent of adults and more than 50 percent of people aged over 55. It is 5 times more frequent in women.

Causes and conditioning factors

This insufficiency occurs because the valves in the veins are incompetent, either because they have been destroyed (rerouting of a thrombus, injury, etc.), or because of a defect of unknown cause in the wall of the vein, leading to the excessive venous dilatation and the separation of the valves. This valvular fault allows the blood to pass from the deep system to the surface system, with

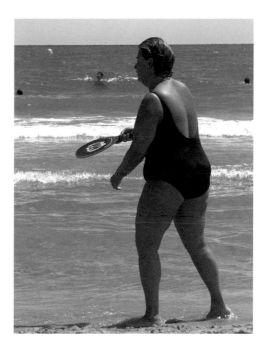

The veins of the legs carry blood through the vena cava to the heart, so they contain opposed pairs of valves which makes the blood flow upward and from the surface system to the deep system. This encourages the blood to move against gravity by the contraction of the leg muscles that act as a pump squeezing the veins.

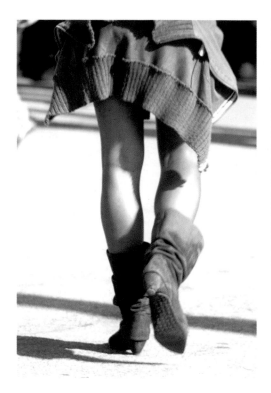 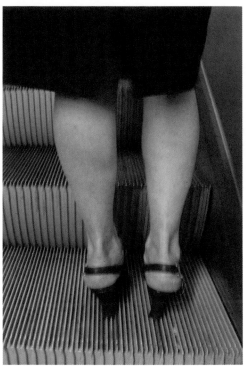

an increase in pressure and the subsequent appearance of varicose veins. The increased pressure damages capillary circulation and increases the pressure in the capillary vessels, leading to the exudation of liquid, swelling, and poor oxygenation of the surrounding tissues.

All these changes encourage inflammation, infection, thrombosis, and tissue necrosis, giving rise to the complication of the disease.

Classification of varicose veins

According to their shape, varicose veins are classified as follows::

1. Spider or thread veins. Dilations of capillaries or small veins. This type of varicose vein is only an esthetic problem, although it can cause a feeling of tightness and heaviness in the skin, as well as tiredness, especially in the evening and during the summer, and a general feeling of heat and burning.

2. Reticular varicose veins. Dilatations of small veins that form networks, usually on the outer side of the leg and in the popliteal cavity (the area behind the knee). In addition to the above-mentioned symptoms, they can cause phlebitis in the surface of the skin which is very painful.

3. Trunk varicose veins. Dilatations of the saphe-

The principal conditioning factors

- Varicose veins are not inherited. What really happens is that people with varicose veins have inherited structural problems in the valves of their veins.

- Age. They occur more often in people aged over 50.

- Sex. They are more frequent in women.

- Pregnancy. They are more frequent in women who have given birth.

- Standing up for prolonged periods.

- Obesity. They are more frequent in obese women. There is no difference in their frequency in obese men.

CVI can manifest itself as: heaviness, itching, pain, tiredness, cramp, or swelling, which improve when the sufferer lies down and when the temperature is cold, and worsen when the sufferer is standing and when the temperature is hot. There is no correlation between the size or length of varicose veins and the severity of the symptoms. They are more marked in women, in whom they are aggravated during menstruation and pregnancy, and when taking oral contraceptives and hormone replacement therapy during menopause.

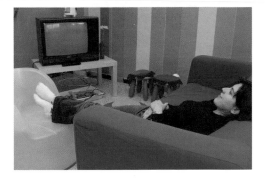

nous veins (thick surface veins) or their tributaries. They are a serious risk for the sufferer and absolutely must be treated, because of the complications they can lead to, which range from superficial phlebitis to deep vein thrombosis (DVT).

Medication and treatment

• Compression. This improves the return of blood through the veins and reduces venous pressure. It lessens symptoms and swelling, delaying the development of the condition. It is indicated in all patients suffering CVI symptoms or varicose veins with an ankle/arm index >0.9.

• Elastic support stockings. These stockings exert decreasing pressure from the ankle to the

During the summer, the side-effects of varicose veins increase the feeling of heaviness in the legs, cramp, and swollen ankles. However, although it is true that heat makes them worse, they can appear all year round.

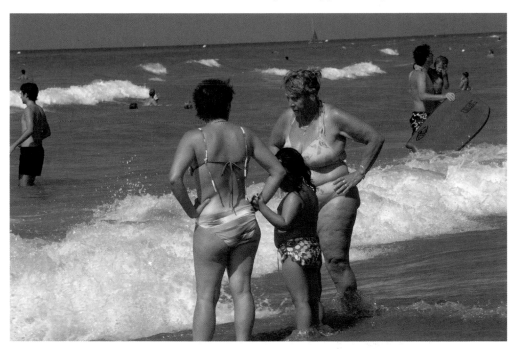

Treatment

Healthy living

- A balanced diet rich in fruit, which contains flavonoids that help constrict the veins.
- Losing weight in the case of obesity.
- Avoiding standing or sitting for long periods.
- Taking physical exercise, such as walking.
- Wearing comfortable shoes. Avoiding high heels.
- Doing ankle flexion exercises.
- Sitting with the feet raised to heart height for 15–30 minutes several times a day.
- Sleeping with the foot of the bed raised by about 6 inches (15 cm).
- Avoiding heat.
- Avoiding constipation.
- Alternating warm and cold water when you take a shower.

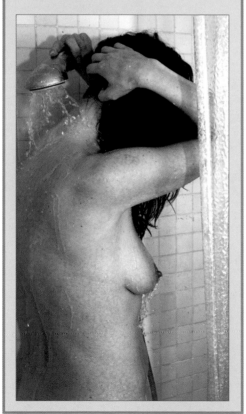

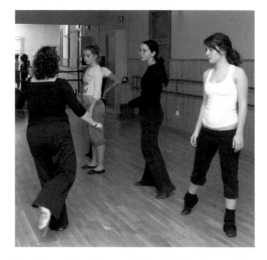

Standing or sitting for long periods makes blood accumulate in the veins of the leg. A little exercise every day, especially walking, helps the veins to contract, empty themselves, and send the blood to the heart, counteracting varicose veins.

waist or knee. According to the pressure they apply to the ankles, they are classified into: light to moderate compression, normal compression, and strong compression. The use of each type is directly related to the severity of the condition. The more symptoms that are experienced or the greater the severity of the complications, the more pressure needs to be applied.

- Sclerotherapy and other relatively noninvasive treatments. Several treatments now exist for small varicose veins. The most widespread is sclerosis, which consists of injecting a chemical substance into the opening of the varicose vein that irritates the vascular wall. The vein then closes, becoming a string that is reabsorbed, thus eliminating the varicose vein.

Other ways of treating this type of minor varicose vein are mesotherapy, or surgical laser treatment, electrocoagulation, cryocoagulation, cryosclerosis, etc.

- Phlebectomy. Moderately sized, or reticular, varicose veins, can be treated by phlebectomy, a procedure not requiring hospitalization, which consists of removing the varicose veins through small incisions under a local anesthetic. At present, this is the most suitable treatment. Sclerosis has sometimes been tried for reticular veins, but the procedure is very complicated.

• Phleboextraction. In the case of large varicose veins, trunk veins, no remedy is more effective than a surgical operation which, like those already mentioned, need not require a stay in hospital and is performed under a local anesthetic. The procedure that gives the best result is out-patient phleboextraction with ligature of the communicating veins.

At present, the removal of the varicose veins through small incisions, extraction of the trunk varicose veins, and sclerosis of the small ones are combined. Ten years after the operation, some 20 to 30 percent of patients develop varicose veins again.

Advice

It is difficult to determine what to do to avoid varicose veins, but the following advice may be useful:

• If, because of the type of work you do, you have to stay on your feet for hours on end every day, you should wear special elastic stockings that

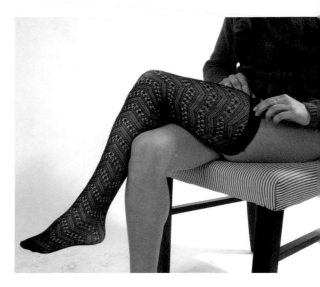

are sold in drugstores or specialist stores.

• It is also important to release any pressure there may be on the abdomen, as pressure will hinder the proper functioning of the circulation.

Varicose veins are permanent dilatations of the surface veins of the legs because of the malfunction of the valves inside those veins. Because of this valvular incompetence, the blood flows back, causing it to accumulate, making the wall of the vein dilate and thicken, and producing the twisting so characteristic of varicose veins.

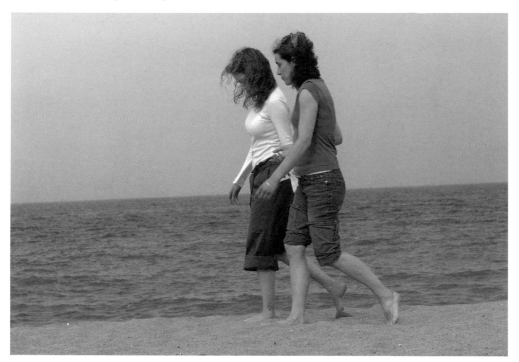

Any activity that increases blood pressure in the legs, such as standing for a long time, increases the pain. Therefore, any activity that reduces blood pressure and counteracts gravity will help alleviate the pain of varicose veins.

• Maintaining a reasonable weight is also fundamental, as is not crossing your legs when seated.

• Direct heat, from stoves, radiators, etc., on the legs is not recommended, because it can make varicose veins worse. Oral contraceptives are totally prohibited for women with varicose veins.

• Avoid constipation.

Complications

• Phlebitis and thrombophlebitis. Phlebitis is an inflammation of a vein accompanied by the formation of a blood clot that obstructs it. Conversely, thrombophlebitis is inflammation due to the formation of a thrombus that sticks to the wall of a vein. Its cause is lack of muscular exercise and being obliged or forced to remain in a horizontal position. To begin with, or in the phlebothrombosis phase, the signs of phlebitis are minimal: sensitivity to pressure, pain caused by flexing the back of the foot, slight fever. At a more advanced stage, called thrombophlebitis, the leg is very painful and is swollen throughout its length by a large edema. The prevention of phlebitis requires strict vigilance of postoperative patients, women who have recently given birth, and anyone who has had to keep their legs still for a long time (in a plaster cast, etc.). Mobilization, leg massage and, above all, allowing the patient to get out of bed as soon as possible have considerably reduced cases of phlebitis.

• Varicose ulcers. Lesions with loss of substance that occur on skin damaged by dermatitis (eczema) following venous pressure. This is the principal complication of CVI. These lesions appear on the inside of the ankles, but can also appear on the outer side, or slightly above mid-calf level. Their size is variable and, typically, they are not painful (except if infected). They should be treated by qualified staff.

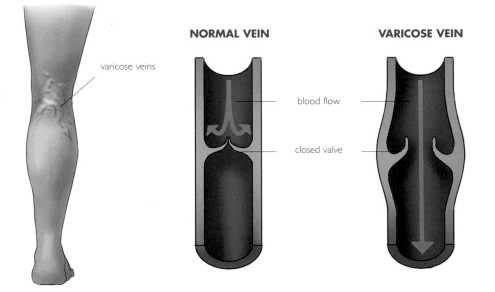

varicose veins

NORMAL VEIN

blood flow

closed valve

VARICOSE VEIN

Dementia

Dementia is a disease of the brain. When a person is suffering from dementia, the cells of their brain deteriorate and cease to function normally. This alteration in the brain cells stops the brain working correctly and these people gradually lose their intellectual capacities and faculties. Some types of dementia are Alzheimer's disease, dementias caused by multiple strokes, or alcoholic dementia. Some degenerative diseases, such as Parkinson's or Huntingdon's diseases, can also lead to dementia.

What is dementia?

For dementia to be diagnosed, a series of shared symptoms must be present that comprise the inability to learn new information because of cognitive damage.

For a person to be considered as suffering from dementia, they must be suffering memory loss.

Perhaps the most terrible thing is that, although these people have suffered some memory loss, they have not lost awareness, so they suffer from being conscious of their illness.

Dementia does not imply a progressive and irreversible disorder. People who have had a severe brain injury, and those severely addicted to drugs, often experience symptoms similar to those of dementia, although their cognitive function improves with the passage of time. However, there are also types of progressive and irreversible dementia, such as Alzheimer's disease.

Simple memory tests are used to diagnose dementia, such as reading a list of words and trying to repeat them, or asking the patient to recount his life story.

Disorders that frequently accompany dementia

Huntingdon's disease. This is a hereditary neurodegenerative disease that starts early but gradually, at about the age of 40. It is characterized by involuntary movements of the arms and legs,

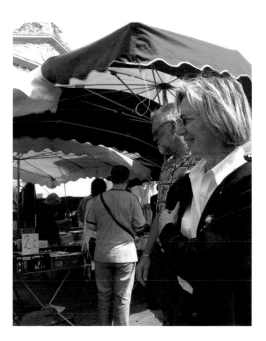

Not all memory losses can be attributed to dementia. There is a condition called benign senile negligence, also known as age-associated memory decline, characterized by a minor loss of memory that is greater than normal. People over the age of 50 complain of day-to-day memory losses, and demonstrate a degree of deviation in memory tests, but this does not amount to dementia. There is also a pathology called pseudodementia, which is dementia caused by a series of depressions. Those affected are indecisive, have difficulty in concentrating, and process information slowly. They also suffer lack of pleasure (anhedonia) and constantly complain.

Vascular dementia

This is the second most frequent type of dementia and is caused by cerebral blood deficiency. Its most frequent causes are usually chronic high blood pressure and arteriosclerosis of the blood vessels that carry blood to the brain. In this type of dementia, numerous small strokes occur, cutting off the blood supply to some parts of the brain. To make the disease progress more slowly, blood pressure and adequate sugar levels must be maintained and smoking must be avoided.

Although no cure is yet available for Alzheimer's disease, adequate medical and social planning can alleviate the burden for patients and their families. Drugs are available that reduce agitation, anxiety, and unpredictable behavior, make sleep more regular, and treat depression. Physical exercise and social activities are important, as are adequate nutrition and the maintenance of general good health.

lack of coordination, and a clear decline in memory, difficulty in concentrating and paying attention, and problems with planning activities. It affects the judgment and reasoning, and causes marked changes in moods and emotions. The memory is considerably affected by Huntingdon's disease, but the recognition of things and people is less affected.

Parkinson's disease. This is a slowly progressing neurodegenerative disease that affects movement, muscular control, and balance. Part of the pathological process develops as the cells are destroyed in certain parts of the brainstem, especially the mass of half-moon shaped cells known as the black matter. The nerve cells in the *black matter* send fibers to the tissues on both sides of

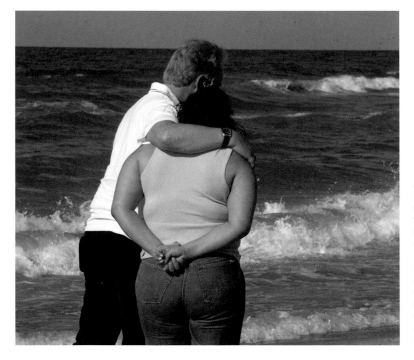

Alzheimer's disease affects about 22 million people worldwide, and is the commonest of the diseases that cause dementia. More than 100,000 people die every year as a result of Alzheimer's disease, making it the fourth most important cause of death among adults, after heart disease, cancer, and strokes.

Symptoms of dementia

- Progressive memory loss.
- Inability to concentrate.
- Reduced capacity to resolve problems and make decisions.
- Confusion.
- Hallucination, illusions.
- Sensitivity or altered perception.
- Deterioration in recognition:
    - Not recognizing familiar things or people.
    - Deterioration in recognition using the senses.
- Altered sleep patterns:
    - Insomnia
    - Increased need to sleep.
    - Disturbance or change in the pattern of sleeping and waking.
- Deterioration in the motor system:
    - Deterioration in the motor response.
    - Inability to draw, imitate gestures, or even get dressed.
    - Changes in walking.
    - Uncoordinated movements.
- Disorientation.
- Specific disorders regarding learning and solving problems:
    - Inability to generalize.
    - Loss of abstract thought.
    - Deterioration in the ability to calculate.
    - Inability to learn.
- Memory deficiency:
    - Short-term memory problems (inability to remember new things).
    - Long-term memory problems (inability to remember the past).
- Absence or deterioration of linguistic ability:
    - Inability to understand speech.
    - Inability to read.
    - Inability to write.
    - Inability to speak fluently.
    - Inability to form words.
    - Swearing and talking gibberish.
    - Inability to repeat a sentence.
    - Persistent repetition of sentences.
- Personality changes:
    - Irritability.
    - Deficient character control.
    - Anxiety.
    - Depression.
    - Indecision.
    - Egocentricity.
    - Inflexibility.
    - Inappropriate mood or behavior.
    - Withdrawal from social interaction.
    - Reduced ability to take care of oneself.
    - Reduced interest in vital daily activities.
- Lack of spontaneity.

the brain and there the cells release essential neurotransmitters that help control movement and coordination. In 30 percent of cases, symptoms of dementia appear, such as slowness of thought, memory loss, disorientation, loss of movement, etc.

Alzheimer's disease. This is the most frequent cause of dementia among the old, accounting for between 50 and 80 percent of all dementias. It is a progressive and degenerative brain disease that causes deterioration in memory, thought, and behavior. The symptoms of Alzheimer's disease include gradual loss of memory, reduced ability to carry out routine tasks, inability to discriminate, disorientation, personality changes, difficulties in learning, and loss of verbal skill. The speed with which these changes occur varies from person to person.